Oxford Medical Publications

Reconceiving Schizophrenia

International Perspectives in Philosophy and Psychiatry

Series editors
K. W. M. (Bill) Fulford
Katherine Morris
John Z. Sadler
Giovanni Stanghellini

Other volumes in the series:

Mind, Meaning and Mental Disorder, 2e
Bolton and Hill

Postpsychiatry
Bracken and Thomas

Dementia
Hughes, Louw, and Sabat (Eds)

Nature and Narrative
Fulford, Morris, Sadler, and Stanghellini (Eds)

The Philosophy of Psychiatry
Radden (Ed)

Values and Psychiatric Diagnosis
Sadler

Disembodied Spirits and Deanimated Bodies
Stanghellini

Oxford Textbook of Philosophy and Psychiatry
Fulford, Thornton, and Graham

Trauma, Truth and Reconciliation: healing damaged relationships
Potter (Ed)

Forthcoming volumes in the series:

Body Subjects and Disordered Minds
Matthews

Empirical Ethics in Psychiatry
Widdershoven, Hope, McMillan, and van der Scheer (Eds)

Reconceiving Schizophrenia

Edited by

Man Cheung Chung

K. W. M. (Bill) Fulford

and

George Graham

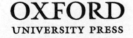

OXFORD

UNIVERSITY PRESS

OXFORD
UNIVERSITY PRESS

Great Clarendon Street, Oxford OX2 6DP

Oxford University Press is a department of the University of Oxford.
It furthers the University's objective of excellence in research, scholarship,
and education by publishing worldwide in

Oxford New York

Auckland Cape Town Dar es Salaam Hong Kong Karachi
Kuala Lumpur Madrid Melbourne Mexico City Nairobi
New Delhi Shanghai Taipei Toronto

With offices in

Argentina Austria Brazil Chile Czech Republic France Greece
Guatemala Hungary Italy Japan Poland Portugal Singapore
South Korea Switzerland Thailand Turkey Ukraine Vietnam

Oxford is a registered trade mark of Oxford University Press
in the UK and in certain other countries

Published in the United States
by Oxford University Press Inc., New York

© Oxford University Press 2007

The moral rights of the authors have been asserted

Database right Oxford University Press (maker)

First published 2007

A catalogue record for this title is available from the British Library

Library of Congress Cataloging in Publication Data
Reconceiving schizophrenia / edited by Man Chung, Bill Fulford and George Graham.
    p.; cm.—(International perspectives in philosophy and psychiatry)
    Includes bibliographical references and index.
    ISBN-13: 978–0–19–852613–1 (pbk: alk. paper)
    ISBN-10: 0–19–852613–X (pbk: alk.paper)   1. Schizophrenia.   I. Chung, Man Cheung,
1962–   II. Fulford, K. W. M.   III. Graham, George, 1945–   IV. Series.
    [DNLM: 1. Schizophrenia.   2. Delusions—psychology.   3. Schizophrenic Psychology.
WM 203 R3105 2006]
    RC514.R4322 2006
    616.89′80019—dc22   2006022881

Typeset by SPI Publisher Services, Pondicherry, India
Printed in Great Britain
on acid-free paper by
Biddles Ltd., King's Lynn.

ISBN 0–19–852613–X (Pbk.)   978–0–19–852613–1 (Pbk.)

10 9 8 7 6 5 4 3 2 1

Contents

Contributors

RICHARD P. BENTALL is Professor of Experimental Clinical Psychology at the University of Manchester, UK. His main areas of research concern the psychological mechanisms involved in psychotic symptoms such as hallucinations and delusions, and also the development of novel psychological interventions for people either experiencing psychosis or at risk of developing a psychotic illness. He has published widely in academic journals and is the author of *Madness explained: Psychosis and human nature* (Penguin Press, 2003).

MAN CHEUNG CHUNG is Reader of Psychology in the Clinical Psychology Teaching Unit, School of Applied Psychosocial Studies at the University of Plymouth. His research interests include philosophy of psychology and health/ clinical psychology. He has published some 100 articles and chapters in the foregoing areas as well as on other diverse topics. In addition to the present book, he has also edited *Psychoanalytic Knowledge* with Colin Feltham (Palgrave Macmillan, 2003), *Psychology of Reasoning* with Ken Manktelow (Psychology Press, 2004), and *Phenomenology and Psychological Science* with Peter Ashworth (Springer, 2006).

K. W. M. (BILL) FULFORD is Professor of Philosophy and Mental Health in the Department of Philosophy and The Medical School, University of Warwick, where he runs a Masters, PhD and research programme in Philosophy, Ethics and Mental Health Practice. He is also an Honorary Consultant Psychiatrist in the Department of Psychiatry, University of Oxford and Visiting Professor in Psychology, The Institute of Psychiatry and King's College, London University. He is the founder and Co-Editor of the first international journal for philosophy and mental health, *PPP – Philosophy, Psychiatry, & Psychology*, and of a new book series from Oxford University Press on International Perspectives in Philosophy and Psychiatry. He is currently seconded part-time to the Department of Health in London as Special Advisor for Values-Based Practice in the Care Services Directorate and the Care Services Improvement Partnership.

GRANT GILLETT is Professor of Medical Ethics at the University of Otago in Dunedin, New Zealand. He is also a practising neurosurgeon. His philosophical work is in philosophy of mind and psychiatry, continental philosophy, and bioethics. His most recent books are *The mind and its discontents* (Oxford University Press, 1999) and *Bioethics in the clinic* (John Hopkins University Press, 2004). He works on post-modern and traditional analytic approaches to mind, language, and psychiatry.

GEORGE GRAHAM is the A. C. Reid Professor of Philosophy at Wake Forest University in Winston-Salem, North Carolina, USA. He is the author of many articles in philosophy of mind and philosophical psychopathology and has helped to produce several books. For more than 17 years, he served as chairperson of the Department of Philosophy at the University of Alabama at Birmingham. He is a past president of the Society for Philosophy and Psychology.

ANDY HAMILTON is a lecturer in Philosophy at Durham University, where he teaches philosophy of mind, aesthetics, and political philosophy. He has published many articles on philosophy of mind, history of philosophy and aesthetics. He is writing a book on aesthetics and music for continuum, and is completing a monograph on philosophy of mind, *Memory and the Body: A Study of Self-Consciousness.*

ROM HARRÉ is Emeritus fellow of Linacre College, Oxford and presently teaches in Washington DC. His most recent work includes *Cognitive Science: A Philosophical Introduction* (Sage Publications Ltd., 2002) and *Wittgenstein and Psychology* (Ashgate, 2005) with Michael Tissaw. His current research is concerned with further developments of positioning theory.

MIKE JACKSON is a consultant clinical psychologist specialising in psychosocial interventions in psychosis, working in the NHS in North Wales. He has a long standing interest in the relationship between benign and pathological forms of psychotic experiences, and he has written a number of papers and book chapters on this theme.

PETER KINDERMAN is Professor of Clinical Psychology at the University of Liverpool, UK. He is the author of a number of articles and book chapters discussing psychopathology and psychological models of mental disorder.

COLIN KING is a mental health survivor who was misdiagnosed with schizophrenia at 17, who has since worked as a mental health practitioner and completed a PhD in institutional racism in sports management and culture. He is presently working on value based research into mental health work and a book, *They diagnosed me a schizophrenic when I was just a Gemini.*

ALFRED KRAUS is Professor of Psychiatry at the Psychiatric University Clinic of Heidelberg, Germany. He has published mainly psychopathological articles on manic-depressive illness, obsessive-compulsive and anxiety disorders, schizophrenia, trans- and intersexualism, and on basics of diagnostics and classification in psychiatry. Particular interests are phenomenological-anthropological and role–theoretical approaches in psychiatry. He has carried out transcultural comparative empirical studies on manic-depressives in Germany and Japan. His books include *Social Behaviour of Manic-Depressives,*

Leib, Geist Geschichte (Hüthig, 1978), *Brennpunkte anthropologischer Psychiatrie, Schizophrenie und Sprache* (Thiema, 1991).

ERIC MATTHEWS is Emeritus Professor of Philosophy and Honorary Research Professor of Medical Ethics and Philosophy of Psychiatry in the University of Aberdeen, Scotland. He has written many articles on the philosophy and ethics of psychiatry, and is currently working on a book applying Merleau-Ponty's concept of the 'body-subject' to problems in mental illness. He is a member of the Committee of the Royal College of Psychiatrists Philosophy Special Interest Group.

JOSEF PARNAS, is Professor of Psychiatry at the University of Copenhagen, medical director at the Department of Psychiatry at Hvidovre Hospital and co-leader of the National Danish Research Council's Center for Subjectivity Research. He has published extensively in the domains of epidemiology, genetics, neurodevelopment and psychopathology of schizophrenia and is currently trying to integrate phenomenological and empirical approaches in the study of subjective experience in psychosis.

JEFFREY POLAND has degrees in philosophy of science and clinical psychology, and he has extensive clinical experience in inpatient psychiatric rehabilitation. He is author of *Physicalism: The Philosophical Foundations* (Oxford University Press, 1994) and a co-author (with William Spaulding and Mary Sullivan) of *Treatment and Rehabilitation of Severe Mental Illness* (Guilford, 2003). He has held academic positions at Colgate University and the University of Nebraska-Lincoln, and he currently teaches in the Department of History, Philosophy, and Social Science at the Rhode Island School of Design.

JENNIFER RADDEN received her graduate training at Oxford University. She is Professor and Chair of the Philosophy Department at the University of Massachusetts, Boston Campus. She is author of articles and chapters on philosophical issues arising out of mental health concepts and policy, and psychiatric practice, as well as *Madness and Reason* (1985), *Divided Minds and Successive Selves: Ethical Issues in Disorders of Identity and Personality* (1996); edited volumes include *The Nature of Melancholy: From Aristotle to Kristeva* (2000) and *Oxford Companion to the Philosophy of Psychiatry* (Oxford University Press, 2004). Between 1997 and 2002 she served as President of the Association for the Advancement of Philosophy and Psychiatry.

LOUIS A. SASS is professor and former chair in the Department of Clinical Psychology at Rutgers, the State University of New Jersey, where he is also a research affiliate in the Center for Cognitive Science. He has published many articles on schizophrenia (and related conditions), phenomenological psychopathology, hermeneutics, psychoanalysis, modernism, and postmodernism;

and is the author of two books, *Madness and Modernism: Insanity in the Light of Modern Art, Literature, and Thought* (Basic Books, 1992, Harvard Paperback, 1994), and *The Paradoxes of Delusion: Wittgenstein, Schreber, and the Schizophrenic Mind* (Cornell University Press, 1994).

MICHAEL A. SCHWARTZ lives in Austin, Texas and is Clinical Professor of Psychiatry at the University of Hawaii. Founding President of the Association for the Advancement of Philosophy and Psychiatry, he is author of numerous articles and book chapters on phenomenological psychiatry, psychopathology and philosophical psychiatry. For over 10 years, he was Professor of Psychiatry at Case Western Reserve University School of Medicine.

GIOVANNI STANGHELLINI is Professor of Dynamic Psychology. He chairs the AEP Section on Philosophy and Psychiatry and co-chairs the WPA Section on Psychiatry and the Humanities. His recent publications in the Oxford University Press IPPP Series (that he co-edits with K. W. M. Fulford, K. Morris and J. Z. Sadler) are *Disembodied Spirits and Deanimated Bodies, the Psychopathology of Common Sense* (2004) and *Nature and Narrative* (2003) (with K. W. M. Fulford, K. Morris, and J. Z. Sadler)

G. LYNN STEPHENS is Professor of Philosophy at the University of Alabama at Birmingham. He has published extensively on philosophical issues connected with psychopathology. He was co-editor of *Philosophical Psychopathology* (MIT Press, 1994), and co-author of *When Self-Consciousness Breaks: Alien Voices and Inserted Thoughts* (MIT Press, 2000), both with George Graham.

OSBORNE P. WIGGINS is Professor of Philosophy and a member of the faculty of the Institute for Bioethics, Health Policy and Law at the University of Louisville in Louisville, Kentucky. He is a recipient of the Margrit Egner Award for his contributions to phenomenological-anthropological psychiatry. With Michael A. Schwartz and others he has published numerous articles in psychiatry and psychopathology.

1 Introduction: on reconceiving schizophrenia

Man Cheung Chung, K.W.M. (Bill) Fulford, and George Graham

This is a book of new essays on some of the most important themes in schizophrenia research. Another book on schizophrenia? It is not to be wondered that this is another book on schizophrenia. Schizophrenia is the most devastating disorder seen by psychiatrists (Frith 1998, p. 388). We do not *really* understand it. Books are needed. Some helpful ones have recently appeared (e.g. Heinrichs 2001; Green 2002). However the condition continues to elude satisfying comprehension. Consider, briefly, the following sketch of what it means to be a victim of the illness.

The victim of schizophrenia. This is a person who is subject to a diverse range of disturbances of perception, thought and cognition, emotion, motivation, and motor activity. It is a range in which episodes of dramatic disturbance are set against a background of chronic disability. The disability may consist of mild inability to cope with work or interpersonal relations, to profound inability to manage daily affairs and to care for oneself. Delusions of thought and cognition are a hallmark of schizophrenia. Perceptual hallucinations (including the subject's mistaking his or her own inner speech for voices), as well as disorders of emotion (including flattened affect), motor disorders, disorganized speech, and disjointed or weakened motivation, are elements of the disorder.

One victim, possessed, unlike many others, with recognition that he has the illness, remarked (Davis 1998, p. 138, p. 144):

> My schizophrenia filled my life with danger. . . . I am convinced that I have schizophrenia, and I am pretty sure that I will be taking medications for the rest of my life. I am 42 years old. I've never married and I have no children. I have no love in my life. I have no relatives . . . except my parents. I am . . . concerned about growing old alone.

In addition to its power to devastate, schizophrenia may be the most theoretically complex and controversial of the mental disorders to which we human beings are vulnerable. Its complexity arises not just from its myriad symptoms, but from the huge variability in genetic susceptibility, age of onset, clinical course, and responsiveness to treatment. Controversy surrounding schizophrenia stems not just from the welter of theories of the origins and course of schizophrenia (more than twenty are mentioned in Sahakian 1986, pp.110–125), but from the explosion of new information relevant to understanding its symptoms from genetics, brain imaging, post-mortem and experimental studies. The recent proliferation of symptom-based information has prompted some theorists to claim that schizophrenia is not a discrete illness but a collection of illnesses. It is not a disorder but a set of disorders. We take no stand on such an iconoclastic charge, but its existence is symptom of the contestability that surrounds the illness.

Philosophical questions might be supposed to be distinct from such symptom complexities and medical-scientific controversies, insulated in a priori armchair interrogatives, but distinctness is a myth about the discipline of philosophy. Real philosophers like to wrestle with a mix of conceptual and empirical perplexities and there is little that is more mixed, conceptually and empirically, than schizophrenia. At least four kinds of questions about schizophrenia have attracted the attention of philosophers and philosophically informed mental health professionals.

1. *Questions of conceptual analysis of symptoms.* Concepts of delusion, hallucination, psychomotor activity, and blunted affect are among the concepts that have played prominent roles in the description of the symptoms of schizophrenia. These concepts and others help to characterize the ways in which the course of schizophrenia often leads to personality disintegration and poses problems of explanation, prediction, and treatment. What do such concepts mean? How are their meanings and conditions of proper application best understood, explicated, or regimented? Take, for instance, the concept of delusion. DSM-IV and related literatures speak of delusion as a type of false belief (American Psychiatric Association 1994, p. 765; Marshall and Halligan 1996, p. 8). Clinicians, however, often describe non-beliefs as delusional. Young (1999) remarks that 'the issues involved in determining the conceptual status of delusions are tricky—one can draw attention to delusions that seem pretty convincing examples of false beliefs, or one can draw attention to delusions which seem like . . . empty speech acts' (p.238). So, how is the concept of delusion best understood? Belief? Non-belief?

2. *Questions of categorization.* The impulse to categorize arises with urgency in the theory and practice of schizophrenia research. Two categorical impulses are among the most prominent. One is the impulse to sort and label not just schizophrenia's symptoms (as mentioned above) but alleged types of the illness and other illnesses similar to schizophrenia. These include paranoid schizophrenia, delusional disorder, and

schizoaffective disorder among others. The second impulse is the effort to place schizophrenia into our conception of the impersonal physical or natural world: to categorize it in impersonal terms. Here the tendency is to try to explain the symptoms of schizophrenia wholly on the basis of physical or mechanical processes that do not themselves refer to the subjective experience of the person with the symptoms and who otherwise may be a 'respected partner with the power to influence his treatment' (Hobson and Leonard 2001, p. 186). What are the different varieties of schizophrenia? What disorders are similar to schizophrenia? What are the strengths and weaknesses of attempts to categorize schizo-phrenia in impersonal terms, absent direct reference to the person suffering from the illness?

Impersonal understanding is a tool of great power, revealing itself in the theoretical and technological successes of physics, chemistry, and the natural sciences. However impersonality also is potentially a blunt and disrespectful instrument. Loss of reference to the person who is the subject of the illness can be psychologically harmful and morally offensive.

3. *Questions of neurobiological models*. Given, in part, the impulse to treat schizophrenia as part of the impersonal natural order, neurobiological models are coming to dominate the medical-scientific picture of schizo-phrenia. It is worth pausing to clarify this trend towards the dominance of the specifically neurobiological. Ignoring differences among neuro-biological models in this context, there is a very effective way of seeing why such models are popular.

Open up and examine any major scientific study of schizophrenia and you will note that in addition to medical psychiatry there are several sciences that purport to contribute to understanding the condition: anthropology, sociology, cognitive psychology, genetics, neurobiology, and so on. Each science or discipline has its own characteristic theoretical vocabulary and domains of objects, relations, and properties, which it describes and to which it refers. With such multiple vocabularies and commitments, one wonders how order and prioritization can be achieved among them. Preference for the neurobio-logical proposes a programme of order and prioritization by privileging neurobiology and its domain, by assigning to brain science explanatory and metaphysical priority over other fields. Privileging the neurobiological is a proposal with economic incentives, too, of course, such as reinforcing the commercial interests of drug and insurance companies (which are taken up by some of our contributors).

To illustrate the pattern of neurobiological preference, suppose that our universe of concern is confined to two scientific hypotheses about the causes of schizophrenia. One of these, say, is the psychologistic non-neuroscientific *double-bind hypothesis* of Gregory Bateson and his colleagues (1956), and the other is, say, the neuroscientific *brain circuitry disruption hypothesis* (our label) of Nancy Andreasen and her colleagues (1998). To the first, schizophrenia is said to be due to a pattern of disordered or mixed-message communication of parents of pre-schizophrenic children, which makes it hard for a child to coherently process, co-ordinate, and respond to messages from parental authorities. To the second, schizophrenia is said to be due to a type of poor information transfer between the prefrontal cortex, the thalamus, and the cerebellum, which makes it hard for the central nervous system to process, and so on, perceptual information from a patient's natural and social environment.

If we believe that schizophrenia is due either to a failure of parent–child communication or to a failure of communication across brain regions, there is no reason to say that such a disjunction is exclusionary. We may be inclined to say: 'Good news; these two hypotheses are compatible'; 'On the one hand, parent–child miscommunication causes brain region miscommunication'; 'On the other hand, brain region miscommunication produces schizophrenia'. However, we may well have qualms about resting anything about the origins of neural miscommunication on so notoriously an evidentially infirm and culturally parochial a hypothesis as the double-bind hypothesis. So, we may be tempted to constrain our ecumenical sympathy for the pair of hypotheses by re-reasoning as follows.

The brain circuitry hypothesis (or something like it) may well be true, even if the double-bind hypothesis is false. Just which environmental or family history factors, if any, cause brain circuits to be disrupted is an issue perhaps for sociology or psychology to consider. It may be double-bind family communication. It may be something else entirely or perhaps no such environmental matters are germane to the onset of schizophrenia. Either way, presumably schizophrenia occurs if the brain is relevantly disrupted. The final pathway of schizophrenia is through the brain and so it is the brain that needs to be studied before or above all else.

Call such a view 'neural preferentialism'. It is the view that neurobiological processes are the proximal or most direct or immediate causes of schizophrenia (and of mental illness in general) and therein should hold causal-explanatory privilege in our understanding of schizophrenia. Neural preferentialism is an immensely popular view. However 'methodological ecumenism' (as preferentialism's generic contrary may be called), now often pronounced unhelpful, still emerges every so often. It is a good thing that it does so, too. Nelson Goodman has remarked, in a completely unrelated context, 'We do not make stars as we make bricks; not all making is a matter of moulding mud' (Goodman 1984, p. 42). So, too, to appropriate Goodman's metaphor, not all mental illness is a mere matter of moulding proximal neural causes. Human beings are environmentally situated and engaged creatures. The brain is a social organ, not a solipsistic one. Extensive causal or influential chains of various sorts, some of them wider and more complicated in environmental embedding and personal historical reach than current physical science can fathom, intersect with the neural and constitute explanatory strata or variables, reference to which, arguably, is and should be a major interest in the study of schizophrenia. Scenes from the life of St. Joan of Arc, for example, may be read both as the dances of neuromodulators and as temptations resisted, courage informed, and persecutions suffered at the admonition of her verbal auditory hallucinations (Joan's notorious 'voices'). These are matters for cultural anthropology, as well as for knowledge of Joan's personal history, to address (see Spence 2004).

Ecumenism, like all 'ism's', should have its limits and its defence clearly requires more systematic discussion and analysis, but the background choice is clear: It is between neural preferentialism or methodological ecumenism Which is it? The ecumenical embraces the neural, but the attitude of neural preferentialism towards non-neurobiological understanding tends to be much less conciliatory and encouraging. It is a form of order that often is epistemologically authoritarian. In any case, the relevance of non-neural explanatory frameworks for schizophrenia needs to be more carefully scrutinized and better understood. That is certainly a topic on which philosophers and philosophically informed mental health professionals like to exert their energies.

4. *Questions of faculty dissection.* The philosopher Alvin Goldman (1993) points out that 'the history of philosophy is replete with dissections of the mind, its faculties, and its operations' (p. xi). Epistemologists write of cognitive and perceptual acts and processes, such as judging, conceiving, introspecting, categorizing, and synthesizing. Ethicists write about the appetites, the passions, the sentiments, and the will. Aestheticians speak of the imagination, sense, sensibility, and apprehension. And so on. The study of schizophrenia has the potential for enriching exercises of dissection and helping to uncover the basic principles by which the human mind is organized. One characteristic of schizophrenia, for example, is that the description and analysis of its symptoms tend to cut across entrenched scientific and everyday categories of mental faculties and operations. Schizophrenic auditory hallucinations, for example, seem to involve as much cognition as perception, as much semantics and interpretation as sound and audition. Schizophrenic delusions mix judgement about self or the first-person with representation of the world: subjective sensitivity with objective apprehension, each interpenetrating the other.

One of the most important lessons of recent research in schizophrenia has been that aspects of our normal experiences of thinking and acting may be underpinned by sub-personal mechanisms of self-monitoring and self-observation. Perhaps these mechanisms are at fault in the formation of some sorts of schizophrenic delusions. So it is important to consider that representing the world may be wrapped up with representing the self-in-the-world or with the embedded self. One certainly does not need schizophrenia to drive home this consideration. Much human cognition expresses the inter-penetration of world and self-representation (Grush 2000). Schizophrenia vividly reinforces the lesson.

Thus there are four—at least four—sets of questions about schizophrenia with philosophical significance or purport. In one form or another they help to constitute the conceptual terrain of this book.

Each author in this book undertakes both to reform some current notions about schizophrenia or its symptoms or neighbouring or related conditions and to focus on one or more of the sets of questions mentioned above. The essays faculty dissect, categorically indulge, model, wrestle, and symptom conceptu-alize, some addressing one or two such tasks, some as many as all four. Given the underlying disposition to reform, thematically the book is a medley on reformative themes associated with schizophrenia rather than a motley set, nominally organized around schizophrenia. So, we have entitled our book *Reconceiving schizophrenia*. Unity among the chapters is sought not in dogmatic allegiance to a single doctrine or hypothesis, however, but in interest in conceptual change and revision. 'We don't really understand schizophre-nia', as we noted above, and some changes or advances certainly must be made in our conception of schizophrenia and related matters in order to address that insufficiency or inadequacy in understanding.

We begin the book with the powerful voice of someone who was diagnosed as a schizophrenic. Colin King describes his upbringing, his experience of being black and suffering racism, and his journey to the diagnosis of schizo-phrenia. He reflects on the inadequate theories explaining race and mental illness, and describes his struggle working for the other side, as a social worker, whose remit is to sign and declare someone mad and in need of compulsory admission to hospital.

In the second paper in the collection, Man Cheung Chung launches our investigation by mapping some of the conceptual terrain within a broadly sketched review of recent work on schizophrenia and the philosophy of schizophrenia. The methods and procedures of Chung's chapter express the commitment of many theoreticians of mental illness to locate their examin-ations in diverse theoretic traditions, as well as clinical materials.

Diversity is the order of the day in the next few papers. Highly suspicious of the neglect of the subjective experience of schizophrenic victims in the study of schizophrenia's conditions of onset and variation, in 'Explaining schizophrenia: the relevance of phenomenology' Louis Sass and Josef Parnas develop a picture of the causal contribution of subjective ex-perience to schizophrenia. Sass and Parnas succeed in reviewing much of the literature on the phenomenology of schizophrenia in their search for a more adequate description of the explanatory relevance of phenomenology to the illness.

Staying with the phenomenological approach, Alfred Kraus argues that we need to take seriously the expressions of schizophrenic victims as descriptions of their experience. We should interpret them as indicative of disruption of their usual experience of being in the world. For the schizophrenic victims to express their self-understanding in terms of, say, machine control, is a true account of the way in which they experience their world. Their existentialia are being experienced in a way which is different from ours.

Similarly, Osborne Wiggins and Michael Schwartz argue that to understand schizophrenia or schizophrenic hallucinations, we need to go beyond our own way of experiencing and expressing the world. A schizophrenic is a particular kind of human being-in-the-world in which ordinary human experience has been transformed in a way that affects space, time, causality, and the nature of objects, i.e. the most basic ontological constituents of the world.

In 'Schizophrenia and the sixth sense' Giovanni Stanghellini offers an account of the phenomenology of the social isolation of victims of schizophrenia, which, he claims, is due in part to the failure to integrate sensory experiences and to undergo them, subjectively, as one's own. Lessons, he claims, about both integration and self-attribution may be learned from a variety of historical sources including Aristotle. Grant Gillett, too, in his discussion of what he calls 'The paralogisms of psychosis' is concerned with the social isolation of victims of schizophrenia, in which, he says, subjects experience a breakdown in a common sense or, more specifically, common patterns of reasoning shared with and nurtured by other persons. Victims therein fall to 'walk in step' with others.

The next four papers are efforts at explicit reform. Jeffrey Poland examines the case for saying that schizophrenia is not a discrete illness but an aggregation of conditions, which are best comprehended and treated by jettisoning the category of schizophrenia—hence, the title, 'How to move beyond the concept of schizophrenia'. The paper by G. Lynn Stephens and George Graham tries to reverse a popular definition of delusion as a type of pathological belief and to replace this conception with a concept of delusion that more adequately corresponds to clinical practice. Delusions, the authors argue, are multi-level conditions that involve a failure of epistemic self-management. Andy Hamilton leads his reader through similar worries to Stephens and Graham, with his paper 'Against the belief model of delusion'. However, rather than seek a general account of the nature of delusion to replace the belief-orientated conception, as in the paper by Stephens and Graham, Hamilton draws a more sceptical conclusion about whether delusion admits of general or broad-based characterization. In 'The clinician's illusion and benign psychosis' Mike Jackson argues that the delusional component in schizophrenia is often treated with a pathologizing or clinical bias and that, in general, delusions or psychoses are best approached with openness to the possibility that they are, in many cases, either benign or even constructive and helpful for their subjects.

In 'Defining persecutory paranoia', Jennifer Radden takes a look at the roles of theme and content in delusional attitudes typical of schizophrenics and victims of similar illnesses—foremost themes of persecution or paranoia. Radden argues that reference to a paranoid theme serves not just to classify a type of delusion but also to identify its neural implementation architecture and significance to the more general contours of schizophrenia.

Peter Kinderman and Richard Bentall in 'The functions of delusional beliefs' seek to rescue the classification of delusions from the category of being unintelligible and irrational, and to re-orient therapy for delusion so that co-operative reasoning with delusional subjects becomes an increasingly popular form of treatment. The authors confront questions about the rationality of a paranoid worldview and whether equipped with a suitably ecumenical or loose understanding of the concept of belief, delusions such as paranoid worldviews might be regarded as global hypotheses or theories with personal functions for their subjects that helpfully might be examined by both subject and therapist.

Rom Harré in 'The logical basis of meta-narratives' and Eric Matthews in 'Suspicions of schizophrenia' explore aspects of the following two widely discussed facts about schizophrenia. One (already noted by Gillett and others) is that certain victims have difficulty fitting into normal human society. The other closely related fact is that medicine must be cautious lest it further marginalize such victims by treating them as broken brains or 'file' persons (to adopt one of Harré's critical metaphors) rather than as human subjects.

The authors of these papers, of course, do not agree with one another on all points. But there are two points on which they do agree. One is on the importance of finding a conception of schizophrenia or its symptoms that respects the personal experience and the reasoning capacity, suitably assisted, of its victims or subjects. The other is on the need to lighten the heavy and imperial hand of the impersonal and, in particular, neurobiological understanding of schizophrenia, which can be corrosive of respect for the personal experience of a subject. These are two points on which, we as editors trust, there will be much more work done by philosophers and non-philosophers alike as schizophrenia continues to be reconceived.

References

American Psychiatric Association. (1994). *Diagnostic and statistical manual of mental disorders*, (4th edn). Washington, DC: American Psychiatric Association.

Andreasen, N.C., Paradiso, S., and O'Leary, D. (1998). 'Cognitive dysmetria' as an integrative theory of schizophrenia: a dysfunction in cortical-subcortical cerebellar circuitry. *Schizophrenia Bulletin*, **24**: 203–218.

Bateson, G., Jackson, D., Haley, J., and Weakland, J. (1956). Toward a theory of schizophrenia. *Behavioral Science*, **1**: 251–258.

Davis, A. (1998). I feel cheated having this illness. In: *Abnormal psychology in context: voices and perspectives* (ed. D. Sattler, V. Shabatay, and G. Kramer), pp. 138–144. Boston, MA: Houghton Mifflin Company.

Frith, C. (1998). Deficits and pathologies. In: *A companion to cognitive science* (ed. W. Bechtel and G. Graham), pp. 380–390. Malden, MA: Blackwell.

Goldman, A. (1993). *Philosophical applications of cognitive science*. Boulder, CO: Westview Press.

Goodman, N. (1984). *Of mind and other matters*. Cambridge, MA: Harvard University Press.

Green, M.F. (2002). *Schizophrenia revealed*. New York: Norton.

Grush, R. (2000). Self, world, and space: the meaning and mechanisms of ego- and allocentric spatial representation. *Brain and Mind*, **1**: 59–92.

Heinrichs, R.W. (2001). *In search of madness: schizophrenia and neuroscience*. New York: Oxford University Press.

Hobson, J. A. and Leonard, J. (2001). *Out of its mind: psychiatry in crisis*. Cambridge, MA: Perseus.

Marshall, J. and Halligan, P. (1966). Towards a cognitive neuropsychiatry. In: *Method in madness: case studies in cognitive neuropsychiatry* (ed. P. Halligan and J. Marshall), pp 3–11. Hove, East Sussex, UK: Psychology Press.

Sahakian, W., Sahakian, B.J., and Sahakian Nunn, P.L. (1986). *Psychopathology today: the current status of abnormal psychology*, (3rd edn). Itasca, Illinois: Peacock.

Spence, S. (2004). Voices in the brain. *Cognitive Neuropsychiatry*, **9**: 1–8.

Young, A. (1999). Delusions. *The Monist*, **82**: 571–589.

2 They diagnosed me a schizophrenic when I was just a Gemini. 'The other side of madness'

Colin King

Introduction

> I like to introduce myself as Mr insane, subnormal and psychotic.
> In England I'm Mr Dangerous, difficult and threatening.
> In my Family, I am brother, son, Father, Uncle and friend.
> At school I'm educationally subnormal, delicate and confused.
> At college, I'm angry, distant and maintain a white free zone.
> In my dreams I'm brave, famous, knowledgeable and articulate.
> In my writing, ineligible and badly presented.
> In my verbal, mumbled, soft and inarticulate.
> In public spaces, I'm your potential mugger, your fitness instructor.
> At police stations, abused, heart problems, potential death case.
> With black people, approachable, loved, appreciated and understood.
> With white people, a cultural misfit, colourless and maladjusted.
> With white women, a sexual objectification of pleasure.
> With white men, masculine, penis orientated, feared.
> In hospital, overtly medicated, controlled and misunderstood.
> On the ward, no rights, no identity, an object of theory.

At 17 years of age I wrote this poem whilst reflecting on my arrival from prison, handcuffed to a Police Officer I was taken to a lock ward hospital after being placed on a Section of the 1959 Mental Health Act. I was told that I was suffering from schizophrenia and manic depression, and that I would be on mediation for the rest of my life. During the last 27 years, since passing my O-level English in hospital and completing my doctorate at Goldsmiths College, University of London, I have witnessed two family deaths, had two children, and suffered two further breakdowns. More significantly, I have read a proliferation of theories and research studies that never came near to understanding what it meant to be diagnosed or misdiagnosed as a black man in English society.

The aim of this paper is to show that the most authentic research comes from the user, those diagnosed as 'mentally ill'. The experiences that are free from the object of theory, research, or the prisoner of the multidisciplinary eye, who often pathologize and make irrational. Consequently, in the first part of this paper I will look at how current theories have explained the relationship between mental illness and racism. The alleged Eurocentrics, Foucault (1967) and Goffman (1967), against the black theorists such as Fanon (1967), Harris and James (1993), and Welsing (1987), who have all sabotaged my claim as just another Gemini. My concern is to see how a theory can help the individual understand their mental illness and reclaim their self-determination. In the context of this paper I am using the metaphor of my own zodiac sign, being a Gemini, as a challenge to the label of schizophrenia, in order to demonstrate that I was misunderstood. That I could simply be Colin with multi-identities, with the liberty to walk the streets without white people feeling they have to cross over, or hold on to their handbag because of the fear of black men.

I believe that the claim to be ordinary, to challenge the powerful fears of mental illness can only be achieved by allowing the users to tell their stories. In the second part of this paper I will analyse how I see my life as a black man trying to survive the damaging labelling that takes place within the school and the hospital settings. I will examine how Gilroy's (1983) idea of 'double consciousness' is useful to understanding the relationship between mental illness and being black and English. More specifically, what Fanon's (1967) idea of the 'white mask' means for black people coping with a system that cannot be sure where racism starts and mental illness ends. I suggest that the biological notions of race and mental illness have been replaced by cultural genes through procedures that pathologize black men through the notion of schizophrenia.

Consequently, in the third part of this paper I will analyse my experiences as a practitioner and researcher, and the problems of colluding with a system that once diagnosed me as mentally ill. I will examine the tensions between spying, empathy, and advocacy, and the ethnical issues of researching the needs of black people. More specifically, whether the practitioner can examine how their practices contain elements of schizophrenia, being out of reality with the subject they are looking at. The ultimate aim of this paper is to encourage those constructed as mentally ill to challenge the professionals who do not tell their stories on any authentic level. In trying to empower the user to challenge racism, I will assess how useful Macpherson's approach to institutional racism, and the recommendations from the 2000 Race Relation Amendment Act, has been to the disillusioned black patient.

Theorizing the dogma

Like death, you always wonder what the cause is, why at that moment life ended. Understanding mental illness, for example schizophrenia, is similar. The reason for why one part of your life terminates is never clear. The idea that mental illness is like a death that needs explanation can be seen by how it has been diagnosed. This is often by people who exempt themselves from being part of the process, for they have never been dead, they have never been diagnosed as mentally ill. As a survivor I attempted to read why the notion of mental illness is so persuasive. The exercise of making sense of the dead theorist is difficult. The word on the page divorces itself from the actual experiences of being seen and told you are different, more critically that you are mad.

On the plane home from my Grandad's funeral I attempted to make sense of Foucault's (1967) book on madness and civilization. Ironically, Foucault's (1967) work seemed as confused as the topic he is trying to discuss. What is interesting is the way that mental illness reflects the concerns of the age, the deviant, those seen as biologically, socially, or politically different. What emerges is that from the fifteenth century to the eighteenth century, madness becomes the symbol of unreason.

The clearest point from Foucault (1967) is that madness is about truth and knowledge, the power to observe and classify, as science becomes a social event. In this respect I do not believe Freud, Bowlby, or Erickson have correctly observed or understood my historical journey from Africa to the context of a cell in an English hospital. I am enlightened when I read Fanon's (1967) argument that European ideas of family strengthen the social order of whiteness, which has been central to rendering me as pathological and mad, as reflected in this quotation from his work (Fanon 1967, p. 15):

> When the Negro makes contact with the white world, a certain sensitizing action takes place. If his psychic structure is weak, one observes a collapse of the ego. The black man stops behaving as an actional man. The goal of his behaviour becomes the other (in the guise of the white man) for the other alone can give him worth.

What I find appealing from Fanon's (1967) comment is that his goal as an Algerian psychologist was to show that the unreasonableness in mental illness that Foucault describes is made more unreasonable when it comes into contact with racial differences. Fanon (1967) helps me to understand that the period of slavery and post-colonialism was vital in taking away the potential for black men like me to define ourselves.

I also wanted to know if there was a relationship between what happened 400 years ago when black men like me were chained, lynched, and brutalized to the way I was overtly medicated, locked up, and injected by white men who replaced their white sheets with white medical coats. I can only speculate about the echo of slavery and its impact upon how theories of race are disconnected from theories of mental illness. Part of this echo of slavery in terms of my own biography of the disordered patient, is represented by what Harris and James (1993) referred to as the 'noble savage'. If, as Foucault (1967) says, mental illness is about unreason, the fact that black men are similar to the savage, tests the reason of those who construct this idea. More painfully, the implications for the control of black men who find their body is divorced from their mind, is that it is unreasonable to assume they do not have any reason. Consequently, the biological notions of race expounded by Darwin, Burt, and Eysenck de-intellualize and de-humanize black men so that they cannot threaten the nature of European order. More specifically, the status of being an individual is denied; it means that the first impression of me as a physical being then influences the allocation of the title of madness.

The perennial struggle is to confront whether theories of mental illness can make explicit black experiences without hiding behind statistics of seeing white men as evil and nasty people. I suggest that the processes and procedures that lead to individuals being assessed as mentally ill take on a race dimension in their application to black men in British society. What is needed is a theory that sees British society as the wider psychiatric ward in which black men are stereotyped. If British society is the psychiatric ward, which makes black people vulnerable to a range of pathological assumptions, the actual ward of the hospital becomes the mirror.

When I read Gilroy's (1983) book on the transatlantic journey from Africa to the Caribbean to British society, I began to see how my life as a mental health survivor could be understood through my father's experiences and his father's. The idea that our consciousness, or what Gilroy (1983) refers to as our 'double consciousness' as both African and English, is shaped by history gives me license to free myself from the stigma of being told that my mental illness, my disorder, was nothing to do with my past.

I believe being defined as a schizophrenic was a way of showing to me that I was simply confused about my identity. When I left hospital and started the first of three degree courses I was forced to read Goffman (1961). I became jealous of the privilege given to him to walk on to a ward and produce a book on what he considered to be the essential components of an asylum. What I found useful in the work of Goffman (1961) was the outcomes of being defined as mad. The processes of mortification, being categorized and enduring the ceremonies of a ward setting, having to accept one's status as mad. What angered me about Goffman (1961) is this naïve assumption that the ward gave me access to people I would not have encountered in the outside world, to the privileged domain of whiteness, as reflected in this quotation (Goffman 1967, p. 165):

> Another group were Negroes, those who so wished were able to some degree to cross the class and colour line, cliquing with and dating white patients and receiving from the psychiatric staff some of the middle class professional conversations and treatment denied to them in the outside world.

Goffman (1956) makes apparent the arrogance of whiteness, as a set of negative beliefs about the other. He enables the white researcher, unmonitored, to make implicit forms of knowledge about mental illness that had profound implications for my life as a black patient. It suggests that by acting the big, mad, and bad patient, black men are rewarded by being brought closer to whiteness. It is a correctional form of whiteness, it strips you of your identity as a black man, it 'deculturalizes' and exposes you to the contamination of the therapies, medication, and procedures of the white man.

By reading Goffman's (1961) ideas of stages and performances, I began to see schizophrenia was a drama, a script that I could act out, but I could not challenge the rationale of the script writers. The whole notion of schizophrenia began to make sense as a process of several agencies. The historical agency that suggested it was about being out of reality. Lastly and most importantly the agency that suggested that the crucial factor of diagnosis was about interpretation, as Goffman alludes to in this statement (Goffman 1961, p. 127):

> What we discover is the self-system of a person undergoing schizophrenia change or schizophrenia process is then in its simplest form, an extremely fear-marked puzzlement, consuming up the use of rather generated and anything but exquisitely refined referential processes in an attempt to cope with what is essentially a failure at being human—a failure of being anything that one could represent as worth.

Goffman (1956) shows that there is an inhumanity in the process of being seen as a schizophrenic. What he fails to do, in terms of my own personal and specific issues as a black man, is show how the European, those who diagnose, use their theories to construct the other as a real, live, complicated drama. The 'other' in this case is the black man who, despite the complexity of his individual situation, is more likely to be diagnosed with an illness he has had little involvement in constructing.

From the talk of Goffman in the 1960s, many have attempted to explain the high numbers of black young men who occupy beds in the English psychiatric system. The pattern has been to see schizophrenia as a political and moral dilemma for English society, in its dealing with the alien—he who does not act in accordance with the demands of white English culture. The theory that the longer period of adjustment of the cultural alien would lead to greater integration and reduced vulnerability to being diagnosed, has been disproved. His failure has been reinforced by statistical estimates that show that black men are ten times more likely to be diagnosed as schizophrenic (Mental Health Foundation 1998).

The school of thought from Littewood and Lipsedge (1989) and their notion of the alien and the alienist, point crucially to the need to examine how mental illness is constructed. When two white men suggest the obvious, that Western psychiatry mirrors what they refer to as 'cultural schizophrenia' as a clash between two cultures, the culture of the white psychiatrist is never made transparent (Littlewood and Lipsedge 1989, p. 29):

> We are still white, male doctors, discussing the private experiences of patients who are frequently black male, working class; part of what Foucault calls the monologue of reason about madness.

I suggest this attempt to see the psychiatric profession as the centre of the construction of the pathologies of the black man is too simplistic. It is not sufficient compensation to the families and friends of those who commit suicide to be comforted by the fact that their loss was due to some obscure issue of unreason and misconstruction. Whilst the debate about misdiagnosis has moved towards the area of constructionism, centring on the medical and social work profession 'paradigms' of looking at the world, this has not resulted in any radical change of practice.

The process of white professionals suggesting that they may construct pathologies, is their license to exemption similar to what Macpherson (1999) refers to as 'unwitting'. Compared to those who diagnosed, who go through a rigid assessment procedure, the professional who listens and assesses is not subjected to the same procedure in terms of having to justify how they are making sense of their reason. I think Harris and James (1999) show that the white professional who assesses mental illness is unethical if he/she does not see the power of how racism operates in their practice (Harris and James 1993, p. 181):

> Culture is then important to psychiatric diagnosis as part of the routine of what is normal and what is pathological. The psychiatrist, often disguised as the anthologist, then occupies a position of power by being able to delineate the boundaries that define and separate behaviour from madness

This quotation from Harris and James (1993) brings to light the power of the psychiatric profession to reinforce a dominant culture without explaining what culture is in terms of how they act. The danger is that the psychiatrist, like the black man, is constructed as bad; their research opinions and actions ultimately leading to pathologies. Consequently the stereotypes and labelling of black young men cannot be avoided; the delusions and hallucinations expressed by the other, are placed firmly back on the nasty, white, male consultant, who then becomes the 'noble savage'. This position is too general and does not take me much further in explaining the specifics of my own personal biography and my career as a mental health patient.

One of the reasons why it is important to understand how the psychiatric profession and their partners operate in the interface with black men is to show that there is an incoherent theory that underlines their performance. The experience of the black inmate reflects how the institutions in which I was located actually operate and how whiteness manifests itself. In this context I suggest there are forms of whiteness that are performed in different ways in constructing mental illness in relation to black young men. In the next part of this paper I want to go through the processes of being diagnosed in order to provide an insight into how whiteness, as a pattern of action, responds to differences. The voice I use in this context is that of the user's voice, specifically the survivor's voice.

Was he a schizophrenic or just another Gemini?

It seems his present illness started at the beginning of the last year following a series of unpleasant events—his father stabbed him with a chisel in the face and forearm. He was stabbed by a friend of his sister's in the chest and treated at Guy's Hospital. He was expelled from school after attacking a teacher who sent him off the football ground. He changed from a person who was usually jocular and likeable to a sullen, taciturn, and irritable boy. When he was admitted here he said that he had been troubled by thoughts of death, both his own and his mother's, and was unable to stop thinking about it. We found that, although he went to bed early, he was unable to get up in the morning. He also tended to be weepy and very irritable and slept late. His appetite was diminished and he had been constipated. After admission there were several episodes during which, with or without provocation, he lost his temper and became physically aggressive towards patients. Because of his high arousal state he was treated with phenol-thiazine as well as anti-depressant.

His schizophrenia seemed to improve and his thoughts about death receded and he became much livelier. However, he still found it very difficult to control his aggression. He also attempted to disclaim responsibility for his actions and the family colluded in his excuses. In a final effort to maintain a situation in which it was possible to continue treating him, a contract was drawn up. He agreed to the contract but, unfortunately, was unable to keep it. He was therefore discharged as he agreed. We still wish to continue efforts to help alter his behaviour pattern, therefore arrangements have been made for him to be admitted to an open ward with a structured environment.

Doctor X: Maudsley Hospital

A white female consultant wrote this report in 1977 after I had been transferred from remand centre where I had been told after an assessment that I was a schizophrenic and a manic-depressive. After three assessments by professionals I had met only once, I had been deprived of my status as a Gemini; the claim of having a split personality had been medicalized. I have tried for the last eight years to get access to my medical notes; my efforts have failed. They were either lost, not available, or the personnel who could give me access had left. In this part of the paper, I want to reveal the journey from being diagnosed to moving towards being a survivor and activist.

First, I can tell my own story, do my own assessment, to show how inadequately theories of race and mental illness had analysed my life, thus redressing the pathologies that have become important in English psychiatry.

Second, I want to inspire other individuals to engage in their own person-centred research, to empower them to become their own advocate. Last, I want to assist professionals in their assessment of their practice, theorists in the management of their interventions, and researchers in the ethics of looking at race and mental illness.

Throughout these challenges I am indebted to the work of Fanon (1967) and his notion of the 'white mask', which he uses to see how Algerians coped with the intervention of white European society. I think the 'white mask' has been important in enabling me to examine how I have coped with white professionals and the need to act white to avoid being seen as mentally ill. I want to use the mask as a tool that helps me in my internal world to develop a range of strategies to deal with the different professionals who have been involved in my life as a mental patient.

In terms of the historical context, I was born 6 June 1960 (no relationship to the devil), the third of six children. The first eleven years of my life were spent in that memorable arena called Crystal Palace. My mother came from Kingston Jamaica, an only child who attended public school with high aspirations to become a doctor. My father came from a large fishing community, a traditional drinking, smoking, self-abusing, male-dominated culture.

Home in the early days was a rented house, which we shared with some innocent rats, with a hole in the wall and a puffin heater as creature comforts. Sleeping four in a bed with my three brothers seemed an adventure then, regarded as poverty today. My father during this period appeared to be consumed with alcohol and disorientated by pure self-pity and anger. We rarely saw the kind and gentle caring side of him; he was a man pent up with frustrations with little contentment and happiness. He never ever said he loved me or he was proud of me, right to the time he lost his sight, his ability to use the toilet on his own, his ability to shave as he lost his desire to live. I had to do all these domestic tasks, and I never remember him fathering me in this way.

I went to Paxton Primary School, like conscription, to join my two brothers who I had witnessed marching off in the two previous years before me. I hoped that the war at school would be easier than the war at home. School was a funny place; white teachers, white pictures, and white images; white Jack and Jill, black golliwog, white nursery rhymes, and white stories. For the first time I really felt unhappy about being black. School situated this need for a 'white mask'; it was there that I really discovered my blackness as a child, especially when the other white kids used to ask me if my father was a coal miner.

At Sunday school, we were introduced to the Lord through our mother, but we were more excited to be mixing with other children, signing and carrying the flag for the cubs during parade days. What I could not understand was why the church was full of black people on one side, colourfully dressed, full of the blessings of the Lord, praying and signing like it was their last visit to church. On the other side of the church was a group of white people, well dressed, sombre, who seemed to look down on us, controlled and expressionless. It was here I began to establish a consciousness of what it meant to be a black person by these different privileges and methods of separation.

At primary school, being a boy, being in an army, not being girlish, and being good at sports, appeared more important than a racial or cultural identity. Gary Glitter, Peter Osgood, and fish and chips took priority over the pain and suffering taking place in South Africa. I left primary school at the same time that Steve Biko was murdered. I had seen my mother struggle for most of her life to bring us up, to love us, and to value education, whilst our Dad valued the power of drink. I pledged to kill him, but knew later in my life that this was my subconscious telling me that I no longer respected him as a parent, as a man, and as a black person. I realized later on in my academic life how important Richard Wright's (1945) reflection was on how the legacy of violence experienced during the period of slavery infringed upon black families like my own.

By the time I left primary school I felt completely unsure about myself. I hated my large lips, my big broad nose, and the deep brownness of my skin. Our school was split between old, white, colonialist teachers, who thought we were monkeys who could not be taught and should be caned, and a new breed of liberal white teachers, enthusiastic, broad side burns, who thought children should be heard. As black children we were caught in the middle of these two distinct forms of whiteness. It confused the operation of the 'white mask' because it was impossible to assess what type of behaviour was being demanded.

By the time I was 14 years of age, I began to realize that happiness was rare, seemingly inaccessible. As I grew older, expectations of being contented diminished. I still had an inner sense of self, untouched by the white world, expressed through nightly dreams of being rich, the best footballer, and the most intelligent man in the world. Waking up reinforced my disillusionment; looking at the mirror seeing that my nose was not straight, hearing my Dad scream blue murder, and my mother fighting him off as he engaged in another battle. The 'white mask' that once had been a protective coping mechanism began to see the pain of surviving in a white world.

Looking back at my school years, the alleged happiest days of your life, seemed a mirage, a set of unfulfilled dreams, surpassed by a list of painful memories. The first time I was asked 'how are you feeling?' And what is it like to be Colin, the Gemini?, Was when I had my first mental health assessment. I often felt being a black child in this country was like having to endure a series of mental health assessments, from the time you are born, through to leaving school to taking your final breath in this world.

School was like one big mental health institution, set times for classes, meals, and physical activities. You were told how to learn, policed and monitored by teachers in sterile, dark, controlling suits, the same suits worn by consultants, asking questions that placed you in an educationally limited programme. At school truancy was the most important therapeutic option to survive the dangers of this white setting.

I had few contacts with white women; only on Dallas, or a pin-up on page three of The Sun newspaper. Unlike the white men, who had either caned me, controlled me, or told me I was mad. Even then in my early adolescence I had developed an unhealthy dislike for white people, which I now rationalize as a dislike for the privilege of whiteness, unable to challenge the pathological outcomes of their intervention, so I would never feel the need for a 'white mask'.

My experience of white men in schooling seriously affected my ability to trust or see any positive images of them as real people. They looked different, smelt different, and had a whole different orientation to life that seemed to transcend anything I had ever experienced. I am ashamed to say that I always wanted to look white, feel white, and be white; everything around me seemed to be made in their image. All the top football players, all the attractive people, actors, and models were white. I wanted to render the 'white mask' redundant and to fully qualify for the status and privilege of being white.

Suddenly you look in the mirror, and you see all those failed black men, who begin to look just like yourself, your father, and your grandfather. You look for people to blame. I began to realize, as shown in the work of Welsing (1991), how white supremacy as a set of powerful symbols dominated my life. In relation to school, with one year left, you have no chance of success. All you are left with is your masculinity, as you begin to wonder whether anybody in the school system really cares about what happens to you.

At the age of 16 whilst playing in a school match against the teachers I was taken off for no apparent reason. I reacted unreasonably in an incident that led to a fight with a PE teacher. I was jumped on by several teachers, spat in the face, and eventually expelled from school. Suddenly you are left with no structure, no identity, no future, your faith in whiteness further dented.

One year later after defending my sister in a fight against fifteen black young boys outside a youth centre, a broken milk bottle was put in my back. My anger disconnected the pain and in a moment of reflection, looking at the hole in my back, I realized that as black men we had learnt to invert our anger about white society into our own self-destruction. I remember lying in the hospital bed after being questioned by the police, adamant that I was not going to inform on the culprits and make them vulnerable to a legal and medical system that was more intent on the discrimination of black men.

The downhill spiral of life continued, six months later I was in a remand centre after a series of minor and senseless actions. Suddenly you are back at school in a residential setting, same faces as school, same teaching mentality but more penal outcomes. Living in a cell for 23 hours a day is the most depriving and de-humanizing experience, the legacy of slavery apparent, with black boys, numbers written on their shirt instead of on their skin. The days spent sleeping, listening to tales from your room-mate, or reading the bible. It is ironic that the one thing you retreat to in periods of grave despair is the bible, which make you believe that if you put your trust in the Lord, your mental soul still belongs to white people.

After long periods of frustration, the social worker, psychiatrist, and probation officer came to start their multiple questionnaires, their assessment. I wanted to tell them anything to get into the more privilege setting of the prison, the mental hospital. They sat on the opposite side of the table asking questions from their notes, like a job interview seeing if I met the job description of madness specification. They look you up and down like some dangerous animal in the zoo. All the pathologies of you as a black man who is mad are rendered in there non-verbally. The cold looks, the strident pen in contact with the form, the look at the door to see if they are safe. They ask the same questions and repeat themselves, look at each other like trying to conduct a performance. You realize that the offer of an open cell with soft toilet paper, not having to shit in a bucket at night, and food without maggots persuades you that it is more suitable to act mad, than eventually become mad through pure deprivation.

I remember looking at the open ward, my acne making me look like I had a second face, mortified, life became morbid, with no purpose, no pride, no joy, and no ambitions, cut off; you begin to think life is like that all the time. What is the use of living if misery and pain are so consistent? We were born to die, so why be born and why live? Some time in the future you will not be here, nor will your family or friends; all will be cold, under ground, pushing up roses.

Madness as a form for a black young man is determined by the perception of the other professionals in the hospital setting. In a mental prison ward, the officers tell you that you are mad, the psychiatrist tells you that you are mad, and the other prisoners believe you are mad; you need some great resolve to be you are the only one who believes in your own sanity.

My mother came to see me regularly in hospital, often in tears. She never hugged me, but I could see by the pained expression on her face that she felt totally helpless. After three months in prison I was deemed clinically mad and moved to a mental hospital, handcuffed to two officers during the short trip to embark upon the next part of my mortifying career as a mental health patient. The locked ward was a very lavish environment compared to the cold walls of a prison. On my first night a disturbed black man tried to strangle me; we later became the best of friends. Although the setting had changed, mental hospitals are far more frightening places than my brief experience of being in prison. They seduce you into the role of the dependent black man by a number of subtle techniques, behaviour therapy, counselling, and group work.

This control is illustrated by the passive aggressive approach of the white female consultant, who excelled at asking me questions about my sense of madness, false nodding, plastic smiles, and tight hands. These actions were often incompatible to the negatives contained in her report. On the ward I was not allowed out until I could walk straight, clean behind my foreskin, and prove that I was not going to hitchhike to Brixton without coming back. Most of my family came to see me regularly but communication was impossible due to too much medication. Most of the day I spent sleeping, trying to fight the dead tongue, the tremors, the shivers, and the inability to walk without assistance.

I had lost my ability to laugh, to be happy; the bad days deteriorated into very bad days. Morbid self-destruction remained paramount to my daily existence; talk was limited as I spent more of the time in the waste of a cocktail of medication. I was restrained on a number of occasions for outbursts. The echo of slavery became more acute, locked up, forced into menial jobs, and threatened not with the whip but a deadly needlefull of medication. White staff in their falseness tried to converse to try to pass the time. My incentive came from my English teacher who somehow got me involved in studying for O-level English. My outbursts gradually subsided as I motivated myself somehow to study whilst hearing people screaming in the background, fights breaking out, staff going home, and watching night turn into day.

I took my O-level English examination in November with the same usual disturbances on the ward, whilst I tried to develop sentences into paragraphs. Somehow I passed; it was meaningless, it represented no achievement, my emotional state stayed the same, my Dad stayed the same, and one day we were all going to die.

I was allowed out for my first weekend. The severity of the medication meant that I could not walk without my mother carrying me down the street, as people laughed. Returning to hospital led to much confusion about what constituted home. The safe institutional setting of a ward, regular meals, fags, a bed, and a patronizing consultant and ward staff continually reminding me of my madness.

The conflict between hospital and home ended very suddenly when I was expelled when one of the inmates tried to sexually assault me in the toilet. I reacted by holding a letter holder to protect me. Suddenly I was out on the streets, offered an out-patients' appointment, with some consultant who could not give a damn how I would manage. I simply replaced the hospital routine with one at home, waking up late, watching television all day, making the occasional trip to sign on, buying fags or food, and disappearing at night when my father returned home. Most of my friends were either unemployed, in hospital, dead, or entertaining school fantasies that were never going to be realized.

Suddenly one day I decided that I had had enough of squandering my already pathetic life, with images of my father, twenty years on, angry and frightened. I was an ugly sight at 18 years of age, unemployed, with a record, no partner, languishing in second-floor council accommodation on one of the worst estates in London, North Peckham. I somehow managed to motivate myself to get to a college with no financial backing. I had to walk to college and back, six miles a day, studying on the toilet as my dad would not allow me to go to college, he had plans for me to go on the building site along with my other brothers.

I committed myself one-hundred per cent to the rigour of college. It felt like primary school, personified by the presence of rich, middle-class kids. I managed to pass O-levels and A-levels and went on to do a degree and social work course. I managed to get through college years, made no friends, and speedily left the lecture room to avoid contamination with liberal, right-on, young socialists. But on reflection I had realized through the use of my 'white mask' that no matter how I demonstrated I could be white to be accepted as normal, I could not change or alter the static minds of those who assess through their polluted notions of whiteness. The report from the white female consultant reflects the dogma contained in the theories discussed in the first section of this paper that lead to the cold portrayal of black men like me. These caricatures that become rigid can only be made sense of when one travels to the other side, in the role of the mental health professional.

Working for the other side: institutional madness

In this part of the paper I want to show how Goffman's (1956) notion of the back and front stages help us to understand the two sides to the diagnosis of schizophrenia. The front stage is the interaction between the client and the professionals, and the back stage where the client is constructed in their absence. I believe the idea of stages is vitally important to the research of misdiagnosis because from a user perspective they can understand the dangers that exist in professionals operating in a contradictory manner. More specifically, when we begin to examine the ethnical dishonesty between the stages, where practitioners or researchers talk to the client to how they behave in the back stage, behind the client's back, institutional madness becomes more transparent. These forms of institutional madness become apparent in two fundamental ways. First, in the manner in which whiteness as sets of actions that operate through individual and collective beliefs and practices. Second, the 'cultural schizophrenia' that Littlewood and Lipsedge (1987) suggest, becomes evident in the multidisciplinary context, in the ways that social workers, psychiatrists, and doctors behave in the back stages of the institutions of mental illness.

I was able to look at these beliefs and practices that lead to diagnosis and the power of whiteness when I qualified as a social worker and began to specialize as a mental health practitioner. I became an approved social worker, now empowered to sign and declare somebody I had never known as mad and needing to be compulsorily admitted to hospital. I could now analyse the demons of my mental health career and how it was constructed by procedures and the ways the professionals acted. I had been given privileged access to the back stages, where the actors and the professionals were situated and performed.

To access some of the conspiracies that I felt operated on a patient, which I was now colluding with, I want to describe one assessment that revealed some of the dilemmas for me as a black man working for the other side. A phone call had come through to the duty desk, a desk where professionals take calls from people in the community about people who may be acting in a dangerous manner. It was apparent that the person was known to the service. I went to the patients' records, with thousand of files with numbers; I wondered if my file was there. The file was read by a white female social worker. The person was known, he was of African origins but described as black—'that mad person who we have sectioned so many times it looks like he needs to come in again, I'll give the police, ambulance and the other doctor a call'.

Despite the apparent madness of assuming madness before it was assessed, it had lead to professionals coming out under the pretension that a section (a compulsory admission) would take place. This shows how these backstage presumptions have profound implications for the drama that takes place in the front stage. After hearing the brief story of this person's recent situation, all professionals decided to come out immediately, only if the police were available. The construction of the black man from the reading of the notes, to the telephone conversation, led to somebody who was aggressive, acting bizarrely, who may not be taking his medication. More importantly he had a diagnosis, he was described as not *suffering* from schizophrenia, he *was* a schizophrenic, and he had an ongoing identity as being mentally ill.

I had learnt in my training that it is best to take the less restricted alternative, that hospitalization should be the last resort. In the context of this black man, perceived as dangerous, the institution now operated in the opposite way, 'if in doubt knock them out' was a cliché that became institutional. Like an SAS operation it was decided that we had got a bed, and we were going to get the body into hospital. Outside this person's home was a scared-looking GP in a shabby suit, pen in hand, informing us that we had to be quick, he had just left his practice. He was accompanied by God, the omnipotent presence of the psychiatrist, also a white man in his fifties. The SAS staffing was completed by two young police officers who wanted to break down the door before we had even entered and one ambulance with two white men who wanted to know if the sections papers had been completed and where we would be taking the body.

The white social worker knocked on the door, with no answer; she knocked again, again no answer; she knocked harder. Eventually a very thin, young, innocent-looking black male answered, in his boxer shorts, tired looking with a blanket around him. He could have been my younger brother. In this context you face a number of moral and political dilemmas, you immediately know on a humane level that the behaviour of these professionals is wrong; powerless to challenge, you painfully watch the drama unfold. The young man tells the professionals to go away, they all follow him into the bedroom where he attempts to go back to bed, shouting 'I am tired, can't you come back another time'. The response is that 'you need to come into hospital and sort your self out, look come now the ambulance is here' like being invited to a trip to the zoo.

The young man runs into the bedroom, his front door is open as spectators from the surrounding estates arrive, he locks himself in, as one of the police officers says, 'Stand back, let me break it down'. The more mature officers advise him that he might be behind the door. In the background the consultant and GP sign their forms; they make no association that this intrusion might have contributed to this person's actions, as they leave. The young man comes out of the bedroom, after a period of bargaining, almost as if we are trying to get a terrorist to come out. He runs into the front room, and I hear the social worker say, 'Just put a blanket over him and get him into the ambulance'. He is brought out of his home with a grey blanket, shouting and screaming, thrown into the ambulance. I feel a silent tear, a pain of disbelief, a revisit to the roots episode, and my own personal biography, like a slave naked, taken away. The 'white mask' used during my own journey into hospital, is now a collusive and submissive mask, failing to speak out against the injustice witnessed. I walk again down the same corridor where I was once chained, now party to a man who looks like me and was equally defiant towards his imprisonment. The ward causes a confusion of roles; on entry I am asked if my bed is ready, as I feel further disorientated, had I come home or was I just part of the conspiracy in which black men are imprisoned?

To examine my role in this drama and how I was contributing to these institutional processes of racism, I refer to Macpherson's (1999) definition of institutional racism, as the most current and most persuasive in British society on several levels. First through the failure to challenge the theories discussed in section one that led to a belief system about black men as the unreasonable, noble savage. Second in the failure to use my own experience as a point of empathy to challenge the practices of the professionals acting in the same ways as they had acted towards me. Third, and most crucially, can we trust whiteness, the ignorance, and lack of self-analysis of the white practitioner to engage in research about the other, without perpetuating the same pathologies. Macpherson's (1999) definition of institutional racism says:

> The collective failure of an organisation to provide appropriate, professional services to people because of their culture, colour or ethnic origins. It may be detected in processes, attitudes or behaviours that amount to discrimination through unwitting prejudices, ignorance and thoughtlessness and racist stereotyping that disadvantage racial and ethnic groups.

This one assessment illustrates the danger of the professionals, mainly white, producing a series of actions and words in which the outcomes lead to the diagnosis of schizophrenia. Once the body is locked away in the setting on the ward, the opportunity to collectively and individually examine one's prejudices and thoughtlessness does not take place. The opportunity to challenge the processes, attitudes, or behaviours of the professional that amount to discrimination is left to the patient, who must apply to a mental health tribunal. The patient must be their own advocate, whilst this role is neglected by the professional, because advocacy, as a political and emotional approach, would lead to questioning of the whole ethos on which the diagnosis is based.

For professionals to maintain their sanity they have to avoid seeing how madness operates in their practice in the diagnosis of schizophrenia. Consequently the only way it was possible to examine the feelings of those who have become the victim of their disordered pathological eye, was to talk to those who had been sectioned, outside of my role as an approved social worker. I was able to do this when employed by the Mental Health Foundation as a researcher, to talk to people with a history of mental illness, to look at what helped them to cope. I did not want to replicate again being the 'black spy' for the purposes of a white organization but to ensure that the confidentiality of black users was preserved and that the information obtained should not be used to reinforce historical stereotypes around black people in mental health and psychiatry.

I talked to six black users, two women and four men, about their potential stories and the specific ways that they faced the potential of further mental health breakdowns. The interviews took place in a small room attached to the main project. It had two seats, quite close together, grey carpet, and light grey walls and pictures of significant black icons (Bob Marley, Nelson Mandela, and Diane Abbott). It was a room of warmth, symbolic of a black space away from the clinical setting of a mental health hospital.

All the users waited to see me, to be heard, but more essentially to be paid. Each was given fifteen pounds for their time; asked questions about their diagnosis, their family, and personal support, their community, the specific therapies that enabled them to survive. Themes were of a disabling sense of loss of a life, as if dead, and life that could not be returned to. The statutory procedures that made them feel de-humanized in terms of their diagnosis had objectified their reality under rigid labels. A few spoke of a sense of being dragged, pulled, arrested, in the process of being taken to hospital. The echo of slavery rings loud again, in the ways these painful encounters were discussed. Most talked as if this was normal and internalized the actions as justified by saying 'maybe it was something wrong with me'.

Some talked as if family and friends had died, they were seen as abnormal and diseased, potentially infectious. The professionals they encountered became symbolic of their vulnerability, people who could do them damage, people who came into their home once a month, insincere in their static questioning, invading them with a needle, medication, and then threatening them with a return to hospital if they deteriorated. I realized that the next step was to challenge these processes that had destroyed their lives; to redress the theories that have pathologized them; that a black perspective to research and diagnosis was important.

Conclusion

As a conclusion to this paper, the black researcher has to analyse his or her own pain in representing the voices, histories, and cultural experiences of the 'black schizophrenic'. The researcher must also censor those who act in unethical ways. The black researcher, in giving information to white institutions, must also ensure that the professionals and the theories that pathologize are exposed. I strongly believe that the user is best positioned to understand the impact of the other, those who theorize and those who intervene into and judge their world. More specifically, whiteness must not escape structural scrutiny.

No longer do I want to go into the homes of black men, as a researcher or a practitioner, and understand their lives through tools that bear no resemblance to their world. When I left the project in Birmingham, when I left that black man in hospital, and when I think of my life in this setting, it reinforces the need to assess how they are understood by the other. There is now an imperative to introduce ethnical standards in the assessment of mental illness. Users should not only be an essential part of this process, they should be part of the ethnical board that examines the practice of the theorist, the practitioner, and the researcher. More specifically in the arena of racism, the black user should be encouraged and activated to use the new Amendments to the Race Relation Act 2000 to ensure that they are consulted with and to monitor all interventions, legal, political, theoretical, and economic that may affect the relationship between racism and mental illness. The alternative is that the establishment will continue to use Christopher Clunis, who stabbed and killed whiteness, as the indicator of how black men are as the noble savage.

References

Fanon, F. (1967). *Black skin, white mask*. London: Pluto Press.

Foucault, F. (1967). *Madness and civilisation*. London: Routledge.

Goffman, E. (1961). *Asylums*. London: Penguin books.

Littewood, R. and Lipsedge, R. (1989). *Aliens and alienist, ethnic minorities and psychiatry*. London: Routledge.

Welsing, F.C. (1991). *The Isis papers. The key to the colours*. Chicago: Third World Press.

Wright, R. (1945). *Black boys*. USA: Pans books.

3 Conceptions of schizophrenia

Man Cheung Chung

Introduction

Philosophy has a special role to play in understanding psychiatry and abnormal psychology, as Karl Jaspers (1923/1963, pp.769–770) remarked:

> Many a psychiatrist has said that he did not want to burden himself with a philosophy and that this science had nothing to do with philosophy.... But the exclusion of philosophy would nevertheless be disastrous for psychiatry.... If anyone thinks he can exclude philosophy and leave it aside as useless he will eventually be defeated by it in some obscure form or other.... Only he who knows and is in possession of his facts can keep science pure and at the same time in touch with individual human life which finds its expression in philosophy.

Indeed, to advance our understanding of psychopathology, the importance of the partnership between philosophy, psychiatry, and psychology cannot be ignored.[1] The International Perspective in Philosophy and Psychiatry book series, of which the present book is part, symbolizes the success of this partnership.[2] This is a partnership in which psychiatrists and psychologists, through philosophical analysis, can learn to reflect critically on the assumptions embedded within classificatory systems, on the way in which the complexity of various mental disorders is understood, on the science and practice of psychiatry and abnormal psychology, and indeed on the ways in which patients experience, perceive, feel, think, and act. At the same time, through investigating different mental disorders, philosophers can raise important philosophical issues and confront the challenges of theoretical constructs in, for example, philosophy of mind (Graham and Stephens 1994; Radden 1996; Wallace et al. 1997; Sass et al. 2000). As a result of this partnership, a new, innovative and challenging way of exploring, describing and indeed understanding mental disorders, including schizophrenia, has come into being.[3]

In relation to schizophrenia, the topic that is the focus of this book, we may ask, 'What are the issues raised thus far through the joint effort of the partnership?'. My survey seems to suggest that, broadly speaking, the issues are as follows. One is concerned with classification and diagnosis in which some have pondered on the validity, usefulness and indeed the problems of classifying mental disorder including schizophrenia. Another issue concerns understanding the subjective experience and meaning of schizophrenics. How can we access this experience and meaning? Some would argue, certainly not through modern diagnostic classifications. Other issues are pertaining to the notion of self in schizophrenia, in particular, the disorder of the self, and the specific symptoms manifested in schizophrenia. In this chapter, my intention is to give an overview of some of the work that has been carried out to address these issues.

Classification and diagnosis of schizophrenia

First and foremost, before we embark on this review, let us remind ourselves briefly of some of the clinical features of schizophrenia. According to DSM-IV, a current, well-recognized, and widely-used means of classifying mental disorders, schizophrenia can typically be divided into positive symptoms, negative symptoms, and disorganized symptoms. To fulfil the diagnosis of schizophrenia, patients would need to present two or more positive, negative, and/or disorganized symptoms for at least one month. Generally speaking, positive symptoms include delusions and hallucinations. Delusion is a false belief that is fixed and firmly held by the patients despite explicit contradictory evidence. That is, it is a disturbance in the content of thought. Patients with delusional beliefs may believe that their thoughts, feelings, or actions are being controlled by external forces or agents (alien control), that their private thoughts are being broadcast (thought insertion), or that their thoughts are taken away by some external forces or agents (thought withdrawal). They may also believe that they are very famous or important people (e.g. Jesus Christ, a delusion of grandeur), that people are plotting against them (delusion of persecution), or that certain environmental events (e.g. television programmes) bear special, significant meanings for them (e.g. delusion of reference).

Hallucinations are sensory or perceptual experiences, which occur without perceptual stimulus in the external world. They can manifest in the form of auditory hallucinations in that they may hear voices uttering single words, brief phrases, or whole conversations, giving commands to patients, talking aloud patients' thoughts, discussing the patients with each other, or commenting on patients' actions. Patients may also experience visual hallucinations in which they see flashes of light or complex images (e.g. the figure of a person). They may also experience tactile hallucinations in which they feel some superficial sensations of being touched, pricked, or strangled. They may also experience hallucination of smell and taste, whereby they experience an unpleasant smell or flavour never experienced before.

Negative symptoms include deficits in normal behaviour, which include emotional and social withdrawal, apathy, and poverty of thought or speech. Patients may become unmotivated in carrying out basic daily tasks such as maintaining personal hygiene and being careless in ensuring personal safety. They may lack an ability to choose or decide things (avolition) and lack interest in having a conversation with people, responding to questions very briefly, without much content and with much delay (alogia). They may also lack certain pleasures in that they feel indifferent to certain activities (e.g. eating, sexual intercourse) that are usually considered to be pleasurable (anhedonia). They can also communicate with others without showing the emotional reactions that it is normal to show in certain situations (flat affect).[4]

Disorganized symptoms include disorganized speech in which patients have problems in communicating with others by, for example, jumping topic and talking illogically (cognitive slippage) or even creating new words (neologisms). They may also display inappropriate affect in which they laugh or cry inappropriately and display disorganized behaviour in which they act in an unusual or bizarre manner in public.

Schizophrenia can also be classified into different subtypes. The paranoid type consists of, for example, patients with persecutory delusions who complain that they are being watched, followed, poisoned, etc., by their enemies. The disorganized type (also called hebephrenic schizophrenia) tends to start from an earlier age and have a gradual onset in which patients display disorganized speech, disorganized behaviour, and flat or inappropriate affect. The catatonic type consists of patients who display unusual motor responses by remaining in fixed positions (waxy flexibility) for a long period of time. They may also imitate others' actions (echopraxia) or repeat their phrases (echolalia). They may also change from extreme stupor to extreme excitement. The undifferentiated type covers patients who do not fit neatly into the above subtypes of schizophrenia. That is, they display the major symptoms of schizophrenia but do not fulfil the criteria for paranoid, disorganized, or catatonic types. Finally, the residual type would be those who have had at least one episode of schizophrenia but who no longer display any major positive symptoms (e.g. hallucinations or delusions). Instead, they display mostly negative symptoms (e.g. flat affect) and some mild positive symptoms (e.g. strange behaviour or eccentric behaviour).

Given the above brief reminder of the way in which schizophrenia is classified according to DSM-IV, one philosophical issue that has been raised and discussed by philosophers, psychiatrists, and psychologists is, ironically, concerned with the problem of classifying mental disorders including that of schizophrenia. The emergence of DSM gave rise to a new paradigm in psychiatry.[5] This paradigm was based on Carl Hempel's views on psychiatric classification in which he argued that psychiatric taxonomy should rely on operational definitions and that it should be seen as serving a descriptive function (i.e. describing symptoms and syndromes) as opposed to a theoretical one.[6]

(To Hempel, this psychiatric taxonomy should only include more theoretical and etiological concepts when sciences progress and scientific knowledge increases). Indeed, DSM is composed of diagnostic criteria according to strict operational definitions, emphasizing its function of describing symptoms.

The validity or the usefulness of the diagnostic classification of mental disorders including schizophrenia is not without conceptual, taxonomic, and clinical difficulties, alongside many controversies and debates. One of the debates, for example, is concerned with the very basic issue of how mental disorder should be defined.

Wakefield (1992a, 1992b), for example, argued that mental disorder, schizophrenia included, should be defined in terms of 'harmful dysfunctions', which means the failure of a mechanism in patients to carry out a particular natural function when the mechanism for such a function was determined by natural selection. In other words, the notion of malfunction, defined in terms of the Darwinian viewpoint, is a necessary component for mental disorder.[7]

One argument against this harmful dysfunction hypothesis is that disorders can nevertheless exist when there is no failed function (i.e. no malfunction or dysfunction). Also, some critics have argued that there are methodological problems embedded with the harmful dysfunction hypothesis, including some of Wakefield's unwarranted and dubious assumptions about the nature of mental mechanisms and their functions (Murphy and Woolfolk 2000).[8]

Furthermore, for Wakefield, while 'harm', in his notion of 'harmful dysfunction', contributes the value-element to disorder concepts, dysfunction, understood in terms of evolutionary biology, implies a value-free foundation. However, the critics have argued, for example, that Wakefield has failed to define function and dysfunction independent of value terms. Also, some would argue that to claim that the grounding of dysfunction is value-free has in fact no practical application for contemporary psychiatric nosology (see Sadler and Agich 1996; Fulford 1999, 2000).

Starting from a different angle, Poland *et al.* (1994) challenged the presupposition of nomological connections between the syndromes that one can observe and aetiological or pathological conditions, which will support the diagnosis and treatment. They argued that such presupposition is often empirically unsupported. They also argued that mental disorders vary considerably across psychological, biological, behavioural, and environmental dimensions, and that these variations are context-dependent. Such notions of heterogeneity and context-dependency are those with which the present forms of the syndrome-based nomological connections found in DSM are incompatible.

Follette and Houts (1996) vented their criticism by arguing that the theory-neutral nosology embedded within DSM is scientifically unprogressive because of its increased number of categories and the lack of a unifying explanatory theory. To reply to the foregoing view, Wakefield (1999a) argued that an increase in taxonomy's categories is not inconsistent with scientific progress and that a unified theory of mental disorders is very unlikely simply because of the diverse ways in which the functions of the mind can go wrong.

Follette and Houts further proposed that instead of following the diagnostic approach characterized by the DSM, a competing theory-laden diagnostic approach should be put in place. That is, instead of one shared theory-neutral manual, different theoretically driven taxonomies should compete with each other so that people can see for themselves which ones can produce the most scientific progress. They believe that the science in psychiatry would advance more effectively if these theory-driven models of diagnosis are allowed to compete with each other. One might argue that the foregoing view is hardly novel in that much of the research in the arena of mental health is in fact composed of theory-based research programmes looking at issues relating to aetiology and treatment. However, the main point that Follette and Hout are making is that such competition should be extended to the very definitions of the disorders that the theories are competing to explain, and that different theories with their own concepts should be the basis for formulating diagnostic categories. Wakefield (1999a) replied to this argument by saying that in the arena of mental health, theoretical integration, which is advocated by the DSM's theory-neutral nosology, is in fact scientifically more progressive than competition.[9]

What has been presented so far represents only a glimpse of the kinds of complex debates and controversies surrounding the diagnostic classification of mental disorders, in which philosophers, psychiatrists, and psychologists engage. Further debates and controversies have been recorded in Philosophical Perspectives on Psychiatric Diagnostic Classification (Sadler et al. 1994).[10]

The primary aim of the volume is to reveal the conceptual difficulties, omissions, success, and failure, and indeed the naive philosophical assumptions embedded within psychiatric diagnostic classifications. Some of these critical views suggest that mental disorder should be defined in terms of ideal types (Wiggins and Schwartz), that the basis of psychiatric concepts should take into account the hermeneutic nature of the diagnostic processes (Spitzer), that the development of a classification should comprise evaluative and descriptive elements (despite the fact that the psychiatric classifications of DSM and ICD are predominantly descriptive in their overall structure) (Fulford), that DSM concentrated too much on psychiatric nosology and not enough on context-dependent psychopathology and personal life history context (Sadler), and that psychiatric diagnostic classification should be multi-theoretical rather than atheoretical (Goodman).

Suggestions were also made in this collection that a phenomenological approach, which is useful in describing patients' subjective experiences, should form part of psychiatric diagnoses (Kraus; Mishara). The concept of situated subjectivity (Caws) might be useful in classifying mental disorders, i.e. to classify disorders in terms of one's failure of embodied subjectivity, failure of interpersonal subjectivity, failure of positional subjectivity, and failures of reflexive subjectivity. The concept of active self-consciousness is also thought to be a valuable theoretical tool for psychiatric classification. Hearing voices, for example, should be reclassified as disturbances of the sense of self of patients or disturbances of self-representation (Stephens and Graham).

In the midst of such debate and controversy is the feeling that while using DSM categories may increase the confidence with which clinicians can proceed with their clinical work, such confidence is in fact false and could be potentially harmful because the categories are essentially unclear, confusing, messy, and composed of too many 'unquantified criterial attributes, which, in turn, means that DSM does not in fact reduce clinical uncertainty' (Poland *et al.* 1994).[11] DSM, to some researchers, is the reason for the general lack of scientific progression in the area of mental disorders, and, as such, should be abandoned (Follette and Houts 1996).[12]

Various attempts have been made to demonstrate (by, for example, revealing the problematic way in which psychiatric concepts such as schizophrenia were constructed by such influential figures as Kraepelin, Bleuler, and Schneider) why the diagnostic approach, characterized by DSM, should be relinquished (e.g. Bentall 1990, 2004; Boyle 1990).[13]

Instead, emphasis should be placed on understanding specific symptoms of psychosis and how patients' cognitive organization and environmental events would make the symptom worse or better as Bentall remarked (2004, p. 141):

> We should abandon psychiatric diagnoses altogether and instead try to explain and understand the actual experiences and behaviours of psychotic people. By such experiences and behaviours I mean the kinds of things that psychiatrists describe as symptoms, but which might be better labelled complaints, such as hallucinations, delusions and disordered speech. I will argue that, once these complaints have been explained, there is no ghostly disease remaining that also requires an explanation. Complaints are all there is.

A recent suggestion is that, given the conceptual difficulties surrounding the classification of mental disorders outlined earlier, one should perhaps define particular clinical symptoms of mental disorders in terms of the philosophical concept of intentionality and the appropriateness of intentional objects of mental states. That is, mental disorders could be conceptualized in terms of the breakdown of intentionality, as opposed to physical lesion or disease (Bolton and Hill 1996; Bolton 2001, 2003).

Schizophrenia and subjective experience and meaning

For some people, one fundamentally important reason for engaging in the foregoing debate or controversy is to ensure that patients' subjective experience, cultural experience, life history, and subjective meanings attributed to their mental disorders have not been ignored, undermined, or obscured by these diagnostic classifications. Some researchers, however, have expressed their concern that the fundamental relationship between patients' experience and their mental disorders is often under-explored. Modern diagnostic classifications, in their view, have not paid enough attention to patients' beliefs and values, the deep significance of their subjective experience, and the way in which patients organize, experience, and express their mental disorders (Wallace *et al.* 1997).[14] The fact is that to record merely patients' symptoms without considering their subjective and cultural experiences should never be the basis for diagnosis. This is because psychotic phenomena (e.g. spiritual experiences) are very much embedded within the structure of patients' subjective values, meanings, and beliefs (Jackson and Fulford 1997).

This lays the foundation for the next issue pertaining to schizophrenia with which philosophers, psychiatrists, and psychologists are concerned; How does one understand schizophrenic patients' subjective meanings and experience (i.e. the first-person data)? One approach that is often thought to be appropriate for examining subjective meanings and experiences is that of phenomenology.[15]

One recent claim, for example, suggests that the phenomenological approach can be used as the fundamental basis for psychiatric diagnosis, as can be seen in Kraus's (2003) phenomenological-anthropological (P-A) diagnosis, which is different from the symptomatological-criteriological (S-C) diagnosis. The P-A diagnosis is oriented toward exploring patients' life world, subjective experience of disturbance, and existential relationship with themselves, with others, and with the world, while S-C focuses on reducing the phenomena of disturbance into some definable and reliable criteria, characterized by inclusion and exclusion criteria, which, in turn, do not necessarily relate to subjective meanings. Instead, to be able to objectify different aspects of behaviour is more important. In other words, the P-A diagnosis focuses on the notion of 'being' while the S-C diagnosis focuses on the notion of 'having'.[16]

Also, there is a claim that Husserl's (1900/1970; 1973) phenomenology has provided some basic concepts of normal mental life in the light of which schizophrenic experiences can be understood (Depraz 2003). Husserl's phenomenology on the activity and passivity of consciousness can obtain for us an understanding of schizophrenic experiences. Our experience completely depends on, in Husserl's term, the synthetic activity of consciousness (the idea that things we become aware of are constituted by the activity of the mind). There are two kinds of activity. One depends on the subject (the ego) and requires their initiative, i.e. active synthesis. The other happens automatically and is elicited by the object, i.e. passive synthesis. According to Husserl, the activity of consciousness is never a pure activity but happens against a background of passivity (e.g. our behaviour is often a response to prior stimulation given passively. Through such behaviour, the 'I' realizes itself as a subjective centre, reacting to the givens passively). Similarly, consciousness is never a pure passivity either. Such passivity is also affected by the act of the ego. In the light of this phenomenological viewpoint, one could see certain schizophrenic experiences (such as 'passivity experiences': delusions of control, alien thoughts, etc.) as consciousness being in the passivity of consciousness. That is, patients do not consider themselves to be initiating their acts or thoughts. Instead, the object itself is thought to be leading or triggering the experience. Consequently, consciousness seems to be alienated from its object. The experience is then felt to be determined from outside (Wiggins *et al.* 1990; Pachoud 2001).

It was Karl Jaspers (1923/1963, 1968) who started the phenomenological movement in psychiatry and attempted to develop his clinical method of describing patients' subjective experiences or states of consciousness, essentially describing mental disorders phenomenologically, following Husserl's phenomenology (for example, Husserl's notions of intuition, description, and presuppositionlessness integrated with Diltheyian and Weberian methods of self-transposal (empathy) and understanding (*Verstehen*)) (Langenbach 1995; Wiggins and Schwartz 1997).[17] That is, he was concerned with the patients themselves and their mental symptoms (e.g. hallucinations and delusions), as opposed to viewing them in terms of brain structures or functions (Spitzer 1990).[18] His main task in his General Psychopathology was precisely to organize or assess patients' internal experiences around a core of meaningfulness, regardless of nosographical attributions.[19] Thus, psychopathology is seen as patients' attempts to describe themselves or express their own experiences (Rossi Monti and Stanghellini 1996).

Jaspers distinguished between subjective symptoms (i.e. patients' symptoms can only be understood by empathy, by transferring oneself or 'feeling into' the psyche of the patients) and objective symptoms (i.e. patients' movement, speech, and the like can only be understood by psychiatrists' rational thinking, as opposed to empathy).[20] For Jaspers, to rely on the objective approach in order to understand objective symptoms would lead to no understanding of the importance or significance of patients' experiences. Only a systematic pursuit for a subjective psychology would allow psychiatrists to understand their patients.[21]

It is worth noting that in a series of articles, Walker (1994a, 1994b, 1995) has revealed in some detail the relationship between Jaspers's psychopathological phenomenology and the early philosophical phenomenology of Husserl and the notion of phenomenology in Kant's philosophy. With regard to the relationship that Jaspers had with Husserl, while Jaspers was clearly indebted to Husserl's philosophical insights for his understanding of psychopathology, Jaspers in fact mistakenly believed that a change occurred in Husserl's philosophy: that Husserl had changed from phenomenology as an empirical 'descriptive psychology' to phenomenology as an 'intuition of essences' (*Wesensschau*) and as a philosophical 'rigorous science' (*strenge Wissenschaft*). In fact, according to Walker, no such change had occurred, and Jaspers had simply failed to understand Husserl's phenomenology.

Walker then went on to argue provocatively that Jaspers's phenomenology in fact did not originate in Husserl's phenomenology but in Kant's theory of knowledge. This is based on the argument that the Kantian concepts of 'appearance', 'representation', and 'form and content' are crucial to Jaspers's phenomenology. In his phenomenology, Jaspers used the concepts of appearance (*Erscheinung*), representation (*Vergegenwärtigung*), and form and content (*Form und Inhalt*), which appear to be absent in Husserl's phenomenology. To extend the argument further, Walker examined the relationship between Karl Jaspers and Max Weber. For Jaspers, phenomenology is considered an understanding and empathic representation of someone's psychic life. For Weber, phenomenology is considered an 'empathic understanding'. While they both believed that this definition of phenomenology was in line with Husserl's, Walker argued that both were mistaken due to their misunderstanding of Husserl's phenomenology.

More recently, Sass and his colleagues and a few other researchers (Mishara 2001; Pachoud 2001; Sass 2001; Urfer 2001; Zahavi 2001) drew our attention to the works of three phenomenological psychiatrists, namely, Eugene Minkowski (1885–1972), Wolfgang Blankenburg (b.1928) and Kimura Bin (b.1931) who demonstrated successfully how the phenomenological approach can indeed be utilized to help us understand schizophrenic experiences.

In brief, Minkowski (1948, 1997), a French psychiatrist, is one of the first phenomenological psychiatrists and believed in utilizing psychiatric phenomenology to enter into the patient's world, despite the fact that he seldom mentioned Husserl or Heidegger and seldom relied on their concepts or descriptions in his works.[22–24] So, one can say that Minkowski's ideas are not phenomenological in the philosophical sense of the word. Nevertheless, the way in which he described his patients clinically is most certainly based on a phenomenological approach in the sense that he aimed to understand patients' subjective experiences and how their experiences determined their behaviour. Some striking parallels are often observed between his descriptions of patients' behaviour and certain Husserlian ideas, which were, however, ignored by Minkowski.

Minkowski believed that phenomenological investigation primarily aims to explore the central factors that constitute the essence of a disorder (i.e. the trouble générateur).[25] The latter means a generative disorder and the underlying core of patients' manifest symptoms. He conceived that the phenomenological nature of schizophrenia (the trouble générateur) is characterized by an altered existential pattern, a reduced sense of basic, dynamic, and vital connection with the world (i.e. the loss of vital contact with reality (VCR) (élan personnel)) with exaggerated intellectual and static tendencies (i.e.

morbid rationalism, morbid geometrism), and characterized by the manifestation of itself in autistic form. In other words, the decline is not about their
mental capacities or some cognitive faculties.

To elaborate the above a little, in terms of the notion of the loss of vital
contact with reality (VCR), according to Minkowski, schizophrenics behave
without a sense of natural, contextual constraint or worldly demand, implying
a loss of vital contact with reality. Such behaviour is thought to be so
unreasonable at times that people think about it in terms of 'crazy actions'.
Thus, the VCR reflects a sense of relatedness between people and the relationship between the inner and outer worlds. VCR flows from the core of one's
personality and enters into a relationship with the outer fast-moving world.
But the interface between the inner and outer is not definable because they are
not static, but constantly changing, becoming and intertwining simultaneously. Psychopathology is characterized by the distortion of the relationship
between the inner, the subjective, and its outer world. However, according
to Minkowski, schizophrenic attitudes can be seen as 'phenomenological
compensation' in which the healthy or intact part of patients' personality
could attempt to remedy the loss of contact with reality and thus find a new
equilibrium so that they would not forever be trapped in the schizophrenic
world. However, patients seldom achieve the above.[26]

With regard to the notion of autism, Minkowski conceptualized it in terms
of 'rich autism' and 'empty autism' (*autisme riche* and *autisme pauvre*).[27]
Rich autism (also called plastic autism) is characterized by a degree of normal
and vital elements in one's personality being preserved, by imaginary attitudes
and being in a dream or fantasy world.[28] Fantasy seldom contains clear and
distinct ideas and often replaces reality, which then determines patients'
behaviour. The content of the fantasy tends to be rigid, stereotyped, and
sterile. Patients also display sulking, irritability, extreme egotism, obstinacy,
and remorse and regrets, which might last for an inappropriate length of time.
On the other hand, empty autism (also called aplastic autism) is characterized
by a more pure or primary autistic state, i.e. the loss of vital contact with
reality.

Turning briefly to the German psychopathologist Blankenburg's (1969,
1971, 1991, 2001) ideas, he employed Husserl's phenomenological approach
and the *époché* to conceptualize schizophrenia. To Blankenburg, schizophrenics suffer from a 'basic change of existence' in the structure of their
consciousness, which leads to the loss of their ability to grasp what is
significant daily and their ability to be connected with others in a shared
world.[29] That is, patients have lost their usual common sense (i.e. loss of a
normal sense of obviousness or natural self-evidence). Common sense can be
defined as practical understanding or one's capacity to see things in their
right light or to arrive at sound judgement. Saying that the schizophrenics
have lost common sense is to say that they have lost their ability to take

things in the right light, despite the fact that they may still retain their ability to use logic and to engage in abstract discussions. However, their ability to make interpretations and sound judgements has been affected, making it difficult for them to cope with daily practical and social activities.

Blankenburg claims that the vulnerability to the breakdown of common sense is in fact part of being human and that our mental health remains intact precisely because of our resistance to losing our common sense. To resist losing our common sense is to ignore the obvious as obvious. That is, because something is obvious, further exploration of this thing is not required or is resisted. However, when the obvious is lost, patients find the loss of it extremely painful and important, as if they cannot live without it.

Turning very briefly to Kimura Bin's (2001) ideas, schizophrenics should not be seen in terms of their inability of using intellect, logic, judgement or memory. Instead, the psyche of the schizophrenics should be seen in terms of the distortion or profound uncertainty of the sense of the 'I' as personal subject of experience and of action. Consequently, they no longer experience representations of things as 'their' representations (i.e. they no longer see that these things belong to them). This distortion of selfhood also implies a distorted relationship between individual subjectivity and the collective subjectivity to which they belong. That is, they want to resist the self being engulfed by the group subjectivity (they resist the 'I' being affected by living). Thus, for Kimura, schizophrenia is a disorder of the self or self-experience, characterized by fundamental changes in patients' possession and control of their own thoughts, actions, sensations, emotions, feelings, and the like. They feel uncertain about their selfhood and often struggle to restore or maintain their self-identity by means of reflecting upon oneself in an obsessive fashion.

According to Sass (2001), there are similarities between the three phenomenological psychiatrists in terms of understanding schizophrenia. For example, they are all amazed by the defective models that exist in psychiatric theories of schizophrenia. In viewing schizophrenia, their perspective is a holistic one as opposed to the modular approach common in contemporary cognitive science. They all emphasized paradigmatic cases as opposed to statistical generalizations. Although all three psychiatrists were indebted to Jaspers's emphasis on the 'actual conscious psychic events' as the main subject of investigation for psychopathologists, they rejected Jaspers's pessimism about the possibility of understanding schizophrenic experiences.[30]

On the contrary, they believed that combining one's empathy and imagination with conceptual phenomenological tools, such as those provided by Husserl and Heidegger, should enable us to enter into the lived-world of schizophrenia. Finally, all three psychiatrists did not agree with the largely developmental explanation of schizophrenia which is popular in the psychoanalytic tradition.

To understand schizophrenia from a phenomenological angle, one cannot but mention R.D. Laing's (1959, 1961, 1971) phenomenological approach to schizophrenia.[31] Laing conceptualized schizophrenia as an extreme form of existential despair, which can be worked through. He proposed the concept of ontological insecurity, which schizophrenics are believed to experience. This is insecurity in terms of lack of trust in their physical and concrete existence in the world, and in which they feel that their dysfunctioned families have not helped them to integrate with society in an acceptable way. The schizophrenics feel suffocated or engulfed by the family and are not allowed to find their independence, while they are desperate to find ways through which they can be real to themselves and others, preserve their own identity, and indeed prevent themselves losing their own self.[32]

In ontological insecurity, Laing mentioned the types of anxiety that schizophrenics tend to experience. First is the anxiety associated with the fear of engulfment, which basically means the fear of being engulfed, overwhelmed, and indeed destroyed by others. Second is the anxiety associated with implosion, which refers to a feeling of complete emptiness. The schizophrenic feels that they are at risk of disappearing altogether. The third anxiety is associated with the feeling of danger of petrification or depersonalization, which basically refers to their fear of being turned into an object or a thing, wherein their notion of selfhood and autonomy are not acknowledged. They find themselves in a situation where they experience the body as a false self, a self that is being controlled, observed, and manipulated by others, and a self that feels that it can only survive by conforming to the expectations of the outside world, while the feelings associated with this external performance are very much detached or dead.

Laing believed that schizophrenic experiences can be understood and worked through. For example, the delusions or hallucinations that schizophrenics manifest can be understood in terms of how they relate to the world with a great deal of struggle or frustration. Laing believed that the biography of schizophrenics can be changed by means of helping them talk about themselves in a new way. For instance, the schizophrenics may experience a paranoia delusion in which they believe that people want to, say, poison them. According to Laing, instead of dismissing patients' delusions and pathologizing them, it is possible to help them explore why and how they experience other people as dangerous to themselves.

Schizophrenia and the self

One message which is implicit in what has been suggested by the foregoing phenomenologists is the idea that if one wishes to have a good understanding of schizophrenia, the starting point should be patients' concept of self. Indeed, the concept of self is a major preoccupation of philosophers, psychiatrists, and psychologists. Jaspers, as was mentioned in an earlier footnote, thought that we cannot comprehend empathically schizophrenic experiences, because of the fundamental change, distortion or loss of their sense of self (i.e. they have lost their sense of unity, and the ownership or control of their own experiences and actions). However, some people want to understand schizophrenia precisely by understanding the disorder of the self which is thought to be the psychopathological core of schizophrenia.

According to Parnas and Sass (2001), the disorder of the self was studied in some detail at the beginning of the nineteenth and twentieth centuries. For example, the disorder of the self among schizophrenics was described in terms of the affliction (*Spaltung*) of the self (Bleuler 1911; Parnas and Bovet 1991), the disunity of consciousness (orchestra without a conductor) (Kraepelin 1899/1900), an alteration of a basic change in self-consciousness or self-awareness (primary insufficiency) (Berze 1914), the sense of self being affected in, for example, their awareness of their own existence and action, temporal-diachronic identity and the boundary between me and not me (Jaspers 1923/1963), and in terms of the loss of ego-boundaries (Schneider 1959). Of course, the previously mentioned phenomenological psychiatrists, such as Minkowski, Blankenburg, and Laing, essentially talked about self-disturbances in terms of the change of the nature of the self as the primary disorder of schizophrenia.

To continue this line of investigation, several authors, unlike Jaspers, have attempted to understand empathically and conceptually some of the perplexed schizophrenic symptoms by focusing on the disorder of the self. Sass (1994), for example, thought that it is not helpful to understand schizophrenia in terms of traditional assumptions that the schizophrenics project subjective meanings onto the external objective world, while being unaware of the subjective nature of such meanings. Neither is it helpful to understand schizophrenia in terms of the psyche's returning to its primordial condition, of some psycho-analytic regression hypothesis or of the dysfunction of reasoning ability. Instead, Sass and colleagues (Sass 2000; Parnas and Sass 2001) proposed to explore the disorder of the self in the pre-onset stage of schizophrenia and schizotypal disorders (i.e. sub-clinical or non-psychotic forms of schizophrenia). They believe that disturbance of the self can be characterized in terms of the reduction of patients' sense of being present in the world, changes in their experiencing their own body, their feeling alienated or dissociated from thoughts and feelings, transitivism (their inability to distinguish the 'me' from the 'not me'), and solipsism.

In particular, Sass (1994) proposed a 'solipsist' interpretation of schizophrenia, developed through the work of Wittgenstein and a case example of a famous paranoid schizophrenic, namely, Daniel Paul Schreber, as an alterative way of understanding the subjective delusional experiences of the schizophrenic.[33, 34] Also see Ogilvie (2000/2001) who explores Wittgenstein's later philosophical work as a source of insight into the schizophrenic experience.

The doctrine of solipsism states that the whole of reality, which encompasses the external world and other human beings, is only a representation appearing to the individual (such as Schreber himself) who holds the doctrine. So, solipsists would say that only their feelings, emotions, and perceptions are real. Solipsism also implies a mixture of increasing subjectivization (i.e. patients' experiencing experience rather than the external world. After all, the idea of an external world is in fact quite limited in schizophrenic experience since they tend to feel that they are the centre of the universe) of the world and self-dissolution and implies a specific type of grandiosity.[35] These experiences are forms of self-deception which is, however, derived from rationality itself rather than from the loss of rationality.

In the light of this doctrine of solipsism, schizophrenia is seen as the manifestation of a 'pervasive sense of subjectivization'. This means that schizophrenics are unable to regard others as subjects and engage with them by means of normal forms of communication, exchanging reasons and developing interpersonal relationships. This is because to engage in such communication implies a relation of reciprocity or co-operation, which the solipsists (i.e. the schizophrenics) are unable to do. This has implications for explaining schizophrenic delusions of alien control in that patients' inability to engage in normal communication and interpersonal relations affects their ability to engage with their own thoughts and impulses. That is, their lack ability to engage with others (in terms of giving and receiving reasons) would lead them to lose their ability to determine whether their own thoughts and impulses contain reasons. In other words, patients would become unable to exert control over their own thoughts (Roessler 2001).

According to this doctrine of solipsism, the difficulty for schizophrenics is that while they are unable to communicate with others, they find themselves part of the external world, with other human beings. In other words, the 'personal or private world' of the schizophrenics is constituted socially with others in the external world. This is why we find it difficult to comprehend the symptoms of schizophrenia. As Japsers (1963) claimed, there could be a community of patients who could understand among themselves. However, what they understand among themselves we cannot understand. They do not find themselves able to communicate with us because we have not shared their experiences (Hoerl 2001).

To elaborate further Sass's exploration of the disorder of the self among schizophrenics, from a phenomenological perspective, Sass and colleagues (Sass and Parnas 2001) believed that schizophrenia is a self of ipseity-disorder characterized by a declined sense of oneself existing as a subject of awareness, by the disappearance of the boundary between the self and the external world, and by an acute self-consciousness and a heightened awareness of aspects of one's experience (i.e. hyperreflexivity).[36]

Ipseity is the pre-reflective modality (i.e. an implicit mental phenomenon) of self-awareness. With ipseity, we can sense ourselves to be the centre of our own experiences, feel our self as that which is separate from the objects that we are perceiving, and feel that our representation of these objects is experienced as that which is different from the object itself (see Stanghellini 2001). With respect to hyper-reflexivity, it is the process in which schizophrenics increasingly monitor or examine their mental lives or mental phenomena, accompanied by a lack of automatic actions.[37] In examining their mental lives, ideas or thoughts have become objects of focal awareness, i.e. they have been objectified as if they existed in an external or outer space. Consequently, the schizophrenics may feel that certain thoughts or ideas can be felt in certain locations of their brains.

While he has accepted the disorder of the self in terms of the ipseity-disorder and hyper-reflexivity, which are thought to be the main phenomena of schizophrenic vulnerability, Stanghellini (1997, 2001) argued that the above conceptualization of the disorder of the self in schizophrenia only shows us limited dimensions of schizophrenic vulnerability. This, he argues, is because the focus is on the pathological changes in the personal or subjective experience of a self, effectively ignoring the fact that the self is not merely a personal or subjective phenomenon. That is, our social existence has been ignored.[38]

To Stanghellini, schizophrenia is considered a resistance to the loss of common sense reality, which is characterized by a socially inherited knowledge and an affective-conative capacity for attunement with others in daily encounters (i.e. intersubjectivity). The latter is that through which we can establish our sense of 'reality' (i.e. one feels familiar with one's surrounding environment) and our sense of 'ipseity' (i.e. we sense that we exist as a subject of awareness). Also, patients have difficulty conforming to conventional rules and norms (antagonomia), remain sceptical of taken-for-granted views, and have no desire to engage in and absorb others' views. To Stanghellini, the lack of attunement with others and the rejection of conventional knowledge is a dangerous way of losing one's own self.

Schizophrenic symptoms

Having discussed the philosophical issues of diagnostic classifications, the importance of grasping the subjective experience and meanings of schizophrenics, and the notion of self of schizophrenics, philosophers, psychiatrists, and psychologists have turned their attention specifically to schizophrenic symptoms, in particular, those known as positive symptoms. Starting from the previously discussed concept of self, some of these researchers have examined positive symptoms in the light of the self as an agent or the action of the self (i.e. agency).

Focusing on the symptom of thought-insertion, for example, Stephens and Graham (1994a, 1994b, 2000) referred to a separability thesis, advocated by Freud. This thesis states that our awareness of our own thoughts (introspection) can be separated from our awareness of ourselves as the subjects (subjectivity) in whom these thoughts occur. In the light of this thesis, schizophrenics may be aware introspectively of their own thoughts but somehow may have mislocated them (or somehow failed to recognize that these thoughts are part of their own psychological history).[39]

For Stephens and Graham, however, this separability thesis was problematic. Instead, they argued for an inseparability thesis with which, they claim, the notion of thought-insertion is compatible. They claim that introspection and subjectivity are inseparable components of self-consciousness and that thought-insertion is not an error of subjectivity. The reason for this argument is that patients who suffer from thought-insertion are often aware of the foreign thoughts occurring within them (e.g. they often say 'someone keeps putting thoughts into my head').

On the contrary, Stephens and Graham argued that thought-insertion should be seen in terms of an error of agency (i.e. certain thoughts occur in the patients but are independent of their intentional stance). That is, patients experience their self as not the agent of their own thoughts or other mental activities. In other words, they give a sub-personal account in terms of non-intentional states. In their experience the thoughts express the agency (i.e. the intention and attitude) of others rather than themselves. Thus, patients conclude that their thoughts are others' thoughts.[40]

To reflect further on the agency-approach to the schizophrenic symptom of thought-insertion, Fulford (1989, 1993, 1994a, 1994b) conceptualized it in terms of the action of the self, more precisely, the 'action failure' of the self. Symptoms of illness, according to Fulford, can be characterized in terms of the feature of the things that patients do and things that are done to them. For example, one can perceive the symptom of pain in terms of something that patients do to themselves (i.e. hurting themselves) and something that is done to them (i.e. they are being hurt). By the same token, in the case of thought-insertion, while other people might conceptualize it in terms of something wrong with the patients, the patients themselves perceive it as something that is done to them (i.e. action failure of the self). That is, instead of understanding thought-insertion and indeed delusion in terms of patients' failure in cognitive functioning, Fulford proposed that one should understand these symptoms in terms of impaired reasons for action (i.e. their inability to do things that they normally can do).[41]

While Stephens and Graham and Fulford focus mainly on the individual experience of schizophrenic symptoms rather than the cognitive or neurobiological explanations of them, some researchers have examined these symptoms in terms of cognitive explanations. For example, one view is that the schizophrenic symptom of thought-insertion should be conceptualized in terms of our intuitive conception of what makes certain thoughts belong to us and the specific cognitive mechanisms involved. For us to say that we are the authors of certain thoughts (that these thought belong to us) is to say that those thoughts stand in a certain causal relation to our background beliefs, desires and interests. We know this through the working of certain cognitive mechanisms in us. Thought-insertion basically results from a malfunction of these cognitive mechanisms which, as a result, fail to help us access the content of our background beliefs, desires and interests (Campbell 2001).[42]

Focusing on a cognitive explanation of the problem of agency in the sense of the action of the self, Frith (1987, 1992) argued that a loss of the sense of agency, in terms of one's intention to act, is an important characteristic of schizophrenia. He distinguishes two ways of forming an intention to act.[43] One is stimulus-driven, in that a particular stimulus (such as ice-cream on a poster) leads people to form their intention to act (e.g. to buy an ice-cream). Frith calls this stimulus-intention. The other is goal and plan-driven, in that, for example, one may intend to buy a German dictionary because one wants to pursue one's goal of learning German. He calls this willed-intention. According to Frith, there is a cognitive monitor in us which is a mechanism of 'metarepresentation'. This monitor aims to keep track of the two kinds of intention (whether stimulus- or willed-intentions) and of the actions that we have actually chosen, as a result of the intentions. For this monitor, to metarepresent an intention would also bring that intention into one's consciousness.[44]

According to Frith, many 'first rank symptoms' (e.g. hallucinations, both auditory and verbal, and thought-insertion) of schizophrenia that involve the loss of the sense of control or possession of one's own thoughts or movements, delusions of persecution, and of reference, in fact result from the dysfunction of the monitor to represent willed intentions.[45]

For example, if we want to pursue our goal of learning German, we form the willed intention to buy a German dictionary. The monitor in us metarepresents that willed-intention and subsequently brings it into our consciousness. After having formed the intention to buy the dictionary, we then carry out the action in the form of buying the dictionary. The monitor in us metarepresents both our action and intention and can confirm that the action that we have carried out has satisfied the relevant intention. For the schizophrenic, due to the dysfunction of the monitor, it fails to represent the intention to buy a dictionary. As a result, they might buy a dictionary without being conscious of the fact that they had formed their intention to do so. That is, they have performed their action, while they had no consciousness or awareness of any intention to carry out such action. To explain this, they might opt for the explanation that some external forces have in fact performed the action, hence, a delusion of control (alien control) (Mlakar *et al*. 1994; Cocoran *et al*. 1995; Cahill and Frith 1996; Currie 2000).

To follow on from this notion of a problem of agency to explain schizo-phrenic symptoms, Spence (2001) attempted to provide a physiological explanation of the disorder of agency in the sense of the action of the self. For example, he argued that patients who suffer from alien control claim that their thoughts, movements, actions, and emotions have been controlled by others. There are apparently physiological mechanisms involved in the initi-ation and control of action. Among patients who report 'made movements', there is a hyperactivation in the right inferior parietal cortex, which serves to programme and adjust limb responses during reaching and grasping move-ments. This hyperactivation may account for the occurrence of the abnormal experience of alien control among these patients.

In recent years, the cognitive and the physiological approaches (in particu-lar, neurophysiological) have combined in order to help us understand more about psychiatric symptoms.[46–49] For example, alien control is one of the 'monothematic delusions' that Martin Davies, Max Coltheart, Robyn Lang-don, and Nora Breen have discussed (2001).[50] Other delusions discussed are the Capgras, Cotard, and Frégoli delusions; the delusion of mirrored-self misidentification; reduplicative paramnesia and delusions sometimes found in patients of unilateral neglect (Young et al. 1992, 1993, 1994, 1996; Gerrans 2000).[51–53] Obviously, it is beyond the scope of this chapter to describe any of these proposals in any detail.

Maher (1974, 1988, 1992, 1999, 2003) is mainly concerned with the role of anomalous experiences in the aetiology of delusions among schizophrenics. He argued that delusions are false beliefs that emerge as normal or rational responses to some unusual or anomalous perceptual experiences. Similar to normal beliefs, he believed that delusional beliefs emerge because of our attempt to explain experiences, that the processes through which people with delusions reason from experience to form beliefs are in fact very similar to the processes that people without delusions tend to go through. In other words, delusions do not stem from aberrant thinking and, to Maher, there is no sharp distinction between normal, non-delusory beliefs and delusional beliefs. He does believe, however, that the origins of anomalous experience may be derived from some neuropsychological anomalies (e.g. some real impairment in sensory functioning, attentional deficit, language disturbances, or motor impairment, etc).[54]

Arguing against Maher's view that delusions are false beliefs which emerge as normal responses to anomalous experiences, Davies et al. (2001) want to argue that delusions result from two factors. One is concerned with a neuropsychological anomaly in perceptual or affective processing manifested in patients' experience. That is, they believe in some neuropsychological anomalies which could produce anomalous experiences which, in tun, may lead to the development of delusions. The second factor is concerned with an abnormality in patients' cognitive systems in which patients seem to have lost their ability to reject such-and-such a belief on the basis of its implausibility and its inconsistency with other things with which patients are familiar (Langdon and Coltheart 2000).[55]

Focusing on Capgras patients (i.e. patients believe that one of their closest relatives has been replaced by an impostor), Ellis and Young (1990; also see Wright *et al.* 1993; Ellis *et al.* 1997; Hirstein and Ramachandran (1997); Stone and Young 1997; Young 1998, 2000) argue that these patients' beliefs are in fact rational responses to highly unusual experiences which are thought to result from brain damage.[56]

To understand this argument, let us refer to those patients who suffer from prosopagnosia. They cannot recognize familiar faces, cannot tell who they are looking at, while some non-verbal forms of response or some affective response to these familiar faces are still intact. So, in other words, the visual system, which is used for overt recognition of faces, has been damaged, while the visual system, which is used for emotional arousal in response to familiar faces, is still intact. In the light of these two visual systems, Ellis and Young claim that the Capgras delusion is characterized by a kind of mirror image of prosopagnosia. That is, Capgras patients' visual system, which is used for overt recognition of faces, is intact but the visual system, which is used for emotional arousal in response to familiar faces, has been damaged. As a result, these patients look at some familiar faces and can see clearly their detailed similarity to the faces that they know well; however, they do not seem to have any affective responses toward them. They then come up with the explanation that the other person with the familiar face is in fact an impostor.[57]

To extend the foregoing idea to patients with Cotard delusion (the belief that one is dead), Young and his colleagues (Young *et al.* 1992; Wright *et al* 1993; Ramachandran and Blakeslee 1998; Gerrans 1999, 2000; Young 2000) suggest that the same kind of damage to the visual system may be responsible for Cotard delusion. That is, Cotard patients also lack affective response in their receptions of others. Partly due to their severe depression, Cotard patients attribute this anomaly to a deficiency in themselves (internal attribution, often with depression) in that they believe that they are emotionally dead, simply dead, or disembodied. Such attribution is different from the Capgras patients in that the latter tend to attribute the anomaly to the presence of impostors (external attribution, often with paranoia) as opposed to themselves. So, the idea is that the underlying basis for both Cotard and Capgras syndromes are in fact similar. One main difference lies in patients' moods. When they are in a suspicious mood, they tend to think that others are impostors; when they feel depressed, they tend to think that they are dead.[58]

One argument against Ellis and Young's approach to Capgras and Cotard is to say that for Capgras patients to keep insisting that the people whom the patients know have been replaced by impostors, patients' delusional belief must imply the statement that the currently perceived person is not that remembered person. That is, Capgras patients seem to look for shared memories from the people with whom they are confronting. In other words, these patients seem to have problems grasping the meaning of the memory demonstrative, as opposed to the perceptual demonstrative (Campbell 2001).

Concluding remark

What I have done is given an overview of the issues raised and discussed thus far by philosophers, psychiatrists, and psychologists, on the subject of schizophrenia. The breadth of the issues investigated reflect a significant step toward understanding or reconceiving schizophrenia. It also reflects the perplexity and complexity of schizophrenia that professionals and academics are facing. In my view, the investigation of these issues has shed new light on the theoretical thinking, which underpins clinical practice and philosophical pursuit. It has also set the stage for further debate and research in the area of schizophrenia.

Endnotes

1. This partnership cannot be ignored partly because many patients of, for example, schizophrenia are in fact preoccupied with philosophical, supernatural and metaphysical problems (Moller and Husby 2000).
2. Some preceding events, including the emergence of the Philosophy Section of the Royal College of Psychiatrists, and the Association for the Advancement of Philosophy and Psychiatry, which set the basis for the present book series, are briefly outlined in the opening chapter of Nature and Narrative (Fulford *et al.* 2003).
3. Sass *et al.* (2000, p. 95) stated that studying schizophrenia is philosophically important for different reasons,'...not only because schizophrenic symptoms challenge traditional Cartesian assumptions, but also because their cognitive and experiential abnormalities can cast illuminating light on a wide range of psychological issues, including the general constitution of the objective world and of intersubjectivity, the notion of self-awareness and its different aspects, the corporeal nature of experience and existence, the experience of time, and the general existential significance of temporal experience. Schizophrenics show interesting abnormalities in all these domains'. Apart from schizophrenia, they also discussed autism and dissociative identity disorder.
4. Positive and negative symptoms can also be conceptualized in terms of Type 1 and Type 2 syndromes (Crow 1985; Tsuang 1993). Type 1 syndrome refers typically to the acute symptoms of delusions, hallucinations, and disorders of thinking. Type 2 syndrome typically refers to the negative symptoms of poverty of thought and speech, decreased motor activity, apathy, lack of spontaneity, and diminished interpersonal interactions. These two Types seem to emphasize the biological correlates and speed of onset of schizophrenia.
5. Despite this new paradigm in psychiatry, the underlying effort to classify mental disorders has a long history. For example, Radden (1996) has argued that Kantian

faculty psychology in fact influenced not only the nineteenth-century doctrine of phrenology, which mapped the functions in the brain but also influenced Kraeplin's nosological division between manic-depression and dementia praecox. Of course, this division has influenced the present-day diagnostic classification systems of DSM and ICD. Many present-day features of mental disorder are thought to have been pointed out by Kant. That is, his philosophical ideas might have been relevant to our understanding of schizophrenic symptoms (Spitzer 1990; Dawson 1994).

6. Carl Hempel (1984), a philosopher of the logical empiricism tradition, was critical of Rümke's phenomenological approach to assessing patients' subjectivity. Hempel found this approach to be unscientific and some 20 years later, DSM-III adopted Hempel's critique of subjectivism in its diagnostic system (see Belzen 1995).

7. In other words, psychiatric disorders should be conceptualized in terms of natural kinds characterized by inherent properties. However, claims have been made that this natural kind view of mental disorders is, in fact, inconsistent with the medical understanding of diseases and with the evolutionary biological understanding of species. A suggestion has been made that the concept of practical kinds, as opposed to natural kinds, may be more helpful, productive and consistent with a scientific view of the world (Zachar 2000).

8. Wakefield (2000), however, argued that the foregoing argument was simply based on a misinterpretation of the harmful dysfunction hypothesis.

9. More debates between Wakefield and Follette and Houts can be found in Wakefield (1999b), Houts and Follette (1998).

10. Also see Radden's (1994) review on psychiatric nosology.

11. Poland et al. (1994) believe in the importance of quantified and well-controlled studies which, they believe, will promote scientifically acceptable research. Unfortunately, to them, DSM categories simply involve too many unquantified criterial attributes.

12. Some researchers would also argue that the lack of scientific progression in the area of mental disorders could be due to the fact that mental health professionals accept too readily the findings of influential biological and genetic studies on schizophrenia, despite the fact that the scientific validity of these studies remains highly questionable (Jenner et al. 1993).

13. See Wing's (1988) (a strong believer in classification and categorization) response to Bentall's idea of abandoning the concept or classification of schizophrenia.

14. Meanwhile, from the viewpoint of patients, they are concerned with what the symptoms really mean for them and often ask, 'Will I (ever) be well? Will I (always) be sick?'.

15. Phenomenological approaches are believed to be important in helping us to understand patients' subjective experience of psychopathology and the distinctive variations in disturbance across different disorders (e.g. De Koning and Jenner 1982; Mishara 1997; Schwartz et al. 1997). Recent research has also suggested that we can combine the approaches of phenomenology and cognitive neuroscience in order to help us understand much more effectively the subjective experience of schizophrenia (see, for example, Parnas et al. 1996; Mishara et al. 1998). For example, cognitive neuroscience can reveal for us the work of neurotransmitters, and disclose our mental structure and the brain and nervous system, etc., which, in

turn, gives us clues for investigating the complexities of subjective psychological experiences from a phenomenological perspective (Kopelman 1996; Spence 1996; Spitzer 1997). Some researchers have claimed that phenomenology has undoubtedly made contributions, not only to psychiatry, but also to psychotherapy; in particular, self-psychological psychotherapy (Gupta and Kay 2002). However, there are claims that have challenged whether phenomenological ideas can really help us understand, for example, experience of hallucinations. For example, while Heidegger's ontology may help us to understand what it is to be a human with intentional characteristics, one may challenge whether it can help us to understand what it is to be a human who can hallucinate. It is not clear if the experience of hallucination can indeed be accommodated within Heidegger's ontology (McManus 1996).

16. Thus, the S-C approach is characterized by a certain distance from patients and by an objectifying function (i.e. patients are seen as people who possess symptoms, the object of an illness), whereas the P-A approach is characterized by an engaged function, which aims to help patients describe the subjective meanings of their disturbance in as much detail as possible (i.e. patients are seen as people who are able to initiate behaviour, to act, and to reflect upon themselves).

17. Jaspers also extensively discussed with Binswanger (1963) the idea of applying empirically Husserl's phenomenology to psychiatry. Binswanger was influenced by Heidegger's existential philosophy and contributed significantly to our understanding of schizophrenia and manic-depression. To Binswanger, Jaspers used far more intuition, characterized by Husserl's phenomenology, than he had acknowledged. Also, Jaspers did not seemingly appreciate adequately Husserl's eidetic method through which the scientific foundations of psychiatry can be clarified (Mishara 1997).

18. Meanwhile, Kraepelin was interested in what disorder is characterized by specific symptoms such as hallucinations and delusions. Freud was hoping to arrive at the first comprehensive psychological explanation of these symptoms (Spitzer 1990).

19. Schneider's clinical psychopathology, on the other hand, aimed to identify symptoms that are important in terms of nosological distinctions. Roughly speaking, there are two camps of post-Schneiderian psychopathologists. The first camp comprises those who have abandoned the notion of nosology (the 'singles'), the second comprises those who still believe in it (i.e. the 'nostalgics').

20. Jaspers used the term '*einfühlen*' (feeling into) to refer to a process in which people participate in the experience of the other person.

21. Chalmers (1996, 1997) argued that subjective experience of consciousness (phenomenological) goes beyond any explanation offered by the materialists. Even if we can explain all the structures and functions of our minds, there will still be subjective experience of consciousness which remains unexplainable. Varela (1996) has proposed a neurophenomenology (i.e. a pragmatic tool for a phenomenological science of consciousness), which aims to address Chalmers's 'hard problem' (i.e. how a physical system could give rise to the subjective experience of consciousness).

22. Minkowski's views are significantly different from those of Kraepelin (1899), Bleuler (1911), and Jaspers (1923). He is probably considered one of the first phenomenological psychiatrists along with Ludwig Binswanger (1963). He studied in depth

Husserl's (1900) 'Logical Investigations' and Max Scheler's (1913) work on emotions. He challenged the psycho-analytic tradition and Jaspers's approach of descriptive phenomenology, which were very common at the time. Minkowski was influenced by Bleuler (1911) and Kretschmer (1922). The latter modified the Kraepelinian distinction between the schizophrenic and affective psychoses to a more general distinction between the schizoid and cycloid types of personality. While the cycloids always retain their contact with the outer surrounding world, the schizoids are unaffected by it and remain in very superficial contact with it (see Urfer 2001).

23. R.D. Laing (1959) claimed that Minkowski was the first person in psychiatry to make a serious attempt to reconstruct patients' lived experience. His views on schizophrenia are thought to stimulate clinical and theoretical interests in contemporary psychiatry (e.g. Cutting 1985, 1997; Parnas and Bovet 1991; Sass 1992).

24. In fact, Minkowski often referred to the works of Bergson, a non-phenomenologist, and used his concepts. For example, Minkowski examined schizophrenic experiences in the light of Bergson's descriptions of consciousness.

25. According to Minkowski, psychiatric disorders can be characterized by affective and cognitive contents (i.e. ideo-affective) and by the spatio-temporal structure of one's experience through which the foregoing contents manifest themselves. Of course, different people manifest these contents differently. However, what is important is that the trouble générateur shapes the symptoms. To access the essence of a disorder, i.e. the trouble générateur, requires one's intuitive effort, i.e. a direct grasping of patients' way of being and experiencing.

26. Also see Minkowski and Targowla (2001) for their discussion on autism in terms of 'contact with reality' (i.e. the attitude that can be seen as a compensation mechanism, a way to maintain some minimal contact with the world).

27. To Minkowski, the term autism is an anthropological term which describes patients who complain about being unable to feel and who contradict the dynamism of life. Such contradiction manifests itself in feelings of emptiness, of fragmented personality, and of immobilization. Patients' autistic thinking is not oriented towards specific goals or future outcomes (unlike realistic thinking which is oriented towards some pragmatic goals). Patients' autistic communication is not oriented towards communication with others but remains private and subjective.

28. Rich autism is similar to Bleuler's (1911) notion of autism, which states that it is a withdrawal from external reality to an unconstrained fantasy life. Minkowski, however, disagreed with Bleuler's conceptualization of autism as a morbid retreat that is accompanied by a predominant inner life. To Minkowski, there are extroverted schizophrenics and there are schizophrenics with a poverty of inner life. Both groups are nonetheless autistic. Also, Minkowski thought that Bleuler's 'fundamental symptoms' (i.e. disturbance of affectivity or the idiosyncratic nature of thinking) did not define autism exhaustively.

29. To an extent, this is similar to Kant's idea that the most striking feature of mental disorder is the loss of the sensus communis (i.e. the loss of ability to connect with others and to relate their understanding to the understanding of others).

30. For Jaspers, due to the profound distortions of the most fundamental features of human subjectivity among schizophrenics, it is impossible for normal people to comprehend empathically (understand) the schizophrenic experience. The best we

can hope for is to attempt to 'explain' them by way of searching for underlying physical causes in the brain and nervous system.

31. Laing, in conjunction with Cooper and Esterson, started the anti-psychiatry movement, which was, to a large extent, based on the phenomenological or existential philosophies of Heidegger and Sartre, mixed with some influential ideas from other traditions. For example, there is a degree of integration between object relations theory (e.g. Winnicott's approach) and existentialism in Laing's work. Laing's the Divided Self led to the development of Kingsley Hall, the Philadelphia Association and the Arbours Association, in which people were free from medical intervention and were allowed to experience their disturbance in a free and unique environment.

32. Laing, at the Tavistock Institute, spent a great deal of time investigating or observing the pathogenic dynamics within families. Laing argued that families, especially mothers, through double-bind interactions (i.e. contradictory messages) between the family and the schizophrenic, can make it impossible for the schizophrenic to find their own identity, to achieve independence and a sense of self, and to live accordingly. In other words, schizophrenia resulted from the dysfunctional interactions between the schizophrenics and their families.

33. Wittgenstein was concerned with solipsism, and his obsession and exploration with this topic, according to Sass, can help us comprehend the inner logic or the struggles of the strange world in which many schizophrenics live. To Wittgenstein, solipsism was a good example of the kind of philosophical disease that many traditional philosophers (e.g. those who are concerned with metaphysics, idealism or sense data phenomenalism) suffer. Such a disease does not result from ignorance but from abstraction, self-consciousness, and disengagement from daily practical and social activities, and indeed common sense. For Wittgenstein, these kinds of philosophical diseases, or the diseases of intellect, essentially correspond to the experiences of schizophrenics such as Schreber. For example, both the solipsists or other metaphysicians and Schreber were convinced by their own profound or special version of reality which was derived from special insights they had, insights that other, ordinary, people do not have.

34. Schreber was a judge in Dresden in 1893 with a high level of intelligence and articulation but suffered from several paranoid schizophrenic episodes. His 'madness' was recorded in his autobiographical book, Memoirs of My Nervous Illness. He suffered from delusions, for example, in which he believed that he was being transformed into a woman and that some supernatural cosmos of 'nerves', 'rays', 'souls' and 'gods' were constantly interacting with one another and with himself. Schreber also thought that he had gained a kind of deep insight that other people did not have. He also thought that his book was the most interesting book written since the beginning of the world.

35. Sass argued that Schreber did not experience his delusions as being literally true but experienced them as having a certain 'subjectivized' quality.

36. Sass and Parnas believe that the phenomenological approach would help psychiatrists to improve criteria for diagnosis and distinguish schizophrenic symptoms.

37. Sass (1992) initially illustrated this notion of hyper-reflexivity as a schizophrenic experience and expression, by means of examining modernist and post-modernist art and literature (e.g. the works of artists and writers including Franz Kafka, Paul Valéry, Samuel Beckett, Alain Robbe-Grillet, Giorgio de Chirico, and Marcel

Duchamp, Friedrich Nietzsche, William James, Martin Heidegger, Michel Foucault, and Jacques Derrida). Through this notion of hyper-reflexivity, he criticized the commonly held assumption that schizophrenics are incapable of self-awareness.

38. Indeed, various studies have already shown the link between schizophrenia and social dysfunctions in interpersonal relations, the problem or the lack of social competence, a disorder of social cognition, a disorder of accurate perception of other people's intentions, and interpersonal difficulties (e.g. Dworkin *et al*. 1993; Dworkin *et al*. 1994; Malmberg *et al*. 1998).

39. This is similar to the argument that schizophrenic delusion is a type of irrationality that results from a violation of a condition of thought called egocentricity. Such violation leads to delusional irrationality. To violate egocentricity means to violate one's property of thought, which allows the person of that thought to recognize it as having come from his or her own mind. The violation of egocentricity is then people's inability to recognize such and such a thought as having originated from their own minds. Schizophrenic thoughts are considered to violate egocentricity and to originate outside of their own minds (e.g. delusion of alien control in nature). The violation of egocentricity then produces strange experiences that form the basis of delusional beliefs and irrationality (Gold and Hohwy 2000). Research has suggested two types of rationality (procedural and epistemic), each of which can break down in different ways in different delusional psychiatric disorders. Procedural rationality is characterized by reasoning that conforms to the principle of the logic of consistency and the principle of inference. Epistemic rationality, on the other hand, is characterized by one's ability to reason in accordance with the norms of good reasoning. It is based on people's perception of how beliefs relate to evidence and how beliefs need to change in the light of changes in evidence (Bermúdez 2001).

40. Also see Chadwick's (1994) commentary on the argument of Stephens and Graham. A recent review examines two important concepts of self, namely, the minimal self (i.e. a self devoid of temporal extension) and the narrative self (i.e. a self involving personal identity and continuity across time). The minimal self is characterized by a distinction between the sense of self-agency and the sense of self-ownership for actions. Schizophrenia is considered to be a disorder of this sense of self-agency. The second concept of self, the narrative self, is discussed in the light of Gazzaniga's left-hemisphere 'interpreter' and episodic memory (Gallagher 2000).

41. This account of schizophrenic symptoms, such as thought-insertion or delusions, involves the notion of intentionality or, more precisely, a failure of intentionality. For example, patients' delusional beliefs are similar to normal beliefs in that they are 'about things' (intentionality) but what the delusional beliefs are about seems to be 'off-target' or mis-directed.

42. Some critics would argue that to search for the underlying clinical processes or the essence of disorder of thought is not a fruitful exercise because the notion of thought-disorder is in fact a 'negative normative concept which does not have any essential clinical characteristics. The term 'thought-disorder' is a phenomenon that results from the effect of one's speech on the listener. That is, the text of one's speech cannot be incoherent but it may be incoherent to those who listen to it in particular situations (Parker *et al*. 1995).

43. Frith's notion of intention to act is similar to that defined by Macmurray (1991). Their intentions to act are movements that agents have chosen. Frith's intention is also similar to that defined by Searle (1983), meaning 'prior' intentions (i.e. they precede action).

44. Frith's ideas can be seen as an attempt to build on the central idea of Feinberg (1978) who claimed that psychotic symptoms come into being due to patients' unawareness of main processes, which take place in their brains or minds. This unawareness leads to the emergence of abnormal experiences and false beliefs. To elaborate this a little, Feinberg proposed a corollary discharge model in which he claimed that thoughts and movements involved a 'free forward' component and that their initiation generate a re-afference signal. The latter basically defines for us the thought or movement as being 'internally generated' or belonging to us. If this free forward mechanism breaks down, a psychotic phenomenon will occur in which patients may feel that they have not experienced agency, while a thought or movement might have appeared (see Spence 2001).

45. However, Frith admitted that his theory does not explain the full range of schizo-phrenic symptoms (Frith and Done 1989).

46. It has been suggested that the three approaches of philosophy, psychiatry, and neuroscience (including cognitive-neuroscience) to the mind may be viewed as aspects of a single truth, i.e. a unified theory or a 'synthetic analysis' (Hundert 1989).

47. According to Mishara and Schwartz (1997), the interdisciplinary approaches of cognitive neuroscience and cognitive neuropsychiatry represent attempts to re-solve the mind/body problem in a new way. This effort of course would have important implications for existing psychiatric explanatory models (also see, for example, Varela 1996). More specifically, Spitzer and Casas (1997) claim that psychopathology should be based on cognitive neuroscience, for example, in terms of concepts such as neuronal activation, neuroplasticity, and neuronal death (Spitzer and Casas 1997).

48. While many neuroscientists believe that the mind is rooted in the brain, Andreasen (1996, 1997) argued that in order to arrive at a scientific psychopathology, one should not try to reduce the mind to the brain but to understand the complex interaction between them.

49. Cutting's book is written from a philosophical perspective (Kantian and Bergsonian) and provides descriptions of the link between psychopathological phenomena and neuropsychological dysfunctions (Cutting 1997).

50. Monothematic delusions are thought to result from brain injury and to be circum-scribed. Monothematic and circumscribed delusions can be compared with ploythematic and elaborated delusions, which are characteristics of the schizo-phrenic (Stone and Young 1997).

51. Some delusions can be explained in terms of the basis of anomalously heightened affective responsiveness. That is, as a result of brain damage, patients may experience strong affective responses in most faces, i.e. not simply those they know. As a result, they feel that they 'know' most of the people they see, even though they are strangers. Yet, while they feel that they know them, they cannot recognize them. Patients may attribute the reason for this to the fact that these people are in disguise. The idea here is that these anomalously heightened affective

responses to faces might lead to the Frégoli delusion (i.e. patients feel that they are being followed by people they know who are unrecognizable because they are in disguise) (see Davies *et al.* 2001).

52. Mirrored-self misidentification is when patients have an unusual experience of their own face seen in the mirror. They feel that they are the reflected objects as if they were on the other side of the glass with loss of the ability to interact fluently with mirrors.

53. Patients' with unilateral neglect might deny ownership of one of their limbs. Such delusion can be explained, at least in part, in terms of the unusual experience resulting from paralysis, the loss of kinaesthetic and proprioceptive feedback from the arm (see Davies *et al.* 2001).

54. After all, Maher is, in essence, a dualist who believes that our interaction or dealing with the world can be reduced to some processing of atomistic sensory inputs.

55. Langdon *et al.* (2002) also speak of the way in which the notion of irony has been compromised in some schizophrenics. We have possessed a set of sophisticated domain-specific cognitive processes, which help us to anticipate or predict the kinds of beliefs that others would likely have, in the light of their given situations. These processes, for the schizophrenics, are dysfunctioned, which make it difficult for the patients to interpret irony.

56. More specifically, Stone and Young (1997) explained delusion in terms of the conflict between two opposing principles that govern belief revision. The two principles are that of conservativism (this refers to our ability to maintain consistency with the set of accepted beliefs) and of observational adequacy (this refers to our ability to rely on our perceptual inputs). Stone and Young argue that delusions can be explained in terms of the alteration of perceptual inputs and a cognitive bias which then allows unconventional ideas to be accepted and held.

57. On the basis of four patients with delusions of misidentification, Breen *et al.* (2000) argued that the thesis of Ellis and Young on the loss of normal affective responses to familiar faces is not a key factor in the development of delusions of misidentification.

58. Gerrans (2000, 2002) believed that Cotard delusions are produced by a reasoning deficit as opposed to attributional style. That is, delusions are explained in terms of the rationalizations of anomalous experiences by means of reasoning strategies, which are not, in themselves, abnormal.

References

Andreasen, N.C. (1996). Body and soul. *American Journal of Psychiatry*, **153**: 589–590.

Andreasen, N.C. (1997). Linking mind and brain in the study of mental illnesses: a project for a scientific psychopathology. *Science*, **275**: 1586–1599.

Belzen, J.A. (1995). The impact of phenomenology on clinical psychiatry: Rümke's position between Jaspers and Kraeplin. *History of Psychiatry*, **4**: 349–385.

Bentall, R.P. (1990) (ed.). *Reconstructing schizophrenia*. London: Routledge.

Bentall, R.P. (2004). *Madness explained: psychosis and human nature*. London: Penguin Books.

Bermúdez, J.L. (2001). Normativity and rationality in delusional psychiatric disorders. *Mind & Language*, **16**(5): 457–493.

Berze, J. (1914). Die Primäre insuffizienz der psychischen aktivität (primary insufficiency of mental activity). In: *The clinical roots of the schizophrenia concept* (ed. J. Cutting and M. Shepherd). Cambridge, UK: Cambridge University Press.

Binswanger, L. (1963). *Being in the world*. New York: Basic Books.

Blankenburg, W. (1969). Ansätze zu einer psychopathologie des 'common sense'. *Confinia Psychiatrica*, **12**: 144–163.

Blankenburg, W. (1971). *Der verlust der naturlichen selbstverstandlichkeit: Ein beitrag zur psychopathologie symptomarmer schizophrenien*. Stuttgart: Ferdinand Enke Verlag.

Blankenburg, W. (1991). *La perte de l'évidence naturelle: une contribution a la psychopathologie des schizophrénies pauci-symptomatiques*. Paris: Presses Universitaires de France.

Blankenburg, W. (2001). First steps towards a psychopathology of 'common sense'. *Philosophy, Psychiatry & Psychology*, **8**(4): 303–315.

Bleuler, E. (1911). *Dementia praecox or the group of schizophrenia*. New York: International University Press.

Bolton, D. (2001). Problems in the definition of 'mental disorder'. *The Philosophical Quarterly*, **51**(203): 182–199.

Bolton, D. (2003). Meaning and causal explanations in the behavioural sciences. In: *Nature and Narrative* (ed. B. Fulford, K. Morris, J. Sadler, and G. Stanghellini). Oxford, UK: Oxford University Press.

Bolton, D. and Hill, J. (1996). *Mind, meaning and mental disorder*. Oxford: Oxford University Press.

Boyle, M. (1990). *Schizophrenia: a scientific delusion?* London: Routledge.

Breen, N., Caine, D., Coltheart, M., Hendy, J., and Roberts, C. (2000). Towards an understanding of delusions of misidentification: four case studies. *Mind & Language*, **15**(1): 74–110.

Cahill, C. and Frith, C.D. (1996). A cognitive basis for the signs and symptoms of schizophrenia. In: *In schizophrenia: a neuropsychological perspective* (ed. C. Pantelis, H.E. Nelson, and T.R.E. Barnes). New York: John Wiley & Son.

Campbell, J. (2001). Rationality, meaning, and the analysis of delusion. *Philosophy, Psychiatry & Psychology*, **8**(2–3): 89–100.

Chadwick, R.F. (1994). Kant, thought insertion and mental unity. *Philosophy, Psychiatry & Psychology*, **1**(2): 105–113.

Chalmers, D.J. (1996). *The conscious mind. In search of a fundamental theory*. New York: Oxford University Press.

Chalmers, D.J. (1997). Moving forward on the problems of consciousness. *Journal of Consciousness Studies*, **4**: 3–46.

Cocoran, R., Mercer, G., and Frith, C.D. (1995). Schizophrenia, symptomatology and social inference: investigating the 'theory of mind' in people with schizophrenia. *Schizophrenia Research*, **17**: 5–13.

Crow, T.J. (1985). The two-syndrome concept: origins and current status. *Schizophrenia Bulletin*, **11**: 471–486.

Currie, G. (2000). Imagination, hallucination and delusion. *Mind and Language*, **15**(1): 168–183.

Cutting, J. (1985). *The psychology of schizophrenia*. London: Churchill Livingstone.

Cutting, J. (1997). *Principles of psychopathology*. Oxford, UK: Oxford University Press.

Davies, M., Coltheart, M., Langdon, R., and Breen, N. (2001). Monothematic delusions: towards a two-factor account. *Philosophy, Psychiatry & Psychology*, 8(2–3): 133–158.

Dawson, P.J. (1994). Philosophy, biology and mental disorder. *Journal of Advanced Nursing*, 20: 587–596.

De Koning, A.J. and Jenner, F.A. (1982). *Phenomenology and psychiatry*. London: Academic Press.

Depraz, N. (2003). Putting the époché into practice: schizophrenic experience as illustrating the phenomenological exploration of consciousness. In: *Nature and narrative* (ed. B. Fulford, K. Morris, J. Sadler, and G. Stanghellini). Oxford, UK: Oxford University Press.

Dworkin, R.H., Cornblatt, B.A., Friedman, R. *et al.* (1993). Childhood precursors of affective vs social deficits in adolescents at risk of schizophrenia. *Schizophrenia Bulletin*, 19: 563–577.

Dworkin, R.H., Lewis, L.A., Cornblatt, B.A. *et al.* (1994). Social competence deficits in adolescents at risk of schizophrenia. *Journal of Nervous and Mental Disease*, 182: 103–108.

Ellis, H.D. and Young, A.W. (1990). Accounting for delusional misidentifications. *British Journal of Psychiatry*, 157: 239–248.

Ellis, H.D., Young, A.W., Quayle, A.H., and de Pauw, K.W. (1997). Reduced autonomic responses to faces in Capgras delusion. *Proceedings of the Royal Society: Biological Sciences*, B264: 1085–1092.

Feinberg, I. (1978). Efference copy and corollary discharge: implications for thinking and its disorders. *Schizophrenia Bulletin*, 4: 636–640.

Follette, W.C. and Houts, A.C. (1996). Models of scientific progress and the role of theory in taxonomy development: a case study of the DSM. *Journal of Consulting and Clinical Psychology*, 64: 1120–1132.

Frith, C.D. (1987). The positive and negative symptoms of schizophrenia reflect impairments in the perception and initiation of action. *Psychological Medicine*, 17: 631–648.

Frith, C.D. (1992). *The cognitive neuropsychology of schizophrenia*. Hove: Lawrence Erlbaum Associates.

Frith, C.D. and Done, J. (1989). Positive symptoms of schizophrenia. *British Journal of Psychiatry*, 154: 569–570.

Fulford, K.W.M. (1989). *Moral theory and medical practice*. Cambridge, UK: Cambridge University Press.

Fulford, K.W.M. (1993). Mental illness and the mind-brain problem: delusion, belief and Searle's theory of intentionality. *Theoretical Medicine*, 14: 181–194.

Fulford, K.W.M. (1994a). Value, illness and failure of action: framework for a philosophical psychopathology of delusions. In: *Philosophy psychopathology* (ed. G. Graham and G.L. Stephens). Massachusetts: The MIT Press.

Fulford, K.W.M. (1994b). Mind and madness: new directions in the philosophy of psychiatry. In: *Philosophy, psychology and psychiatry* (ed. A.P. Griffiths). Cambridge, UK: Cambridge University Press.

Fulford, K.W.M (1999). Nine variations and a coda on the theme of an evolutionary definition of dysfunction. *Journal of Abnormal Psychology*, 108: 412–420.

Fulford, K.W.M. (2000). Teleology without tears: naturalism, neo-naturalism, and evaluationism in the analysis of function statements in biology (and a bet on the twenty-first century). *Philosophy, Psychiatry and Psychology*, **7**: 77–94.

Fulford, B., Morris, K., Sadler, J., and Stanghellini, G. (2003). *Nature and narrative*. Oxford, UK: Oxford University Press.

Gallagher, S. (2000). Philosophical conceptions of the self: implications for cognitive science. *Trends in Cognitive Sciences*, **4**(1): 14–21.

Gerrans, P. (1999). Delusional misidentification as subpersonal disintegration. *The Monist*, **82**: 590–608.

Gerrans, P. (2000). Refining the explanation of Cotard's delusion. *Mind & Language*, **15**(1): 111–122.

Gerrans, P. (2002). A one-stage explanation of the Cotard delusion. *Philosophy, Psychiatry & Psychology*, **9**(1): 47–53.

Gold, I., and Hohwy, J. (2000). Rationality and schizophrenic delusion. *Mind & Language*, **15**(1): 146–167.

Graham, G. and Stephens, L. (1994) (ed.). *Philosophical psychopathology*. Massachusetts: The MIT Press.

Gupta, M. and Kay, L.R. (2002). The impact of phenomenology on North American Psychiatric Assessment. *Philosophy, Psychiatry & Psychology*, **9**(1): 73–85.

Hempel, C.G. (1984). Fundamentals of taxonomy. In: *Philosophical Perspectives of Psychiatric Diagnostic Classification* (ed. J.Z. Sadler., O.P. Wiggins, and M.A. Schwartz). Baltimore: John Hopkins University.

Hirstein, W. and Ramachandran, V.S. (1997). Capgras syndrome: a novel probe for understanding the neural representation of the identity and familiarity of persons. *Proceedings of the Royal Society: Biological Sciences*, **B264**: 437–444.

Hoerl, C. (2001). On thought insertion. *Philosophy, Psychiatry & Psychology*, **8**(2–3): 189–200.

Houts, A.C. and Follette, W.C. (1998). Mentalism, mechanisms and medical analogues: reply to Wakefield (1998). *Journal of Consulting and Clinical Psychology*, **66**(5): 853–855.

Hundert, E.M. (1989). *Philosophy, psychiatry and neuroscience: three approaches to the mind*. Oxford: Oxford University Press.

Husserl, E. (1900/1970). *Logical investigations*. London: Routledge & Kegan Paul.

Husserl, E. (1973). *Experience and judgment: investigations in a genealogy of logic*. Evanston: Northwestern University Press.

Jackson, M. and Fulford, K.W.M. (1997). Spiritual experience and psychopathology. *Philosophy, Psychiatry & Psychology*, **4**: 1–14.

Jaspers, K. (1923/1963). *General psychopathology*. Manchester, UK: Manchester University Press.

Jaspers, K. (1968). The phenomenological approach in psychopathology. *British Journal of Psychiatry*, **114**: 1313–1323.

Jenner, F.A., Monteiro, A.C.D., Zagalo-Cardoso, J.A., and Cunha-Oliveira, J.A. (1993). *Schizophrenia: a disease or some ways of being human?*. Sheffield: Sheffield Academic Press.

Kimura, B. (2001). Cogito and I: a bio-logical approach. *Philosophy, Psychiatry and Psychology*, **8**(4): 331–336.

Kopelman, L. (1996). Normal grief: good or bad? Health or disease. *Philosophy, Psychiatry & Psychology*, **1**(4): 209–220.

Kraepelin, E. (1899/1990) *Psychiatry: a textbook for students and physicians, volumes 1 and 2*. New Delhi: Amerind Publishing.

Kraus, A. (2003). How can the phenomenological-anthropological approach contribute to diagnosis and classification in psychiatry? In: *Nature and narrative* (ed. B. Fulford, K. Morris, J. Sadler, and G. Stanghellini). Oxford, UK: Oxford University Press.

Kretschmer, E. (1922). *Koerperbau und charakter*. Berlin-Goettingen-Heidelberg: Springer.

Laing, R.D. (1959). *The divided self*. Harmondsworth: Penguin.

Laing, R.D. (1961). *Self and others*. Harmondsworth: Penguin.

Laing, R.D. (1971). *The politics of the family*. London: Tavistock.

Langdon, R. and Coltheart, M. (2000). The cognitive neuropsychology of delusions. *Mind & Language*, **15**(1): 184–218.

Langdon, R., Davies, M., and Coltheart, M. (2002). Understanding minds and understanding communicated meanings in schizophrenia. *Mind & Language*, **17**: 68–104.

Langenbach, M. (1995). Phenomenology, intentionality and mental experiences: Edmund Husserl's logische allgemeine psychopathologie. *History of Psychiatry*, **6**: 209–224.

Macmurray, J. (1991). *The self as agent*. London: Faber & Faber.

Maher, B.A. (1974). Delusional thinking and perceptual disorder. *Journal of Individual Psychology*, **30**: 98–113.

Maher, B.A. (1988). Anomalous experience and delusional thinking. In: *Delusional Beliefs* (ed. T.H. Oltmanns and B.A. Maher). New York: Wiley.

Maher, B.A. (1992). Delusions: contemporary etiological hypotheses. *Psychiatric Annals*, **22**: 260–268.

Maher, B.A. (1999). Anomalous experience in everyday life: its significance for psychopathology. *The Monist*, **82**: 547–570.

Maher, B.A. (2003). Schizophrenia, aberrant utterance and delusions of control: the disconnection of speech and thought, and the connection of experience and belief. *Mind & Language*, **18**(1): 1–22.

Malmberg, A., Lewis, G., David, A., and Allebeck, P (1998). Premorbid adjustment and personality in people with schizophrenia. *British Journal of Psychiatry*, **172**: 308–313.

McManus, D. (1996). Error, hallucination and the concept of ontology in the early work of Heidegger. *Philosophy*, **71**: 553–575.

Minkowski, E. (1948). Phénoménologie et analyse existentielle en psychopathologie. *L'évolution Psychiatrique*, **11**: 137–185.

Minkowski, E. (1997). *Au-delà du rationalisme morbide*. Paris: Ed L'Harmattan.

Minkowski, E. and Targowla, R. (2001). A contribution to the study of autism: the interrogative attitude. *Philosophy, Psychiatry & Psychology*, **8**(4): 271–278.

Mishara, A.L. (1997). *Phenomenology and the unconscious. The problem of the unconscious in the phenomenological and existential traditions*. The Hague: Kluwer Academic Publishers.

Mishara, A.L. (2001). On Wolfgang, Blankenburg, common sense and schizophrenia. *Philosophy, Psychiatry & Psychology*, **8**(4): 317–322.

Mishara, A.L. and Schwartz, M.A. (1997). Psychopathology in the light of emergent trends in the philosophy of consciousness, neuropsychiatry and phenomenology. *Current Opinion in Psychiatry*, **10**(5): 383–389.

Mishara, A.L., Parnas, J., and Naudin, J. (1998). Forging the links between phenomenology, cognitive neuroscience, and psychopathology: the emergence of a new
discipline. *Current Opinion in Psychiatry*, **11**: 567–573.

Mlakar, J., Jensterle, J., and Frith, C.D. (1994). Central monitoring deficiency and
schizophrenic symptoms. *Psychological Medicine*, **24**: 557–564.

Moller, P. and Husby, R. (2000). The initial prodrome in schizophrenia: searching for
naturalistic core dimensions of experience and behaviour. *Schizophrenia Bulletin*,
26(1): 217–232.

Murphy, D. and Woolfolk, R.L. (2000). The harmful dysfunction analysis of mental
disorder. *Philosophy, Psychiatry & Psychology*, **7**(4): 241–252.

Ogilvie, J. (2000–2001). On self-conceiving: philosophical yearnings in a schizophrenic context. *Creativity Research Journal*, **13**(1): 87–94.

Pachoud, B. (2001). Reading Minkowski with Husserl. *Philosophy, Psychiatry &
Psychology*, **8**(4): 299–301.

Parker, I., Georgaca, E., Harper, D., McLaughlin, T., and Stowell-Smith, M. (1995).
Deconstructing psychopathology. London: Sage.

Parnas, J. and Bovet, P. (1991). Autism in schizophrenia revisited. *Comprehensive
Psychiatry*, **32**: 7–21.

Parnas, J. and Sass, L.A. (2001). Self, solipsism, and schizophrenic delusions. *Philosophy, Psychiatry & Psychology*, **8**(2–3): 101–120

Parnas, J., Bovet, P., and Innocenti, G. (1996). Schizophrenic trait features, binding and
cortico-cortical connectivity: a neurodevelopmental pathogenetic hypothesis.
Neurology, Psychiatry and Brain Research, **4**, 185–196.

Poland, J., von Eckardt, B., and Spaulding, W. (1994). Problems with the
DSM approach to classifying psychopathology. In: *Philosophy psychopathology*
(ed. G. Graham and G.L. Stephens). Massachusetts: The MIT Press.

Radden, J. (1994). Recent criticism of psychiatric nosology: a review. *Philosophy,
Psychiatry & Psychology*, **1**(3): 193–200.

Radden, J. (1996). Philosophy of mind and mental concepts. *Current Opinion in
Psychiatry*, **9**: 364–367.

Ramachandran, V.S. and Blakeslee, S. (1998). *Phantoms in the brain: human nature
and the architecture of the mind*. London: Fourth Estate.

Roessler, J. (2001). Understanding delusions of alien control. *Philosophy, Psychiatry &
Psychology*, **8**(2–3): 177–187.

Rossi Monti, M. and Stanghellini, G. (1996). Psychopathology: an edgeless razor.
Contemporary Psychiatry, **3**: 196–204.

Sadler, J.Z., and Agich, G.J. (1996). Diseases, functions, values and psychiatric
classification. *Philosophy, Psychiatry and Psychology*, **2**: 219–231.

Sadler, J.Z., Wiggins, O.P., and Schwartz, M.A. (1994) (ed.). *Philosophical Perspectives on Psychiatric Diagnostic Classification*. Baltimore: The John Hopkins University Press.

Sass, L.A. (1992). *Madness and modernism*. New York: Basic Books.

Sass, L.A. (1994). *The paradoxes of delusion*. Ithaca: Cornell University Press.

Sass, L.A. (2000). Schizophrenia, self-experience, and the so-called 'negative symptoms.' In: *Exploring the Self: Philosophical and Psychopathological Perspectives on
Self-Experience* (ed. D. Zahavi). Amsterdam: John Benjamins.

Sass, L.A. (2001). Self and world in schizophrenia: three classic approaches. *Philosophy, Psychiatry & Psychology*, **8**(4): 251–270.

Sass, L.A. and Parnas, J. (2001). Phenomenology of self-disturbances in schizophrenia: some research findings and directions. *Philosophy, Psychiatry & Psychology*, **8**(4): 347–356.

Sass, L.A., Whiting, J., and Parnas, J. (2000). Mind, self and psychopathology. *Theory & Psychology*, **10**(1): 87–98.

Scheler, M. (1913). *Zur phänomenologie und theorie der sympathiege gef?ble und von liebe und hass*. Halle: Niemeyer.

Schneider, K. (1959). *Clinical psychopathology*. New York: Grune and Stratton.

Schwartz, M.A., Wiggins, O.P., and Spitzer, M. (1997). Psychotic experience and disordered thinking: a reappraisal from new perspectives. *Journal of Nervous and Mental Disease*, 185(3): 176–187.

Searle, J.R. (1983). *Intentionality: an essay in the philosophy of mind*. Cambridge, UK: Cambridge University Press.

Spence, S.A. (1996). Free will in the light of neuropsychiatry. *Philosophy, Psychiatry & Psychology*, **3**: 75 93.

Spence, S.A. (2001). Alien control: from phenomenology to cognitive neurobiology. *Philosophy, Psychiatry & Psychology*, **8**(2–3): 163–172.

Spitzer, M. (1990). Kant on schizophrenia. In: *Philosophy and psychopathology* (ed. M. Spitzer and B.A. Maher). New York: Springer-Verlag.

Spitzer, M. (1997). A cognitive neuroscience view of schizophrenic thought disorder. *Schizophrenia Bulletin*, **23**: 29–50.

Spitzer, M. and Casas, B. (1997). Project for a scientific psychopathology. *Current Opinion in Psychiatry*, **10**: 395–401.

Stanghellini, G. (1997). For an anthropology of vulnerability. *Psychopathology*, **30**: 1–11.

Stanghellini, G. (2001). Psychopathology of common sense. *Philosophy, Psychiatry & Psychology*, **8**(2–3): 201 218.

Stephens, G.L. and Graham, G. (1994a). Voices and selves. In: *Philosophical perspectives on psychiatric diagnostic classification* (ed. J.Z. Sadler., O.P.Wiggins., and M.A.Schwartz). Baltimore: The John Hopkins University Press.

Stephens, G.L. and Graham, G. (1994b). Self-consciousness, mental agency and clinical psychopathology of thought-insertion. *Philosophy, Psychiatry & Psychology*, **1**(1): 1–10.

Stephens, G.L. and Graham, G. (2000). *When self-consciousness breaks. Alien voices and inserted thoughts*. Cambridge: MIT Press.

Stone, T. and Young, A.W. (1997). Delusions and brain injury: the philosophy and psychology of belief. *Mind & Language*, **12**: 327–364.

Tsuang, M.I. (1993). Genotypes, phenotypes and the brain: a search for connections in schizophrenia. *British Journal of Psychiatry*, **163**: 299–307.

Urfer, A. (2001). Phenomenology and psychopathology of schizophrenia: the views of Eugene Minkowski. *Philosophy, Psychiatry & Psychology*, **8**(4): 279–289.

Varela, F.J. (1996). Neurophenomenology: a methodological remedy for the hard problem. *Journal of Consciousness Studies*, **3**: 330–349.

Wakefield, J.C. (1992a). The concept of mental disorder: on the boundary between biological facts and social values. *American Psychologist*, **47**: 373–388.

Wakefield, J.C. (1992b). Disorder as harmful dysfunction: a conceptual critique of DSM-III-R's definition of mental disorder. *Psychological Review*, **99**: 232–247.

Wakefield, J.C. (1999a). Philosophy of science and the progressiveness of the DSM's theory-neutral nosology: response to Follette and Houts, part 1. *Behaviour Research and Therapy*, **37**: 963–999.

Wakefield, J.C. (1999b). The concept of disorder as a foundation for the DSM's theory-neutral nosology: response to Follette and Houts, part 2. *Behaviour Research and Therapy*, **37**: 1001–1027.

Wakefield, J.C. (2000). Spandrels, vestigial organs and such: reply to Murphy and Woolfolk's 'the harmful dysfunction analysis of mental disorder.' *Philosophy, Psychiatry & Psychology*, **7**(4): 253–269.

Walker, C. (1994a). Karl Jaspers and Edmund Husserl-I: the perceived convergence. *Philosophy, Psychiatry & Psychology*, **1**(2): 117–134.

Walker, C. (1994b). Karl Jaspers and Edmund Husserl-II: the divergence. *Philosophy, Psychiatry & Psychology*, **1**(4): 245–265.

Walker, C. (1995). Karl Jaspers and Edmund Husserl-III: Jaspers as a Kantian phenomenologist. *Philosophy, Psychiatry & Psychology*, **2**(1): 65–82.

Wallace, E., Radden, J., and Sadler, J.Z. (1997). The philosophy of psychiatry: who needs it? *Journal of Nervous and Mental Disease*, **185**(2): 67–73.

Wiggins, O.P. and Schwartz, M.A. (1997). Edmund Husserl's influence on Karl Jaspers's phenomenology. *Philosophy, Psychiatry & Psychology*, **4**: 15–36.

Wiggins, O.P., Schwartz, M.A., and Northoff, G. (1990). Toward a Husserlian phenomenology of the initial stages of schizophrenia. In: *Philosophy and psychopathology* (ed. M. Spitzer and B.A. Maher). New York: Springer-Verlag.

Wing, J.K. (1988). Abandoning what? *British Journal of Clinical Psychology*, **27**: 325–328.

Wright, S., Young, A.W., and Hellawell, D.J. (1993). Sequential Cotard and Capgras delusions. *British Journal of Clinical Psychology*, **32**: 345–349.

Young, A. W. (1998). *Face and mind*. Oxford, UK: Oxford University Press.

Young, A.W. (2000). Wondrous strange: the neuropsychology of abnormal beliefs. *Mind & Language*, **15**(1): 47–73.

Young, A.W. and Leafhead, K.M. (1996). Betwixt life and death: case studies of the Cotard delusion. In: *Method in madness: case studies in cognitive neuropsychiatry* (ed. P.W. Halligan and J.C. Marshall). Hove, Sussex, UK: Psychology Press.

Young, A.W., Robertson, I.H., Hellawell, D.J., de Pauw, K.W., and Pentland, B. (1992). Cotard delusion after brain injury. *Psychological Medicine*, **22**: 799–804.

Young, A.W., Reid, I., Wright, S., and Hellawell, D.J. (1993). Face-processing impairments and the Capgras delusion. *British Journal of Psychiatry*, **162**: 695–698.

Young, A.W., Leafhead, K.M., and Szulecka, T.K. (1994). The Capgras and Cotard delusions. *Psychopathology*, **27**: 226–231.

Zachar, P. (2000). Psychiatric disorders are not natural kinds. *Philosophy, Psychiatry & Psychology*, **7**(3): 167–182.

Zahavi, D. (2001). Schizophrenia and self-awareness. *Philosophy, Psychiatry and Psychology*, **8**(4): 339–341.

4 Explaining schizophrenia: the relevance of phenomenology

Louis A. Sass and Josef Parnas

Abstract

Is phenomenological psychopathology purely descriptive or can it also have explanatory relevance? This question is addressed in relation to schizophrenia and by focusing on a phenomenological account advocated by the present authors. In our view, schizophrenia is best understood as a disorder of consciousness and self-experience (disturbed ipseity) that involves two key aspects: hyper-reflexivity (forms of exaggerated and alienating self-consciousness) and diminished self-affection (a diminished sense of existing as a subject of awareness or agent of action).

After mentioning some prior views concerning phenomenological description or explanation and also mental causation, we outline several ways in which the subjective dimension of schizophrenia can be relevant for explanatory purposes. We distinguish two explanatory perspectives according to whether the relationships at issue apply to phenomena that occur simultaneously (the synchronic dimension) or in succession (the diachronic dimension). Within the first or synchronic realm, we discuss three kinds of relationship: equiprimordial, constitutive, and expressive—all of which involve not causation but a kind of phenomenological implication. Then we turn to the diachronic dimension. Here we consider primary, consequential, and compensatory processes. All three can play a role in a causal account of the development of schizophrenic symptoms over time.

Introduction

Writers on phenomenological philosophy and psychiatry often characterize phenomenology as a descriptive rather than an explanatory enterprise. This statement can doubtless be understood variously. The general idea, however, is that the purpose of phenomenology is to describe and define the nature and varieties of human experience rather than to give an account of the causal mechanisms or efficacious processes that bring it about. One phenomenological psychiatrist, Wolfgang Blankenburg (1971, p. 4; 1991, p. 27), e.g. explicitly denies that his account of the 'basic disorder' (*Grundstörung*) in schizophrenia is intended to have any aetiological significance; he aims, he says, only to capture the 'essence' of typically schizophrenic abnormalities (see also Buytendijk 1987, p. 130). The phenomenologists who eschew explanatory ambitions should not, incidentally, be understood as arguing for the causal irrelevance (or independence) of conscious experience; typically, they mean to imply a bracketing or setting-aside of all such questions in order to facilitate a purified description of subjective life.

In this paper, we use 'phenomenology' in the standard philosophical and continental sense: that is, to refer to the study of lived experience and of how things manifest themselves to us within and through such experience (Moran 2000; Sokolowski 2000, p. 2). In psychiatric phenomenology, it is, of course, the subjective dimension of mental disorders that is of relevance. The tradition of psychiatric phenomenology derives from Husserl, Heidegger, Merleau-Ponty, and Jaspers; it must be distinguished from the context of mainstream Anglophone psychiatry, where the term 'phenomenology' simply refers to readily observable signs and symptoms.

The identification of phenomenology with description (not to mention the very distinction between description and explanation itself) is not, however, nearly as straightforward or as universally accepted as it may first appear.[1]

At an early phase of his work, Edmund Husserl (1859–1938)—phenomenology's founder—did present phenomenology as a purely descriptive approach that excludes all concern with both genesis and causation (Bernet *et al.* 1993, p. 195). In the classic preface to his *Phenomenology of perception*, Maurice Merleau-Ponty (1962, pp. vii–viii) characterizes phenomenology as:

> ... a matter of describing, not of explaining or analyzing ... (as an attempt) to give a direct description of experience as it is without taking account of its psychological origin and the causal explanations which the scientist, the historian, or the sociologist may be able to provide.

But as Merleau-Ponty also points out, Husserl later adopted a broader and more ambitious view, advocating the need to supplement 'static' or 'descriptive phenomenology' with phenomenology of a 'genetic' or 'constructive' type. Indeed, Husserl (1999) himself came to speak of 'explanatory' phenomenology—a 'phenomenology of regulated genesis' (p. 318). Genetic phenomenology, for Husserl, includes the study of how complex objects and modes of experience come to be constituted, over time, via the synthesis of simpler or more basic processes or 'lived experiences' (1999, p. 319).[2]

In his late work, Husserl (1989) also spoke of 'motivational' relationships or even a 'motivational causality', whose study clearly fell within the province of phenomenology (p. 227; 1999, p. 320). Husserl carefully distinguished motivational causality from causality as understood in a narrower sense—

that is, from the 'natural causality' or 'real causality' of physical nature (which, presumably, involves the efficient form of causality). 'Motivation,' for Husserl, concerns the attitude and orientation of the subject; unlike blind causality, it involves the subject's viewpoint on or interpretation of the world. Husserl described motivation as providing the 'fundamental lawfulness of spiritual life' (1989, pp. 231, 241ff.).[3]

Husserl's concept of motivation is broader than the ordinary concept of motive, disposition, or ground for action. It covers many forms of implicative interdependence between mental acts and experiences that contribute to the coherence and unity of consciousness, both in its synchronic and diachronic aspects (1989, pp. 223–293).[4]

To grasp the mind of another person is to grasp the distinctive form of coherence of that person's consciousness; this requires that one move beyond mere static understanding of mental states toward an understanding of the unity of that person's subjectivity and its development over time. As we shall see below, a phenomenological understanding of a disturbed overall mode of consciousness or lived-world may allow one to make sense out of seemingly bizarre actions or beliefs that might otherwise seem completely incomprehensible. One may, for example, come to see how the person's actions or beliefs are in some respects inspired or justified by the kinds of experiences the person is having, or in the light of general features of the person's experience of time, space, causality, or selfhood.

It is clear, in any case, that Husserl (1989, p. 402) gradually moved away from Wilhelm Dilthey's sharp opposition between description (as the goal of the human sciences) and explanation (as the goal of the natural sciences). In his lectures on phenomenological psychology of 1925 (1977, p. 39), Husserl spoke of:

> ... ultimate unclarities concerning the mutual relation of nature and mind and of all the sciences which belong to these two titles ... what seems at first obviously separated, upon closer inspection turns out to be obscurely intertwined, permeating each other in a manner very difficult to understand.

The concepts of both 'explanation' and 'causation' are problematic, heterogeneous, and 'obscurely intertwined'. Both concepts have been disputed since ancient times and continue to be highly contested in contemporary philosophy (Audi 1999, p. 127; Crane 1999). It is not clear, for example, whether the notion of causation is really a cluster of related but somewhat disparate concepts or whether a single basic concept underlies it (Mackie 1974, p. 117). One prominent candidate for such a basic concept would be 'effectiveness', as when a cause is defined as 'that which can be used for the purpose of making, or bringing it about that, something happens' (R.M. Gale, quoted in Mackie 1974, p. 168n). The Cambridge dictionary of philosophy defines 'explanation' in simple and general terms: as 'an act of making something intelligible or understandable, as when we explain an event by showing how or why it occurred' (Audi 1999, p. 298). The paradigm cases of explanation typically refer to efficient causal mechanisms or processes in the physical world. There are, however, also concepts of both 'motivational' and 'mental' causation (Husserl 1989; Heil and Mele 1993). Indeed, 'causal relevance' can be defined quite broadly—as requiring only that a given attribute or factor (the cause) 'makes a difference' to the probability of the occurrence of a given property (the effect) (Grunbaum 1993, p. 163; Woodward 2003). Further, the possible forms of explanation need not be restricted to causation alone: they can also involve other forms of relationship that reveal the underlying unity or interdependence of a group of phenomena. Indeed, explanatory factors can be said to cover '*all* those things to which any event or process can be ascribed, *anything* in the light of which it can be said to make sense' (Lawson-Tancred 1995, pp. 418–419, emphasis added). Explanation can be defined as 'an apparently successful attempt to increase the understanding of [a given] phenomenon' (Wilson and Keil 2000, p. 89).

Given the problematic nature of these issues, it is hardly surprising there is no consensus about or clear statement of these issues in psychopathology or the more specific domain of phenomenological psychopathology. The classic phenomenological psychopathologists have different attitudes to this issue. Some (e.g. Erwin Straus) think of phenomenology's investigation of the nature of experience as a purely descriptive enterprise, and look exclusively to neighbouring fields—such as psycho-analysis and biological psychiatry— to supply causal or explanatory accounts. By contrast, in his later work, Ludwig Binswanger attempted to apply the later Husserl's 'constitutive phenomenology' to explain the genesis of psychotic worlds, e.g. to explain how delusional worlds come to be constituted and to develop as they do (Spiegelberg 1972, pp. 209, 214, 267ff.; Tatossian 1997, pp. 12–13).

The only extensive treatment, in English, of the nature of description, explanation, and understanding in phenomenological psychopathology, can be found, scattered about, in Jasper's massive text, *General psychopathology*—a classic work that was last revised in 1941 and published in English translation in 1963. Though extremely valuable, Jaspers' presentation is also problematic in various ways.[5]

Another seminal figure in phenomenological psychopathology, Eugene Minkowski, sometimes equivocates as to whether the '*trouble génerateur*' is to be understood as pathogenetically primary (in a causal sense) or as thematically central. In *La Schizophrénie*, Minkowski (1927) describes 'loss of vital contact with reality' as 'not a consequence of other psychical disturbances, but an essential point [or state] from which spring, or at least from which it is possible to view in a uniform way all the cardinal symptoms' (1927/1997, p. 87, translation by LAS). According to the latter interpretation ('view in a uniform way'), the *trouble génerateur* would bring symptoms together in relationships of phenomenological implication.

The purpose of the present chapter is to offer a clear and reasonably succinct, contemporary overview of these issues for use by psychiatrists, clinical psychologists, and other students of psychopathology. Here we cannot claim to offer anything approaching an all-inclusive or fully rigorous classification of the forms of explanation—which have been disputed at least since Aristotle. We do wish to indicate certain important forms of explanation relevant to psychopathology that are neglected in psychiatry, forms that refute the widespread assumption that phenomenological accounts are unimportant because they are 'merely' descriptive in nature.

Our chapter is an attempt to offer a synoptic overview of a great many issues that have been unduly neglected in psychopathology. These issues are disparate and extremely complex. They are, however, also clearly inter-related, and need to be considered together—even at the risk of some inevitable superficiality and oversimplification. In this chapter we attempt to acquaint readers with a range of concepts and theorists in the phenomenological tradition, and to show, using these concepts, how a phenomenological approach can move beyond mere description to play an explanatory role in psychopathology. In the course of doing so, we will touch upon the relationship between phenomenology and neurobiological explanations, and we will address, at somewhat greater length, the differences between phenomenological accounts of experience and the forms of mental causation typically countenanced by analytic philosophers. We also hope to provide a preliminary taxonomy of six forms of phenomenological explanation, each of which fits into one of two general explanatory perspectives. These general perspectives are distinguished according to whether the relationships at issue apply to phenomena that occur simultaneously or in succession. Whereas the first explanatory perspective involves what might be called phenomenological implication, the second has a causal or at least quasi-causal significance.[6]

In this article, we will focus on schizophrenia, and we will use our own, phenomenological account of the disorder to illustrate the above-mentioned issues. We believe, however, that most of our formulations have general application to other forms of psychopathology. The main purpose of this article is to use our account of schizophrenia as a way of illustrating the explanatory relevance a phenomenological approach can have. Our account, which has strong affinities with the work of several other phenomenological psychopathologists (especially Minkowski and Blankenburg; Sass 2001a), has been developed and defended in detail elsewhere (Parnas 2000, 2003; Sass 1992a, 1994, 1998a, 2003a, 2003b; Sass and Parnas 2003). Here we sketch it as briefly as possible, hoping only to indicate its relevance to the broad range of schizophrenic symptoms before moving on to consider a variety of distinct ways in which it may have more than merely descriptive significance. Our concern here is not to prove the correctness of our particular interpretations of schizophrenia, but only to lay out a set of explanatory *possibilities*.

Disturbed ipseity: a phenomenological account of schizophrenia

The purpose of a phenomenological investigation is to give an accurate account of the form and structure of subjective life. (The term 'account' is appropriately vague in this context, since it can refer to both description and explanation.)

To carry out such a project, it is necessary to bracket all ontological commitments and common sense assumptions (the 'phenomenological reduction'), and also to carry out of a series of imaginative variations as a way of specifying the invariant features of the phenomena in question (the 'eidetic reduction'; see Bernet *et al.* 1993). The goals of this kind of investigation are twofold. The first goal (which would seem to be more purely descriptive) is to examine different types of objects and modes of their presentation exactly as they are experienced. The second goal (which is perhaps more explanatory) is to disclose the intrinsic structures of experience that are their conditions of possibility, e.g. the structures of self- and object awareness, of temporality, spatiality, embodiment, and the like. (In the case of phenomenological psychopathology, one is typically dealing not with one's own experience but with a representation of the patient's experience that is built up on the basis of verbal reports and expressive gestures, among other data.) It should be noted that phenomenology is concerned both with the ways objects of awareness are given in experience (Husserl called these 'noematic' aspects, which include the experiential content and mode) and also with the nature of the acts of awareness by which these objects and modes are formed (constituted) in the intentional stream of awareness (the so-called 'noetic' aspects). (*Re* phenomenology, see Moran 2000; Sokolowski 2000; *re* phenomenological psychopathology, see Parnas and Zahavi 2002; Sass 1992a, 1992b.)

According to the view to be presented here, the core abnormality in schizophrenia is a particular kind of disturbance of consciousness and, especially, of the sense of self or ipseity that is normally implicit in each act of awareness. (Ipseity derives from *ipse*, Latin for 'self' or 'itself.' Ipse-identity or ipseity refers to a crucial sense of self-sameness, of existing as a subject of experience that is at one with itself at any given moment (Henry 1973; Ricoeur 1992; Zahavi 1999).) This self or ipseity disturbance has two main aspects or features that may at first sound mutually contradictory, but are in fact complementary. The first is hyper-reflexivity—which refers to a kind of exaggerated self-consciousness, that is, a tendency to direct focal, objectifying attention toward processes and phenomena that would normally be 'inhabited' or experienced as part of oneself. The second is diminished self-affection—which refers to a decline in the (passively or automatically) experienced sense of existing as a living and unified subject of awareness. (Please note that the term 'affection' as used here refers to a process of being affected by something; it has nothing to do with the notion of fondness, or liking of oneself.)[7]

This two-faced disturbance of ipseity disrupts the normal pre-reflective sense of existing as a self-presence that is the 'I-centre' or 'central point of psychic life'—what, in Husserlian phenomenology, could be called the 'source-point of the rays of attention', 'centre of reception', or 'pole of the affections' (Bernet et al. 1993, pp. 209ff.).

These mutations of the act of awareness are typically, perhaps necessarily, accompanied by alteration in the objects or field of awareness—namely, by disruption of the focus or salience with which objects and meanings emerge from a background context; we refer to the latter as disturbed perceptual or conceptual 'grip' or 'hold' on the world (Merleau-Ponty 1962, p. 240; Dreyfus 2002).[8]

Our descriptions of hyper-reflexivity and diminished self-affection, on the one hand, and of loss of perceptual/conceptual 'hold,' on the other, are attempts to characterize, respectively, the noetic and the noematic infrastructures of the schizophrenic's characteristic mode of experience and lifeworld (see Table 4.1).

It should be noted that the hyper-reflexivity in question is not, at its core, an intellectual, volitional, or 'reflective' kind of self-consciousness; nor is it merely an intensified awareness of something that would normally be taken as an object (e.g. in the case of an adolescent's self-consciousness about his or her appearance). Most basic to schizophrenia is a kind of 'operative' hyper-reflexivity that occurs in an automatic fashion. This has the effect of disrupting awareness and action by means of an automatic popping up or popping-out of phenomena and processes that would normally remain in the tacit background of awareness (where they serve as a medium of implicit self-affection), but that now come to be experienced in an objectified and alienated manner (see Merleau-Ponty 1962, p. xviii re 'operative intentionality'—*fungierende Intentionalität*). The writer Antonin Artaud, who suffered from schizophrenia, seems to have experienced this with regard to his own limbs, which he describes in one passage as 'no more than images of bloody old cottons pulled

Table 4.1 A phenomenological account of schizophrenia

The central feature, IPSEITY DISTURBANCE (a disruption of consciousness and self-experience), has three facets:
NOETIC ABNORMALITIES (abnormalities in the constituting *act* of awareness).
1: Hyper-reflexivity.
2: Diminished self-affection (or diminished ipseity).
NOEMATIC ABNORMALITY (abnormalities in the constitu*ted objects* or *field* of awareness—perceptual or cognitive).
3: Disturbed grip or hold.

out in the shape of arms and legs, images of distant and dislocated members' (1965, p. 29; 1976, p. 65).[9]

The self-disturbance being postulated is not fundamentally a disturbance of self-image or social identity; nor does it primarily involve the continuity of identity over time (which is not to say that these aspects of selfhood will not be affected in any way). It pertains, rather, to a more fundamental sense of existing as an experiencing entity of some kind, as a kind of implicit subject-pole that would normally serve as the vital centre-point of subjective life. This fundamental feature of normal awareness—known as ipseity—is especially difficult to articulate in rich descriptive detail precisely because it is such a pervasive, fundamental, and obvious aspect of consciousness. Antonin Artaud was referring to an aspect of this when he spoke of what he called 'the essential illumination' and this 'phosphorescent point,' equating this illuminating centre-point with the 'very substance of what is called the soul,' and describing it as a prerequisite for avoiding 'constant leakage of the normal level of reality' (1965, p. 20; 1976, pp. 169, 82). Another patient with schizophrenia described the condition of lacking this crucial if ineffable self-affection that is essential to normal ipseity: 'I was simply there, only in that place, but without being present' (Blankenburg 1971, p. 42; 1991, p. 77).

Finally, the mutations of the perceptual or cognitive field of awareness (disturbed grip or hold) involve not just any kind of obscurity or disorganization. As we shall see, there are characteristic forms of confusion or 'perplexity' (*Ratlösigkeit*; Störring 1987) that derive from an absence of vital, motivating concerns (which is a concomitant of normal self-affection), and from an emergence into awareness of what would normally have been too self-evident to be noticed.

Our account differs from most contemporary as well as traditional conceptualizations of schizophrenia. These include classic psychiatric (neo-Kraepelinian) approaches that view schizophrenia as a kind of dementia involving a general lowering of the intellectual level, as well as psycho-analytic approaches that view schizophrenia as a regression to infantile or instinct-ridden forms of consciousness. Our emphasis on diminished self-affection and hyper-reflexivity (the two aspects of disturbed ipseity) does, however, have close affinities with the views put forward by several key figures in the tradition of phenomenological psychiatry—especially Eugene Minkowski (1997a), who considered the *trouble genérateur* of schizophrenia to be a 'loss of vital contact' with reality that was bound up with a decline of the core sense of self (affecting what he called 'the seat, or better, the source, of the felt and the lived'; pp. 302, 309), and also Wolfgang Blankenburg (1971, 1991), who described a loss of the normal common-sense grasp of the world that is frequently accompanied by exaggerated awareness of what would normally be taken-for-granted.[10]

Ours is a holistic and unifying approach and, as such, differs from current approaches that trace different schizophrenic symptoms to a variety of distinct and perhaps only loosely related mechanisms or modules, such as efferent copy, working memory, or hypofrontality—or that treat the different syndromes of schizophrenia as resulting from very different underlying mechanisms (Cahill and Frith 1996; Mojtabai and Rieder 1998). We argue that the two-faceted disturbance of the act of awareness (hyper-reflexivity and diminished self-affection) can be shown to be implicated in each of the three major syndromes of schizophrenia recognized in contemporary research: the 'positive', 'disorganization', and 'negative' syndromes.

The most important positive symptoms are the Schneiderian first-rank symptoms, which include experiences in which the patient feels that her thoughts, emotions, bodily sensations, or movements are under the control or possession of some alien being or force. Here the decline of self-affection or ipseity—of the sense of being a subject of experience or agent of activity—is patently obvious. We argue, however, that these experiences of diminished self-affection must be understood to be bound up with a kind of exaggerated reflexive awareness—an awareness that has the effect of objectifying and thereby alienating sensations and processes that would normally be lived in a more tacit or implicit fashion, that is, that would normally serve not as objects but as a kind of medium of self-awareness (see Sass 1992a, Chap. 7; Spence 2001, p. 170). This analysis is consistent with a line of German research on the 'basic symptoms', research that documents a wide variety of mild experiential anomalies that are present in prodromal as well as residual phases and seem to be bound up with a core, trait feature of schizophrenia (Klosterkötter 1992; Klosterkötter et al. 1997). The 'basic symptoms' include various anomalies of thinking, affect, and bodily experience that, in our view, involve focal awareness of processes and sensations that would normally be experienced in a tacit or implicit fashion. Longitudinal research (see below) has documented a progressive development that often leads, via gradual objectification, from mildly anomalous awareness of kinesthetic sensations, thought processes, or states of affective arousal, to more alienated experiences of one's own body, thinking, or emotion, eventuating in experiences of actual dispossession that can attain delusional proportions.

Abnormal reflexive awareness also seems to play a prominent role in the disorders of thought, language, and attention characteristic of the 'disorganized' syndrome. Thus schizophrenic abnormalities of thought and attention often seem to involve a disruptive, hyper-reflexive awareness of processes or phenomena that would normally be part of the 'cognitive unconscious' (Frith 1979); while the confusing quality of schizophrenic discourse often results from abnormalities in managing the complex and shifting relationship between what would normally be asserted and what is presupposed in a conversation. We argue that this loss of an organizing focus is itself bound up with a decline of motivation and vital directedness inherent in diminished self-affection.

The possible role of diminished self-affection in negative symptoms is not difficult to imagine. Patients with so-called negative symptoms are typically anergic, withdrawn, and lacking in the normal level of affective expression, and they often report experiencing a lack of a sense of inner vitality. As we point out, however, research shows that patients who present with negative symptoms generally report experiencing various 'positive' phenomena as well, including many of the above-mentioned 'basic symptoms' as well as forms of disturbing affective arousal (Kring and Neale 1996; Sass 2003b, Sass in press). Perhaps the most extensive phenomenological study of negative-symptom schizophrenia (Blankenburg 1971, 1991) emphasizes the loss of 'natural self-evidence', i.e. a loss of the sense of familiarity and taken-for-grantedness that is a condition for normal thought and interaction. A key feature of loss of natural self-evidence is a hyper-reflexive awareness of issues and presuppositions that would normally remain in the background of awareness.

Now that we have summarized our phenomenological approach to schizophrenia, we can turn to our own main subject: namely, how this sort of account, rather than being purely descriptive, can have explanatory or even causal relevance. To pursue these matters, it is necessary to explore three questions:

1. What general type of relationship can be envisaged between the mental, experiential, or symptomatic domain and a neurobiological level of description—and what implications does this have for the relevance or value of phenomenological description and understanding?
2. What are the various ways in which the experiential features of mental disorders can play an explanatory role? We will first discuss forms of explanation that involve relationships of phenomenological implication, and then turn to relationships relevant to the realm of genesis or causation.
3. How can we comprehend the roles that ipseity-disturbance and hyper-reflexivity in particular play, both in structuring the nature of schizophrenic experience as well as in determining the long-term developmental transformations of schizophrenia?

Here we can give only a relatively brief response to these questions, especially the first. More detailed commentary would take us far beyond the scope this paper, leading into many vexed issues in the philosophy of mind and action.

Phenomenology and the mind–brain relationship

The first issue is the most basic of the three, bearing as it does on the mind–brain or mind-body issues that have long been at the heart of philosophical debate. Opinions vary radically on these matters (Chalmers 1995), not least because of the profoundly enigmatic nature of the physical basis of consciousness—that mysterious event or process whereby something appears for something else or is displayed in the first-person perspective. Despite exaggerated claims of progress by a few philosophers and cognitive scientists, most would agree that we do not, in fact, have '*even a glimmer* [of understanding] of how anything physical could be a locus of conscious experience' (Fodor 1998, p. 83, our italics; see also McGinn 1993; Nagel 1979, p. 175).

From a practical standpoint, however, it seems reasonable to argue that a phenomenological description must, at the very least, act as a constraining condition on the nature of any neurobiological explanation (Gallagher 1997). This simply means that the neurobiological explanation must be compatible with the facts about the subjective dimension. It would, after all, hardly make sense to articulate biological hypotheses that clearly contradict human experience. Even if the realm of human experience or phenomenal awareness (of the so-called 'qualia') were purely epiphenomenal, playing no causally efficacious role, it would surely be one of the explananda or causal consequences that any satisfactory causal explanation would have to account for. And a necessary requirement for any coherent reductionism is that the entity to be reduced be properly described and understood (Nagel 1974); hence, phenomenology is indispensable.[11]

In a pragmatic spirit, one might propose, as a heuristically useful approach to the mind–brain relationship, an attitude called 'indicative isomorphism' (Varela 1996). Indicative isomorphism proposes that a preliminary step in narrowing the explanatory gap must be made through identification of stable correlations between invariants elucidated at both sides of the mind–brain equation. A phenomenological account will here provide certain invariant configurations of the structures of consciousness as the target variables. At the neural level, the target variables might be, for example, patterns of coherent oscillations in the gamma band among neuronal populations distributed in the regions of potential interest.

The adjective 'indicative' in 'indicative isomorphism' simply signifies a claim that certain forms of experiencing, if properly understood, are likely to imply, in quite general ways, the participation of certain neural domains and functions rather than others. This is expressly intended to be a philosophically 'weak' proposal: the presence of actual isomorphism is not assumed a priori, but rather is investigated case by case and without metaphysical commitments to any of the major positions concerning the mind–brain relationship. Indicative isomorphism merely proposes that the experiential invariants elucidated in a phenomenological account may be associated with certain invariant configurations or functional patterns at the neural level, and that the possibility of such correlations should be investigated.

We believe that this philosophical weakness or generality is appropriate given the preliminary status of consciousness research. The purpose of this very general proposal is to help to stimulate more detailed pathogenetic hypotheses and explorations that can eventually lead toward a naturalizing of phenomenology—that is, toward discovering the neurobiological correlates of various forms of abnormal consciousness and, perhaps in the long run, toward fostering real understanding of the relationships between subjectivity and the material or natural order.

Explanatory relevance of the mental or subjective domain: preliminary considerations

Before we attempt to explain our phenomenological position on this issue, it will help to situate our approach in relation to certain traditional as well as contemporary Anglo-American conceptions of the nature of explanation and understanding in psychology and psychopathology.

Traditionally, a distinction has often been made between 'explanation' and 'understanding', with explanation being said to pertain to (causally determined) physical processes, and understanding to be appropriate for the comprehension of human experience, action, and expression (Von Wright 1971). Human actions and experiences have been assumed to be recalcitrant to causal explanation for at least two reasons: first, because they have a particularistic, context-embedded quality that defies the possibility of theoretical generalization; and second, because mechanistic or deterministic causal models are presumed to be inapplicable to the realm of goal-directed activity, which is dominated by motive or reason. In recent years, however, aspects of this traditional dichotomy have been questioned by analytic philosophers who argue (against certain followers of Wittgenstein or of hermeneutics, such as Paul Ricoeur) that reasons are in fact a species of cause. The influential work of Donald Davidson (1980) calls attention to a perhaps intuitively obvious fact: namely that a reason *does* play a role in a causal account of a given action when it is claimed to be the reason why an agent actually did act as he did. In such a case, however, the reason (according to Davidson) must fulfill certain logical requirements such that it can be schematized as part of what is called a 'practical syllogism'. (For critiques of Davidson, see Evnine 1991; Sass 2001b, pp. 264–274.)

On the account offered by Davidson and other analytic philosophers (the belief–desire–intention paradigm; see Cummins 2000, p. 127), mental causality involves a triangulation of desire, belief, and a dispositional belief system. If I desire Italian food, and believe there is a good Italian restaurant around the corner, and if, in addition, my desire or belief is not *in*congruent with my dispositional beliefs (e.g. I believe there are stairs I can use to go down to the street), then this triangular interaction has a possible causal role in explaining my finally going out to have an Italian meal. On this sort of account, the ensuing intentional action is like the conclusion of a syllogism (the 'practical syllogism'): it follows from it logically. 'For a desire and a belief to explain an action in the right way', Davidson writes, 'they must cause it in the right way, perhaps through a chain or process of reasoning that meets standards of rationality' (1980, p. 232ff.). Here a desire, motive, or reason (I want Italian food) is re-described as something that has real causal efficacy.[12]

Many contemporary Anglo-American philosophers and cognitive scientists assume that this is the only way in which mental events could have a causal role; they present it as the only alternative to an account in terms of physical causation (but see Griffiths 1997, p. 244).[13]

It is reasonable to ask, therefore, about the relationship between this sort of account and that which phenomenology has to offer.

It should be noted that this sort of intentional account, in terms of beliefs and desires, presupposes overall intentional rationality. Indeed, it is often argued that overall rationality is constitutive—intrinsic to the very definition—of what it means to have mind or to exhibit meaningful action. Many Anglo-American philosophers have been persuaded by Davidson's claim that mental explanation, or the very possibility of the ascription of mental states in the course of interpersonal understanding, simply requires that one be able to assume the essential rationality of the person being understood or explained, and that, when such an assumption cannot be made (i.e. when the 'principle of charity' in interpretation cannot be applied), the only alternative is to resort to explanation of a physicalistic sort.

This raises the question of what Davidson's claim might imply regarding patients with schizophrenia, persons whose actions and beliefs so often seem to be highly irrational. If one accepts the premise that having mental states presupposes overall rationality, it may seem to follow that such individuals cannot be considered to have mental states at all or, at least, not to have mental states that we could imagine or could meaningfully ascribe to them. Some analytic philosophers seem to have drawn just this conclusion (see Campbell 1999, p. 624). For psychiatrists, such a position about schizophrenia and the limits of mental explanation will be reminiscent of views, long influential in psychiatry, that were put forward by Karl Jaspers early in this century.

In schizophrenia, Jaspers (1963) claimed, there seem to be experiences that are simply incomprehensible, that will not yield to imaginative-empathic comprehension. Either the experiences are too inherently strange to allow empathy, or else their motivation, their evolution from antecedent states, makes no discernible sense. (Jaspers called the former case 'static' un-understandability, exemplified by delusional mood and first-rank self-disturbances; the latter he called 'genetic' un-understandability, exemplified by bizarre actions or responses of schizophrenia patients who may sing or laugh for no good reason or may become excited by a key on the table without being able to explain why (p. 581).) In Jaspers' view, such schizophrenic symptoms simply defy empathic or rational understanding and must therefore be seen (and ultimately explained) as direct morbid eruptions from an underlying organic process.

We disagree with these views of schizophrenia as psychologically incomprehensible or devoid of meaningful mental states and as amenable only to biological explanation. We also disagree with a number of prominent but (in our opinion) ill-considered assumptions about psychological explanation on which they are based.

It should be evident from the above that discussion of mental causation in recent analytic philosophy has focused largely on the question of the rational coherence and potential explanatory significance of individual mental contents, e.g. the belief that there is an Italian restaurant on the corner; the desire that one eat an Italian meal. Only phenomena that can be said to contain (or to be describable in terms of) this sort of 'propositional content' are capable of serving the kind of rationalizing or justificatory function that is required by the practical syllogism (Evnine 1991, p. 11). It is here that the distinctness of the phenomenological perspective becomes important.

Phenomenology does not ignore the content of experience; nor does it deny that some aspects of this may be analysable in terms of sentence-like propositional attitudes. But the emphasis of a phenomenological account, the focus of its description effort, is directed elsewhere—toward formal or structural features that involve more pervasive aspects or infrastructures of human experience (e.g. modes of temporal or spatial experience, general qualities of the object world, forms of self-experience).[14]

These latter have more in common with the phenomena of mood or cognitive style than they do with particular beliefs, perceptual contents, or wishes whose significance could be captured as a sentence or a logical proposition.[15]

Consider, for example, our concepts of diminished self-affection, hyperreflexivity, and loss of cognitive-perceptual 'hold': these are not reasons nor are they causes, at least of a physicalistic kind. In what sense, then, can these three concepts be said to have any explanatory significance or to contribute to a genetic or causal explanation of schizophrenia? Pursuing these questions will lead us in two directions: first toward the question of the relationship between the three just-mentioned aspects; and second, toward an examination of the roles these aspects may play in determining both short- and long-term developmental transformations of schizophrenia.

In the following discussion of the explanatory relevance of a phenomenological account, it will be useful to distinguish two general, explanatory perspectives according to whether the relationships to be described are primarily synchronic or diachronic—that is, whether they apply to phenomena viewed as occurring simultaneously or in succession.[16]

First we consider the domain of the synchronic, where we distinguish three kinds of relationship: equiprimordial, constitutive, and expressive. Although these do not involve either causation or genesis over time, they do involve forms of what might be called 'phenomenological implication'—and thus they perform an explanatory rather than merely descriptive function. Later we turn to the domain of the diachronic. Here we will distinguish primary, consequential, and compensatory processes. All three help to account for the genesis of schizophrenic phenomena, and are potentially relevant to what might broadly be defined as causal accounts of the development of schizophrenic symptoms (see Table 4.2).[17]

Synchronic relationships

Equiprimordial relationships[18]

As we have said, hyper-reflexivity and diminished self-affection involve fundamental distortions of the act of awareness: altered interplay of tacit and explicit components, and a concomitant loss of a grounding sense of existing as a subject of action and awareness. But how, we may ask, are we to understand the relationship *between* hyper-reflexivity and diminished self-affection? Our account clearly suggests that these particular alterations of the mode of experience or intentionality are locked into a fairly intimate complementarity, and that any straightforward, unidirectional model might be overly simplistic. One possibility is to view them as intimately intertwined yet distinct processes that can interact with or even give rise to each other. This process could work in either direction: if something normally tacit became focal, one might, as a result, no longer feel as if one were inhabiting the tacit medium; but if, for some reason, one no longer had a sense of inhabiting the tacit medium, this could lead to hyper-reflexive awareness of what is normally tacit. We do not wish to deny the heuristic usefulness of this way of thinking, or its ability to reveal certain aspects of the complexities that may be involved.

Careful phenomenological investigation suggests, however, that hyper-reflexivity and transformation of ipseity may, in many cases, not best be conceived as outcomes or indices of distinct processes but, rather, as aspects of a single whole that we simply happen to be describing from two different angles of vision. Indeed, it might be argued that these two disturbances are really one and the same phenomenon, the very same distortion of the intentional arc that we are merely describing in different words. Whereas the notion of hyper-reflexivity emphasizes the way in which something

Table 4.2 Forms of phenomenological explanation

SYNCHRONIC RELATIONSHIPS: PHENOMENOLOGICAL IMPLICATION
Equiprimordial
Constitutive
Expressive relationships
DIACHRONIC DIMENSION: PHENOMENOLOGICAL CAUSALITY
Primary
Consequential
Compensatory processes

normally tacit becomes focal and explicit, the notion of disturbed ipseity emphasizes a complementary aspect of this process, the fact that what once was tacit is no longer being inhabited as a medium of taken-for-granted selfhood. Thus neither is more basic than the other; they are equiprimordial aspects of a fundamental (noetic) disturbance of the act of awareness. A clear theoretical grounding for this view is provided by the philosopher Michael Polanyi's (1964, 1967) account of the vector of conscious awareness as a continuum stretching between the object of awareness (what he calls the 'distal' pole), which is known in a focal or explicit way, and that which exists in the 'tacit dimension', i.e. which is experienced in what Polanyi terms a more subsidiary, implicit, or tacit manner. A tacit or subsidiary awareness of kinesthetic and proprioceptive sensations serves as the very medium of pre-reflective selfhood, ipseity, or self-awareness (the 'proximal' pole of the vector of awareness), which, in turn, is the medium through which all intentional activity is realized.

Constitutive relationships

The relationship between this two-faceted noetic transformation of the act of awareness, on one hand, and the loss of perceptual/conceptual 'hold' (a transformation of the noematic object or field), on the other, would also be misunderstood or oversimplified if it were conceived on the model of contingent causation between independent processes. We do conceive of the noetic aspects of the dissolution of intentionality (hyper-reflexivity and diminished ipseity) as the more fundamental or constitutive disturbance; they are aspects of the act of consciousness whereby experience is constituted. In our view, self-affecting notions like 'dissolution of natural experience' (Binswanger), 'loss of natural self-evidence' (Blankenburg 1971, 1991), loss of 'perspectival abridgment' (Sass, 1992a, Chap. 4), and 'loss of hold or grip' are alternative ways of describing the noematic or constitut*ed* aspects of this dissolution—which contribute to the peculiar 'perplexity' (Störring 1987) that is so characteristic of schizophrenia.[19]

It is important to remember that normal ipseity, with its usual self-affection and balance between the tacit and the focal, is not only a condition for the experience of appetite and vital energy. It also provides a point of orientation: it is what grounds human motivation and organizes our experiential world in accordance with needs and wishes, thereby giving objects their 'affordances', their significance for us as obstacles, tools, objects of desire, and the like. In the absence of this vital yet implicit self-affection, and the lines of orientation it establishes, the structured nature of the worlds of both thought and perception will be altered or even dissolved. For then there can no longer be any clear differentiation of means from goal; any reason for certain objects to show up in the focus of awareness while others recede; or any reason for attention to be directed outward toward the world rather than inward toward one's own body or processes of thinking. Without normal self-affection, the world will be stripped of all the affordances and vectors of concern by which the fabric of normal, common-sense reality is knitted together into an organized and meaningful whole.[20]

This, we believe, is the basis of the distinctively schizophrenic 'perplexity' (*Ratlösigkeit*) described in classic German psychopathology.

Perplexity refers to a self-aware, anguishing, and (to the patient) perfectly inexplicable sense of being unable to maintain a consistent grasp on reality or to cope with normal situational demands, which is usually accompanied by withdrawal into the self (Störring 1987, p. 80; also Blankenburg 1971, p. 54; 1991, p. 94). Perplexity involves a 'strange turning in upon one's self': the patient becomes aware that 'his empathic capacity is growing less, that his activity is declining and that he is gradually becoming detached from the world of perception'.

At times schizophrenia patients appear to experience something closely akin to Heideggerian *Angst*: the anxiety born of registering the arbitrariness of any particular way of looking at life and the vertigo this can engender. They may also experience the more nihilistic anxiety that Sartre describes in *Nausea*: the sense of living in a world in which pure matter, devoid of all human meaning or purpose, looms forth as the only realm that truly exists (Sass 1992a, pp. 49, 139).

In emphasizing the foundational role of hyper-reflexivity and diminished self-affection, we are not suggesting that they exist independently of or prior to the noematic disturbance: they are not the cause but the *condition of possibility* for the disturbance of cognitive perceptual hold. This is not to say that one or another aspect may not be more salient at a given moment or in a given patient. But it does suggest there is an intimate relationship between the phenomena of excessive self-awareness and loss of self (hyper-reflexivity and diminished self-affection) as well as between both of these aspects and the practical goal-lessness, disengagement, and disintegration of meaning that are hallmarks of the schizophrenic syndrome. A passage from Artaud (1976, p. 82) seems to link the unity or organization of the field of awareness ('clustering') together with the sense of self-affection ('phosphorescent point'):[21]

> What is difficult is to find one's place and to reestablish communication with one's self. Everything depends on a certain flocculation [coming-together] of things, on the clustering of all these mental gems around a point which has yet to be found ... a phosphorescent point at which all reality is recovered.

This constitutive type of relationship does not, incidentally, conform to either of the two types of explanation that are countenanced by many recent Anglo-American philosophers: it is neither 'a psychophysical link holding between states of affairs or events' nor 'a relationship of making intelligible holding between sentences' (Taylor 1993, p. 326)—the latter being the only form of mental causation accepted by many analytic philosophers (Heil and Mele 1993; Sass 2001b). But, as the philosopher Charles Taylor (1993, p. 326) rightly notes, these two alternatives do not, in fact, exhaust the space of possibilities. Another possibility Taylor mentions is the 'world-shaping relation' between the lived-body or corporeal subject and the world of experience—also an instance of a *constitutive* relationship.[22]

Expressive relationships

We have now described equiprimordial and constitutive relationships; both pertain to ways of linking different aspects of the form of consciousness. A third type of relationship of mutual phenomenological implication—the expressive type—involves situations in which the (noematic) content of mental life seems to represent or express, in a more specific way, what appear to be more general formal or structural characteristics of mental life. (This distinction corresponds, in Heidegger's system, to the difference between 'ontic' facts and 'ontological' dimensions of existence; see Sass 1992b.) Take, for example, a delusion about dissolving, being controlled by an influencing machine, or being constantly recorded by video cameras. This sort of delusion may be understandable, not because it plays a role in a logical syllogism, but because it actually expresses or emblematizes, in relatively concrete form, more general or formal features of the prevailing state or mode of consciousness—in this case, the general state of ipseity-disturbance (see Merleau-Ponty's notion of an 'emblem of being': Merleau-Ponty 1968, p. 270; Dreyfus and Wakefield 1988, p. 280). Here phenomenology clearly plays more than a merely descriptive role. To articulate such expressive relationships provides an integrating vision, an understanding not of patterns of causal interaction but 'of style, of logical implication, of meaning and value', (Geertz 1973, p. 145); and this does serve an explanatory function (see also Minkowski 1997b, *re* relationships of signification and expression).

Apparent logical contradictions in the content of a person's thoughts may become understandable in this way. Consider, for instance, the famous influencing-machine delusion of the patient Natalija (Tausk 1933)—a delusion that implies that Natalija experiences herself as, at the same time, godlike (at the centre of the world, with all other entities existing only for her), but also a mere passive entity within the world (a machine manipulated by others). The fact that the self can be experienced both as a passive mechanism and as a kind of solipsistic deity—sometimes at the same moment—can be understood if one recognizes that both these forms of self-experience are implicit in a hyper-reflexive focus on the functioning of one's own mind and its role in the constitution of the experiential world (see Sass 1998a; also Sass 1992b; Bovet and Parnas 1993). An uncanny, solipsistic passage in which Artaud

(1976, p. 60) describes the universe as dependent on 'the rootlets ... trembling at the corners of my mind's eye' seems to express a similarly paradoxical, hyper-reflexive awareness of his own consciousness as both a material entity and the godlike foundation of the universe (Sass 1994, pp. 96ff.). Many so-called 'bizarre' delusions, pathognomonic of schizophrenia, are not, in fact, psychologically incomprehensible—as Jaspers claimed. The phenomenological approach allows one to understand these bizarre contents of consciousness as arising from and, in a sense, expressing aspects of the profoundly altered form of experiencing that is characteristic of schizophrenia: including blurred Self-World articulation, solipsistic access to the mind's own constituting activity, and mutation of spatial and temporal axioms of experience.[23]

Conclusion: phenomenological implication

In our view, then, the three facets (hyper-reflexivity, diminished self-affection, loss of hold), and also the form and emblematic content of experiential life, are linked together in relationships of necessary implication rather than contingent correlation or causal interaction. The implications in question are not, however, logical (like the practical syllogism) but, rather, phenomenological in nature, with the individual factors being understood as mutually implicative aspects or expressions of mental activity as a whole (Marbach 1993, p. 35). This is what Husserl was pointing to when he described 'conscious life' as 'contain(ing) an intentional intertwining, motivation, mutual implication by meaning ... which in its form and principle has no analogue at all in the physical' (Husserl 1977, p. 26). Similarly, Merleau-Ponty (1962) spoke of 'internal links' between aspects of experience that 'display one typical structure ... standing in a relationship to each other of reciprocal expression' (p. 157).[24]

Phenomenological investigation is, in this way, less a matter of discovering interacting processes or of analysing logical syllogisms than it is of un-folding the different facets of conscious life or activity in order to provide a richer grasp of its lived texture and internal structure.

The diachronic dimension

We turn now to the diachronic dimension, to questions concerning schizophrenia's development over time and the relative causal primacy of various kinds of processes. As we shall see, neither hyper-reflexivity nor diminished self-affection is a singular or fully homogenous phenomenon; each can play what might be termed a primary, consequential, or compensatory role in the generation of experiential abnormalities. Although for brevity's sake we will put more emphasis on hyper-reflexivity in the pages below, most of our points could also be developed with regard to the aspect of diminished self-affection.

Primary hyper-reflexivity

Both Husserl and Merleau-Ponty have described the multi-layered nature of human intentionality. The founding level is an intentionality of a so- called 'operative' or bodily sort; this occurs on a pre-reflective level and is the medium in which habits and dispositions become sedimented (Merleau-Ponty 1962, p. xviii). Operative intentionality happens, phenomenologically speaking, in a passive, non-willed, or automatic mode. It is generated through sensory, sensori-motor, and kinesthetic associations, as well as through equivalencies across sensory modalities, which are realized in the series of spatio-temporal moments or perspectives, instigated by bodily movement (Merleau-Ponty 1962; re Hussserl, see Dodd 1997). In this tacit mode, a person's active response to the world need not be determined by explicit mental content involving mental representations expressed in propositional form. It may involve a more direct response to the thing itself—whose relationship to the self, perceived as a certain tension created by a deviation from optimal Gestalt, leads to a globally attuned response (Merleau-Ponty 1962, pp. 139ff., 153; Dreyfus 2002). One's response to the world may, of course, also be imbued with a sense of activity and volition—as is characteristic of what might be termed 'reflective intentionality' (Merleau-Ponty 1962, pp. x, xviii). But these more active, thematic, or focal forms of intentionality (e.g. acts of judgement or explicit object recognition) will always be embedded in or founded on a more fundamental, pre-reflective, or operative level of intentionality.

What has just been said applies to normal human intentionality. Forms of hyper-reflexive intentionality can, however, also be distinguished according to whether they have an 'operative' as opposed to a more 'reflective' character. Here we use the label 'operative hyper-reflexivity' to denote a process afflicting the more fundamental levels of intentionality—a process in which the normally transparent field of experience becomes increasingly disrupted by unusual sensations, feelings, or thoughts that would normally remain in the background of awareness but that now pop into awareness and come to acquire object-like quality (a kind of spatialization of experience). Patient reports suggest that this is first experienced as a largely passive process, more like an affliction, typically involving cenesthesias, a loss of the automaticity of movement, and certain cognitive and perceptual disturbances—phenomena that, in the 'basic-symptom' research, are designated with the apt term 'basal irritation' (Klösterkötter et al. 1997). At the proximal pole of the vector of awareness, the same phenomenon manifests itself as a fundamentally diminished or altered sense of self-presence and presence to the world.

Certain of the affective-anhedonic or a-volitional disturbances common in schizophrenia are clearly rooted in this kind of primary or basal disruption of the act of awareness. To be moved, to become engaged and inspired to action—in other words to be affected by an object (hetero-affection)—can only be realized in a process involving self-affection or ipseity. There must be a sense in which the experience is felt as happening *to me* and as relevant *to me*, and this requires a sense of being at one with myself and my own acts of awareness. A failure of self-affection necessarily disrupts the flow of affective and conative processes, largely because the condition of altered auto-affection and disturbed tacit-focal structure does not furnish a sensitive milieu in which affection by the object can elicit spontaneous response or channel the intentional flow into purposeful or willed activity.[25]

As a result, emotion loses its spontaneity; and action, deprived of its more automatic or spontaneous grounding, can only take place in a willful and deliberate manner. Levels of action and experience that would normally be tacitly constituted, now require effort; and eventually this can lead to the feelings of fatigue and exhaustion that are so common in schizophrenia (what Blankenburg (1971, pp. 84ff., 101–104; 1991, pp.132ff., 153–156) calls 'schizophrenic asthenia').

In its most primary form, then, this 'irritation' may well occur in a largely passive manner, and therefore represents an 'operative' rather than 'reflective' kind of hyper-reflexivity. This 'irritation' may, in fact, be a rather direct consequence of a neurally based cognitive dysfunction. (The popping-up of normally tacit sensations could, for example, result from disturbances of the hippocampus-based comparator system or from some other disturbance of 'cognitive co-ordination' (Gray *et al.* 1991; Phillips and Silverstein, 2003)— to mention but two of the most plausible of current neurocognitive models.)

Consequential hyper-reflexivity

Primary 'irritation' and ipseity disturbance do, however, attract further attention, thereby eliciting processes of scrutiny and self-exacerbating alienation ('consequential hyper-reflexivity'). Although these may have a somewhat more active or quasi-volitional quality (which is not to say, however, that they are fully conscious or volitional), they occur as by-products of a more primary disturbance. A patient may, for example, find himself paying more attention to odd kinesthetic sensations, or may find himself scrutinizing odd visual appearances in a way that only increases their oddness.

In some interesting self-descriptions, Artaud (1976, p. 293) describes a kind of alienated and possibilitarian, introspective awareness of his own mind that occurs in this consequential way:

> The brain sees the whole thought at once with all its circumstances, and it
> also sees all the points of view it could take and all the forms with which it

could invest them, a vast juxtaposition of concepts, each of which seems more necessary and also more dubious than the others, which all the complexities of syntax would never suffice to express and expound.

Clearly this experience involves a hyper-reflective kind of introspection. But Artaud himself tells us that this form of alienated, intellectual self-consciousness is actually a by-product of something more primary, namely, of an absence of any 'dominant theme'—which Artaud describes as a 'fragility' or 'slackening' and which he associates with what appear to be forms of operative hyper-reflexivity and diminished self-affection. Thus a more primary ipseity-disturbance seems to allow, perhaps to inspire, a more reflective turning-inward and self-alienation of a mind that comes to take itself as its own object. And, in turn, this inwardness and self-reflection seems to contribute to an undermining of the normally tacit sources of self-affection. Thus Artaud goes on to describe a 'mental confusion' whose most characteristic feature, he says, is (1976, pp. 293ff.):

> ... a kind of disappearance or disintegration of first assumptions which even causes me to wonder why, for example, red (the color) is considered red and affects me as red, why a judgment affects me as a judgment and not as a pain, why I feel a pain, and why this particular pain, which I feel without understanding it.

Compensatory hyper-reflexivity

The primary disturbances of ipseity do not merely elicit fairly automatic consequences; they also inspire defensive or compensatory forms of hyper-reflexivity. Patients may attempt, for example, to reassert control and re-establish a sense of self by means of an introspective scrutinizing. Or they may engage in pseudo-obsessive intellectual ruminations in attempting to make up for a more primary sense of unnaturalness and unfamiliarity of the world and other people.

Diminished self-affection can also develop in a compensatory fashion. We know that, in Dissociative Identity Disorder and Post-Traumatic Stress Disorder, patients undergo a loss of the sense of their own reality or existence as experiential subjects that is, at least in part, defensively motivated. Similar developments can occur in schizophrenia-spectrum patients—who may have good reason to seek the escape inherent in self-obliteration. Consider, for example, one schizophrenic patient's description of using prolonged fixation of attention (staring at a spot) to bring about a kind of intentional self-dissolution: 'I hold fast to my spot and drown myself in it down to its very atoms' (Sechehaye 1956, p. 32).[26]

Defensive or compensatory processes often have counterproductive effects, however. The more active or reflective forms of hyper-reflexivity may, for example, serve as the source of further alienations or diminishments of ipseity and perceptual meaning. Introspectionist studies with normal individuals show that a kind of hyper-reflection—in these cases produced in a purely volitional manner—can in fact bring on some alterations of the sense of both self and world that are strikingly reminiscent of what occurs in schizophrenia (Hunt 1985, 1995; Sass 1994, pp. 90, 94, 159, 161). And, we might now add, these further alterations could also inspire still further forms of hyper-reflexivity that can take on a life of their own. The patient may ruminate on his own ruminations to the point of a total loss of meaning. Attention may become devoted to detail, with consequent destruction of the Gestalt field of experience. The inner life may become tortured and painfully self-conscious, ultimately fragmenting itself from within. 'My downfall was insight', explained one young man with schizophrenia, 'too much insight can be very dangerous, because you can tear your mind apart.' 'Well look at the word "analysis" ', he said on another occasion. 'That means to break apart. When it turns in upon itself the mind would rip itself apart.' 'Once I started destroying [my mind], I couldn't stop' (Sass 1992, pp. 337–338).

All this suggests the possibility of a veritable cascade of hyper-reflexivity—of the primary, consequential, and compensatory sort, and involving hyper-reflexivity of the operative as well as the more reflective kind. What can result is a veritable 'centrifuging' of the self—a process whereby phenomena that would normally be 'inner' or tacit are progressively spun outward and away, thereby depriving the individual of the very medium of normal forms of ipseity or self-experience.

Conclusion: phenomenological causality

Longitudinal studies of schizophrenia that begin with premorbid and pro-dromal phases (Klosterkötter *et al.* 1997) clearly demonstrate a progressive shift from basal or primary irritation to full-blown first-rank symptoms through increasing objectification and externalization of normally tacit inner phenomena. They show that particular first rank symptoms are generally preceded (even in early, premorbid stages) by subtle experiential anomalies ('basal irritation') that are suggestive both of hyper-reflexivity and diminished self-affection; and that these anomalies tend to affect the same experiential domain (e.g. bodily sensation, thought, or affect) that eventually becomes externalized and thematized in the form of first-rank symptoms affecting that same domain. Experiences of thought-broadcasting or thought-insertion are, for example, typically preceded by disturbances of concentration or a subtle sense of peculiarity in one's thinking; experiences of imposed actions are preceded by sensations of movement, pulling, or pressure inside the body or on its surfaces (Klosterkötter 1992, pp. 3, 37). Over time, this type of disturbed ipseity will have a progressive detrimental impact on behaviour as well as subjective life: experiences of loss of natural self-evidence, perplexity, and ineffable self-transformation come to be exacerbated but also masked by processes of morbid spatialization and objectification. The lapsing into silence, inaction, or inexpressiveness characteristic of negative-syndrome schizophrenia can be understood not only as a direct consequence of progressive distortion of normal ipseity, but also as a defensive reaction to these disconcerting experiential changes.

It should be obvious, upon reflection, that the forms of symptomatic progression we have been describing cannot be considered to be mere epiphenomena of neurophysiological changes. Indeed, they can be neither understood nor explained without making reference to the subjective or phenomenological dimension. This is not to deny the key role of neurobiological abnormalities. Indeed, these latter may well have ultimate causal primacy—as the main source of the early experiential abnormalities of the 'basal irritation' (see above). Once the field of experience is transformed, however, this gives rise to forms of attention and modes of experience involving developments-from or reactions-to subjectively experienced aspects of both self and world. It is not, for example, neural events *per se* but, rather, the experience of certain kinesthetic sensations as focal objects that elicits ever more intense forms of reflective concentration. In this way, subjective experience can play an important causal role in the progressive experiential transformations of a developing schizophrenic illness. These relevant features of subjective life concern its overall look or 'feel'; they are not analysable in terms of sentence-like propositional contents.

These experiential transformations will certainly be accompanied by changes on the neural plane; indeed, they may be, in large measure, manifestations on the phenomenal level of progressive organic changes occurring on the biological level. Still, these phenomenal changes do not play a purely epiphenomenal role, given that certain irreducible features of subjective life seem to provide both the motivation and the field of possibility for the progressive developments. (There may also be processes of 'downward causation': when alterations on the subjective and psychological level entrain parallel changes on the neurophysiological level.) Here we might speak of a certain 'autonomy of the phenomenological.' As the philosopher McClamrock (1995, p. 42) points out in a book on causal explanation in cognitive science, causal analysis sometimes requires one to specify a set of objects and goals that are a function of the way in which the world is experienced by the patient. In this sense, 'irreducibly subjective' properties are sometimes able to account for a person's behaviour in a way that reference to the state of the nervous system alone could not possibly do; they will sometimes constitute the 'preferred level of explanation'.[27]

Husserl (1989) made the same point when he contrasted 'motivational causality' with the 'natural causality' of the physical world (pp. 227, 241): 'The Object stimulates me in virtue of its *experienced properties* and not its physicalistic ones', wrote Husserl. 'The world [that motivates my action and mental activity] is *my surrounding world*. That is to say, it is not the physic-alistic world but the thematic world of my, and our intentional life (including what is given to consciousness as extra-thematic...my thematic horizon)' (pp. 228, 230).

To clarify motivational causality is (among other things) to specify the person's (or patient's) way of seeing things and to grasp how the (perceived) environment solicits or elicits further forms of action and perception—which, of course, have their own consequences, thereby leading to comprehensible and predictable (but not wholly determined) progressions of behaviour and experiential modes. It is not enough to say, then, that the experiential phenomenology of abnormal experiences merely constrains explanations on the cognitive or neurobiological levels: it can actually provide a key element of the explanations themselves.

Conclusion

We have outlined a variety of ways in which phenomenology, rather than being merely descriptive, can actually have explanatory significance. First we considered an alternative approach to mental causation—one that em-phasizes logical relationships between mental contents (the belief-desire-intention or practical-syllogism paradigm popular in analytic philosophy). Then we discussed a number of ways in which the phenomenological emphasis on formal aspects of subjective life (of the field of experience, and of acts of awareness) can be relevant for explanatory purposes. Within the realm of simultaneous phenomena (the synchronic realm), we discussed equiprimordial, constitutive, and expressive relationships. These involve not causation but a kind of phenomenological implication. Within the realm of successive phenomena (the diachronic dimension), we considered primary, consequential, and compensatory processes. All three are relevant to a causal or developmental account of the genesis of schizophrenic symptoms over time.

Endnotes

1. See, for example, Simon (2000, p. 25): 'The line between descriptive and explana-tory laws is not a sharp one, for we may find all kinds of intermediate cases—especially for qualitative explanations.' As Simon points out, both 'causal' and 'explanation' are terms 'gravid with implications' and highly 'problematic' (p. 22). See Michotte (1963) for experimental demonstration of the difficulty of separating perceptual observation from causal attribution.

2. In 1921, Husserl (1999, pp. 318f)) contrasts ' "explanatory" phenomenology as a phenomenology of regulated genesis [with] "descriptive" phenomenology as

a phenomenology of possible essential shapes (no matter how they have come to pass)'.

3. It is not easy to provide a succinct *précis* of Husserl's complex views on genetic phenomenology and motivational relationships. On these difficulties, see Bernet *et al.* (1993, p. 196). For attempts to clarify these issues, see Steinbock (1995) and Depraz (2001).

4. Motivation can operate through associative and other links among the contents of awareness. These would be analogous to the kinds of links emphasized by analytic philosophers who speak of 'mental causation' or the 'practical syllogism'—see below. Motivation (in Husserl's sense) can, however, also operate through formal or structural aspects of the (noetic) act of consciousness itself—as, for example, when inner time consciousness serves as a necessary condition for the unity of the flux of experiences, or when a distorted mode of self-experience is expressed in specific kinds of delusional beliefs (see below: Expressive relationships) (Husserl 1989, p. 238).

5. Jaspers' (1963) views on phenomenology, description, and explanation require careful examination. Although Jaspers (1963) uses 'phenomenology' to refer to a purely descriptive project relevant to 'static' understanding of psychopathological phenomena, he also recommends pursuing a 'genetic understanding' of 'how one psychic event emerges from another,' which he calls the 'psychopathology of meaningful connections' and considers a form of 'interpretive psychology' (pp. 27, 314; Spiegelberg 1972, pp. 182, 186). The latter would seem to be a subtype of Husserl's 'motivational causality,' and might well be considered a form of phenomenological explanation. Jaspers (1963) acknowledges that we can call this 'genetic understanding or perception of meaningful connection' a process of 'psychological explanation, if we like.' But he prefers to reserve the term 'explanation' for 'objective causal explanation, which is the perception of causal connection in the strict sense'—that is, in the realm of the natural sciences where phenomena are seen from the outside only (pp. 27–28, 301).

6. We are aware that, according to many philosophers, a cause can be simultaneous with its effect (Mackie 1974, p. 161). A future, more fully adequate taxonomy will doubtless need to take this into account.

7. The term 'affection' in 'self-affection' is meant to evoke the notion of both affect and passivity, as against a more active and cognitive, intentional mental process or event. Affection and intention are thus a pair of concepts, with connotations of passivity and activity respectively. To be affected means to be touched, moved, motivated, a process that is primordially linked to emotionality. See Henry (1973).

8. Merleau-Ponty (1962) describes this grip or hold as involving 'a certain culmination and optimum balance in the perceptual process', a perceptual 'field in which richness and clarity are in inverse proportion to each other' (p. 318), 'a spectacle as varied and as clearly articulated as possible' (p. 250). Maximal 'grip' or 'hold' on the world requires a 'certain balance between the inner and outer horizon' (p. 302). If seen from too close, a living body, now divorced from its background, can seem an outlandish 'mass of matter'; if seen from too far away, it may lose its 'living value' and appear as a puppet or automaton (p. 302). Merleau-Ponty describes 'maximum sharpness of perception and action [as] point[ing] clearly to a perceptual *ground*, a basis of my life, a general setting in which my body can co-exist

with the world' (p. 250); this, in turn, requires normal self-affection and an appropriate balance between tacit and explicit modes of awareness.

9. Contrast this with the kind of awareness we normally have of our bodies: 'not ... knowledge in thematized form. [Rather] an inarticulate and indistinct familiarity completely devoid of positional and disclosing consciousness' (Gurwitsch 1964, p. 302, describing Merleau-Ponty's views).

10. Blankenburg speaks of 'loss of natural self-evidence', the *Grundstörung* in schizo-phrenia, as a key 'condition of possibility' for what he terms the 'primary autism' of the schizophrenic form of life (1986; 1991, pp. 201, 230, 232; Parnas and Bovet 1991). Blankenburg clearly states that, when describing 'loss of natural self-evidence' as a '*basic* disorder' or '*Grundstörung,*' he is concerned not with aetiology or causal explanation but with capturing the 'essence' of the transform-ation (1971, p. 27; 1991, p. 4). One might question, however, whether this is entirely true. Blankenburg does go on to use the concept of 'compensation' (1971, pp. 30, 54, 62, 68, 113; 1991, pp. 62, 93, 106, 113, 168), which clearly implies that he is willing to offer interpretations regarding degrees of pathogenetic primacy and kinds of pathogenetic roles.

11. Conscious experience is 'an explanandum in its own right' (Chalmers 1995, p. 209). 'Without some idea ... of what the subjective character of experience is, we cannot know what is required of physicalistic theory' (Nagel 1979, p. 71).

12. Actually, Davidson's position on the causal efficacy of mental contents is very difficult to pin down, as various commentators have remarked (see Sass 2001b, pp. 287–290, for discussion and various references, including Kim 1985). Wake-field and Eagle (1997) is a clear example of a reading that interprets Davidson as ascribing real causal efficacy to 'mental representations' existing 'in the head' (p. 323). Sass (2001b) offers a critique of the coherence of Davidson's position and of its actual relevance for psychological explanation.

13. Griffiths (1997, p. 244) argues that 'many problems in the philosophy of mind have been occasioned by the loss of ... flexibility in our thought about mental contents' that was occasioned by adoption of the philosophical 'propositional attitude' theory. As Griffiths points out, the latter approach (exemplified by Donald David-son) derives from Aristotle's formalized model of action explanation via the 'practical syllogism'.

14. Jaspers (1963), p. 59: ' ... from the phenomenological point of view, it is only the form that interests us'.

15. See Sass (1998b) for an introduction to hermeneutic phenomenology, where the emphasis is on background or 'horizonal' aspects of existence.

16. This is a simplified distinction motivated by pedagogical concerns; all conscious processes are in fact intrinsically temporal in nature. There is at least a rough correspondence between our synchronic-diachronic distinction and Husserl's dis-tinction between static and genetic (including motivational) phenomenology (see Husserl 1999, pp.144, 319). Philosophers have debated the question of the rela-tionship between causation and temporal sequence, with some pointing out that a cause can sometimes be simultaneous with its effect. In this paper, however, we focus on possible causal sequences.

17. Obviously, we are not using 'causal' here in the narrow sense of mechanical efficient causality.

18. The term 'equiprimordial' is taken from Heidegger (1962).
19. In this respect, we follow Husserl rather than Heidegger. Heidegger conceived of human existence as a condition of *being there* (*Dasein*) and questioned what he saw as his mentor, Husserl's, overly subjectivist and Cartesian conception of mind as constituting the experiential world. Although Husserl fully recognized there is no noesis (act of consciousness) without a correlative noema (object of consciousness), he nevertheless gives a special status to the noetic acts, which he describes as 'animating construals' or 'apprehensions' that are responsible for the transcendental constituting of the objects and field of our awareness (Husserl 1983, pp. 226, 238, 277). One may certainly debate the merits of a Heideggerian versus a Husserlian approach (Tatossian 1997, p. 12). It is worth noting, however, that the Husserlian interest in constituting mental processes and the genesis of experiential worlds is probably more congruent with the aspirations of contemporary psychology and cognitive science, which seek to identify mental processes that underlie and in this sense account for the experiential abnormalities.
20. See Dworkin *et al.* (1998, pp. 390, 412) *re* role of the individual's 'concerns' in determining the emotional meaning and general significance of events.
21. Certain findings *re* memory functions can be linked to disturbed ipseity. Several studies show that, rather than demonstrating general deficits of memory, patients with schizophrenia seem to have a focal deficit in the type of remembering that involves mental reliving of their own actions and experiences (Danion *et al.* 1999). Their impaired memory can in fact be improved when they are 'forced to involve the self at encoding'. An ipseity disturbance (diminished sense of personal engagement in the original experience) would seem able to account for these findings.
22. Other types also fall outside this dualism of explanatory types; see below.
23. For another discussion of how thought content can reflect more general, formal aspects, or the nature of an ongoing process, see Silberer's (1951) discussion of 'autosymbolic' phenomena.
24. Merleau-Ponty (1962) uses the concept of 'reciprocal expression' in a broad way—to refer to 'internal links' between whole modes of experience: 'Thus sexuality is not an autonomous cycle. It has internal links with the whole of active and cognitive being, these three sectors of behavior [sexuality, action, cognition] display one typical structure, and stand in a relationship to each other of reciprocal expression' (p. 157).
25. Huber (1986, p. 1140) describes the 'loss of automatic behaviors' that occurs when 'the intended goal of action is not sufficiently effective in eliciting the single steps to achievement of the goal, without increased concentration'.
26. The study by Danion *et al.* (1999), cited in a previous note, illustrates the potential contribution of such self-obliteration to the loss of memory of one's own actions and experiences—a phenomenon that may be relevant both to schizophrenia and dissociative disorders.
27. McClamrock (1995) describes 'the characterizations of the world under which behavior is systematic with respect to it' (p. 4) as 'distal causes', and states that, in causal analysis, these may 'screen off' (i.e. render less relevant) more proximal causes (p. 54). See also pp. 45–53, 178, 187 and *passim* for arguments from philosophy and cognitive science. For related discussion, see Searle (1983), especially pp. 112–140.

References

Artaud, A. (1965). *Antonin Artaud anthology* (ed. Jack Hirschman). San Francisco, CA: City Lights Books.

Artaud, A. (1976). *Antonin Artaud: selected writings* (trans. H. Weaver) (ed. S. Sontag). New York: Farrar, Straus, & Giroux.

Audi, R. (ed.) (1999). *The Cambridge dictionary of philosophy*, (2nd edn). Cambridge, UK: Cambridge University Press.

Bernet, R., Kern, I., and Marbach, E. (1993). *An introduction to Husserlian phenomenology*. Evanston, IL: Northwestern University Press.

Blankenburg, W. (1971). *Der verlust der natürlichen selbstverständlichkeit: ein beitrag zur psychopathologie symptomarmer schizophrenien*. Stuttgart: Ferdinand Enke Verlag.

Blankenburg, W. (1986). Autismus. In: *Lexicon der psychiatrie* (2nd edn) (ed. C. Müller), pp. 83–89. Berlin: Springer.

Blankenburg, W. (1991). *La perte de l'évidence naturelle: une contribution à la psychopathologie des schizophrénies pauci-symptomatiques* (trans. J.-M. Azorin and Y. Totoyan). Paris: Presses Universitaires de France.

Bovet, P. and Parnas, J. (1993). Schizophrenic delusions: a phenomenological approach. *Schizophrenia Bulletin*, **19**: 579–597.

Buytendijk, F.J.J. (1987). The phenomenological approach to the problem of feelings and emotions. In: *Phenomenological psychology: the Dutch school* (ed. J.J. Kockelmans), *pp.* 195–207. Dordrecht: Martinus Nijhoff.

Cahill, C. and Frith, C.D. (1996). A cognitive basis for the signs and symptoms of schizophrenia. In: *Schizophrenia: a neuropsychological perspective* (ed. C. Pantelis, H.E. Nelson, and T.R.E. Barnes), pp. 373–395. New York: John Wiley & Son.

Campbell, J. (1999). Schizophrenia, the space of reasons, and thinking as a motor process. *The Monist*, **82**: 609–625.

Chalmers, D. (1995). Facing up to the problem of consciousness. *Journal of Consciousness Studies*, **2**: 200–219. Reprinted in: Shear, J. (1997). *Explaining consciousness—the 'hard problem'*, pp. 9–30. Cambridge, MA: MIT Press.

Crane, T. (1995). Causation. In: *Philosophy: a guide through the subject* (ed. A.C. Grayling), pp. 184–194. Oxford, UK: Oxford University Press.

Cummins, R. (2000). How does it work? Versus 'what are the leaps?': two conceptions of psychological explanation. In: *Explanation and cognition* (ed. F.D. Keil and R.A. Wilson), pp. 117–144. Cambridge, MA: MIT Press.

Danion, J.-M., Rizzo, L., and Bruant, A. (1999). Functional mechanisms underlying impaired recognition memory and conscious awareness in patients with schizophrenia. *Archives of General Psychiatry*, **56**: 639–644.

Davidson, D. (1980). *Essays on actions and events*. Oxford, UK: Clarendon Press.

Depraz, N. (2001). *Lucidité du corps*. Dordrecht, Holland: Kluwer.

Dodd, J. (1997). *Idealism and Corporeity. An Essay on the Problem of the Body in Husserl's Phenomenology*. Dordrecht, Holland: Kluwer Academic Publishers.

Dreyfus, H. (2002). Intelligence without representation—Merleau-Ponty's critique of mental representation. *Phenomenology and the Cognitive Sciences*, **1**: 367–383.

Dreyfus, H. and Wakefield, J. (1988). From depth psychology to breadth psychology: a phenomenological approach to psychopathology. In: *Hermeneutics and psychological theory* (ed. S. Messer, L. Sass, and R. Woolfolk), pp. 272–288. New Brunswick, NJ: Rutgers University Press.

Dworkin, R.H., Oster, H., Clark, S.C., and White, S.R. (1998). Affective expression and affective experience in schizophrenia. In: *Origins and development of schizophrenia* (ed. M.F. Lenzenweger and R.H. Dworkin), pp. 385–424. Washington D.C.: American Psychiatric Press.

Evnine, S. (1991). *Donald Davidson*. Stanford, CA: Stanford University Press.

Fodor, J. (1998). *In critical condition: polemical essays on cognitive science and the philosophy of mind*. Cambridge, MA: MIT Press.

Frith, C.D. (1979). Consciousness, information processing, and schizophrenia. *British Journal of Psychiatry*, **134**: 225–235.

Gallagher, S. (1997). Mutual enlightenment: recent phenomenology in cognitive science. *Journal of Consciousness Studies*, **4**: 195–214.

Geertz, C. (1973). *The interpretation of cultures*. New York: Basic Books.

Gray, J. A., Feldon, J., Rawlins, J.N., Hemsley, D.R., and Smith, A.D. (1991). The neuropsychology of schizophrenia. *Behavioral and Brain Sciences*, **14**: 1–20.

Griffiths, p. E. (1997). *What emotions really are*. Chicago: University of Chicago Press.

Grünbaum, A. (1993). *Validation in the clinical theory of psychoanalysis*. Madison, CN: International Universities Press.

Gurwitsch, A. (1964). *The field of consciousness*. Pittsburgh, PA: Duquesne University Press.

Heidegger, M. (1962). *Being and time* (trans. J. Macquarrie and E. Robinson). New York: Harper and Row.

Heil, J. and Mele, A. (ed.) (1993). *Mental causation*. Oxford, UK: Clarendon Press.

Henry, M. (1973). *The essence of manifestation* (trans. G. Etzkorn). The Hague: Martinus Nijhoff.

Huber, G. (1986). Negative or basic symptoms in schizophrenia and affective illness. In: *Biological psychiatry 1985* (ed. C. Shagass, R.C. Josiassen, W.H. Bridger, K.J. Weiss, D. Stoff, and G.M. Simpson), pp. 1136–1141. New York: Elsevier.

Hunt, H.T. (1985). Cognition and states of consciousness. *Perceptual and Motor Skills*, **60**: 239–282.

Hunt, H.T. (1995). *On the nature of consciousness*. New Haven, CN: Yale University Press.

Husserl, E. (1977). *Phenomenological psychology* (lectures, summer semester, 1925) (trans. J. Scanlon). The Hague: Martinus Nijhoff.

Husserl, E. (1983). *Ideas pertaining to a pure phenomenology and to a phenomenological philosophy: first book* (trans. F. Kersten. Dordrecht, Holland: Kluwer.

Husserl, E. (1989). *Studies in the phenomenology of constitution: Second book* (trans. R. Rojcewicz and A. Schuwer). Dordrecht, Holland: Kluwer.

Husserl, E. (1999). *The essential Husserl* (ed. D. Welton). Bloomington, IN: Indiana University Press.

Jaspers, K. (1963). *General psychopathology* (trans. J. Hoenig and M.W. Hamilton). Chicago: University of Chicago Press.

Kim, J. (1985). Psychophysical laws. In: *Actions and events: perspectives on the philosophy of Donald Davidson* (ed. E. LePore and B. McGlaughin). Oxford University Press: Blackwell.

Klosterkötter, J. (1992). The meaning of basic symptoms for the development of schizophrenic psychoses. *Neurology, Psychiatry, and Brain Research*, **1**: 30–41.

Klosterkötter, J., Schultze-Lutter, F., Gross, G., Huber, G., and Steinmeyer, E.M. (1997). Early self-experienced neuropsychological deficits and subsequent schizophrenic diseases: an 8-year average follow-up prospective study. *Acta Psychiatrica Scandinavica*, **95**: 396–404.

Kring A.M. and Neale, J. (1996). Do schizophrenic patients show a disjunctive relationship among expressive, experiential, and psychophysiological components of emotion? *Journal of Abnormal Psychology*, **105**: 249–257.

Lawson-Tancred, H. (1995). Ancient Greek philosophy II: Aristotle. In *philosophy: a guide through the subject* (ed. A.C. Grayling), pp. 398–439. Oxford, UK: Oxford University Press.

Mackie, J.L. (1974). *The cement of the universe: a study of causation*. Oxford, UK: Clarendon.

Marbach, E. (1993). *Mental representation and consciousness. towards a phenomenological theory of representation and reference*. Dordrecht: Kluwer Academic Publishers.

McClamrock, R. (1995). *Existential cognition: computational minds in the world*. Chicago: University of Chicago Press.

McGinn, C. (1993). *The problems of philosophy*. Oxford, UK: Blackwell.

Merleau-Ponty, M. (1962): *The phenomenology of perception* (trans. C. Smith). New York: Routledge & Kegan Paul.

Merleau-Ponty, M. (1968). *The visible and the invisible* (trans. A. Lingis). Evanston, IL: Northwestern University Press.

Michotte, A. (1963). *The perception of causality*. New York: Basic Books.

Minkowski, E. (1927). *La schizophrénie*. Paris: Payot.

Minkwoski, E. (1997a). *Traité de psychopathologie*. Paris: Institut Synthelabo.

Minkowski, E. (1997b). *Au-delà du rationalisme morbide*. Paris: Harmattan.

Moran, D. (2000). *Introduction to phenomenology*, London: Routledge.

Mojtabai, R. and Rieder, R.O. (1998). Limitations of the symptom-oriented approach to psychiatric research. *British Journal of Psychiatry*, **173**: 198–202.

Nagel, T. (1974). What is it like to be a bat? *Philosophical Review*, **83**: 435–450.

Nagel, E. (1979). *Mortal questions*. Cambridge, U.K.: Cambridge University Press.

Parnas, J. (2000). The self and intentionality in the pre-psychotic stages of schizophrenia. In: *Exploring the self: philosophical and psychopathological perspectives on self-experience* (ed. D. Zahavi), pp. 115–147. Amsterdam: John Benjamins.

Parnas, J. (2003). Self-disorders in schizophrenia: a clinical perspective. In: *The self and schizophrenia: a neuropsychological perspective* (ed. T. Kircher and A. David). Cambridge, UK: Cambridge University Press.

Parnas, J. and Bovet, p. (1991). Autism in schizophrenia revisited. *Comprehensive Psychiatry*, **32**: 7–21.

Parnas, J. and Zahavi, D. (2002). The role of phenomenology in psychiatric classification and diagnosis. In: *Psychiatric diagnosis and classification* (World Psychiatric Association Series) (ed. M. Maj, W. Gaebel, J.J. Lopez-Ibor, and N. Sartorius), pp. 137–162. New York: John Wiley & Sons.

Phillips, W.A. and Silverstein, S.M. (2003). Convergence of biological and psychological perspectives on cognitive coordination in schizophrenia. *Behavioral and Brain Sciences* **26**: 65–82..

Polanyi, M. (1964). *Personal knowledge*. New York: Harper Torchbooks.

Polanyi, M. (1967). *The tacit dimension*. Garden City, New York: Anchor Books.

Ricoeur, p. (1992). *Oneself as another* (trans. K. Blamey). Chicago: University of Chicago Press.

Sass, L. (1992a). *Madness and modernism: insanity in the light of modern art, literature, and thought*. New York: Basic Books. (Harvard Paperback 1994.)

Sass, L. (1992b). Heidegger, schizophrenia, and the ontological difference. *Philosophical Psychology*, **5**: 109–132.

Sass, L. (1994). *The paradoxes of delusion: Wittgenstein, Schreber, and the schizophrenic mind*. Ithaca, NY: Cornell University Press.

Sass, L. (1998a). Schizophrenia, self-consciousness, and the modern mind. *Journal of Consciousness Studies*, **5**: 543–65.

Sass, L. (1998b). 'Ambiguity is of the essence': the relevance of hermeneutics for psychoanalysis. In: *Psychoanalytic versions of the human condition and clinical practice* (ed. P. Marcus and A. Rosenberg), pp. 257–305. New York: New York University Press.

Sass, L. (2001a). Self and world in schizophrenia: three classic approaches in phenomenological psychiatry. *Philosophy, Psychiatry, Psychology*. **8**: 251–270.

Sass, L. (2001b). Wittgenstein, Freud, and the nature of psychoanalytic explanation. In: *Wittgenstein, theory, and the arts* (ed. R. Allen and M. Turvey), pp. 253–295. London: Routledge.

Sass, L. (2003a). Schizophrenia and the self: hyper-reflexivity and diminished self-affection. In: *The Self in schizophrenia: neuropsychological perspectives* (ed. T. Kircher and A. David), pp. 242–271. Cambridge, UK: Cambridge University Press.

Sass, L. (2003b). Negative symptoms, schizophronia, and the self. *International Journal of Psychology and Psychological Therapy*, **3**: 153–180.

Sass, L. (in press). Contradictions of emotion in schizophrenia. *Congnition and Emotion*.

Sass, L. and Parnas, J. (2003). Schizophrenia, consciousness, and the self. *Schizophrenia Bulletin*. **29**: 427–444.

Searle, J. (1983). *Intentionality*. Cambridge, UK: Cambridge University Press.

Sèchehaye, M. (1956). *A new psychotherapy in schizophrenia*. New York, Grune & Stratton.

Silberer, H. (1951). Report on a method of eliciting and observing certain symbolic hallucination-phenomena. In: *Organization and pathology of thought, selected sources* (ed. D. Rapaport), pp. 195–207. New York: Columbia University Press.

Simon, H.A. (2000). Discovering explanations. In: *Explanation and cognition* (ed. F.C. Keil and R.A. Wilson), pp. 21–60. Cambridge, MA: MIT Press.

Sokolowski, R. (2000). *Introduction to phenomenology*. Cambridge UK: Cambridge University Press.

Spence S. (2001). Alien control; from phonomenology to cognitive neurobiology. *Philosophy, Psychiatry and Psychology*, **8**: 163–172.

Spiegelberg, H. (1972). *Phenomenology in psychiatry and psychiatry: a historical introduction*. Evanston, IL: Northwestern University Press.

Steinbock, A.J. (1995). *Home and beyond*. Evanston, IL: Northwestern University Press.

Störring, G. (1987). Perplexity. In: *The clinical roots of the schizophrenia concept* (ed. J. Cutting and M. Shepherd), pp. 79–82. Cambridge, UK: Cambridge University Press (orig. published 1939).

Tatossian, A. (1997). La phénomenologie des psychoses. Paris: L'Art du Comprendre (Juillet 1997, Numero double, hors série).

Tausk, V. (1933). On the origin of the 'influencing machine' in schizophrenia. *Psychoanalytic Quarterly*, **2**: 529–530. (orig. published 1919.)

Taylor, C. (1993). Engaged agency and background in Heidegger. In: *The Cambridge companion to Heidegger* (ed. C. Guignon), pp. 317–336. Cambridge, UK: Cambridge University Press.

Varela, F. (1996). Neurophenomenology. *Journal of Consciousness Studies*, **3**: 330–349

Von Wright, G.H. (1971). *Explanation and understanding*. Ithaca, NY: Cornell University Press.

Wakefield, J. and Eagle, M. (1997). Psychoanalysis and Wittgenstein: a reply to Richard Allen. *Psychoanalysis and Contemporary Thought*, **20**: 323–351.

Wilson, R.A. and Keil, F.C. (2000). The shadows and shallows of explanation. In: *Explanation and cognition* (ed. F.C. Keil and R.A. Wilson), pp. 87–114. Cambridge, MA: MIT Press.

Woodward, J. (2003). *Making things happen: a theory of causal explanation*. New York and Oxford UK: Oxford University Press.

Zahavi, D. (1999). *Self-awareness and alterity: a phenomenological investigation*. Evanston, IL: Northwestern University Press.

5 Schizophrenic delusion and hallucination as the expression and consequence of an alteration of the existential a prioris

Alfred Kraus

Introduction

This article relates schizophrenic delusion and hallucination to an alteration of categories of being, which here are called existential a prioris. Categories in philosophy are mostly understood in the sense of Aristotle as basic character-istics of beings and in the sense of Kant (1978) as the a priori conditions of every experience. 'A priori' in this context means coming before any kind of experience. Heidegger's (1953) differentiation between categories related to the kind of being of pure *Vorhandenheit*, the being of objects like houses or trees, and categories characterizing the *Dasein*, i.e. the existentiality of hu-mans, called by him *Existenzialien* (existentials), is important in what follows.

Fulford (1989), Spitzer (1994) and others have previously pointed to the immense difficulties with the definition of delusion and hallucination. Even if definitions are founded on the essence of something, essence and definition are not identical. Here only the essence of delusion and hallucination in schizophrenia are considered. Delusions in psychiatry are mostly conceptual-ized intellectually-cognitively; hallucinations mostly sensorily. Both concepts presuppose the comparability of delusional 'reality' and normal reality, of hallucination and normal perception. Thus, the difference in the case of delusion would purely consist of false cognitions or judgements and in the case of hallucination in the lacking of an external object. However, with delusion as well as with hallucination every conceptualization and definition is difficult to objectify. It seems we have here another kind of reality. Every statement a patient makes about the object of her/his experience seems only to adapt it more or less to normal reality. Thus the patient tries in a certain sense to 'normalize' the altered kind of her/his experiencing. K. Schneider (1967) has discussed the problem of the relationship between what the patient really experiences and that which she/he reports, because her/his report has inevitably to adapt to the structure of common language and its logic. In this way Schneider says, the 'reporter transposes the contradictions of his experiences, their floating and shredded character to ordered and sayable things' (p. 134). K. Jaspers (1965), apart from stating his criteria for the definition of delusion, emphasized that in the delusion of people with schizophrenia, a globally altered relationship of their likewise altered personality has taken place. Similar statements were made by K. Schneider (1967). In our view, not only a globally altered kind of experience of the self, but also of others, and of the world, is expressed in the delusions and hallucinations of those with schizophrenia. Without taking into consideration this altered pre-reflective 'being-in-the-world', which shows itself in another kind of 'reality', every objectifying concept and definition of schizophrenic delusion and hallucination is only exploratory and superficial and in the end misses its object.

Our main thesis, therefore, is that delusion and hallucination in people with schizophrenia are secondary phenomena; primary is an alteration of fundamental structures of *Dasein* (Heidegger 1963), of 'categories' of being, which—in their empirical application in psychiatry—we call, with Needleman (1968, p. 23), existential a prioris. The alteration of existential a prioris results in an alteration in the structure of experience of a concrete individual.

We are dealing here with the conditions of the possibility of schizophrenic delusion and hallucination in the essence of humans, with the altered basic self- and world-relationships as a consequence of an alteration of the existential a prioris. This is not to be understood in the sense of cause and effect but in that of the foundation of delusion and hallucination in those alterations. However, even if our description of delusion and hallucination as 'categorial disorders' or alterations of 'categories of being' is not a causal assessment, it could help to pave the way for investigations of their neurobiological as well as psychosocial and psychodynamic causes or conditions.

After explaining the concept of the existential a priori and its application in psychiatry, we will now demonstrate how an alteration of the experience based on an alteration of a priori structures is expressed by patients with so-called 'technical' delusions and hallucinations. These are psychotic symptoms, described by those experiencing them as related to certain influences on them of technical media.

Self- and world-experience in delusion and hallucination

The technical kind of delusion, which is mostly combined with so-called *Ich-Störungen* (disorders of ego), is particularly suitable for demonstrating the alteration of the existential a prioris. An alteration of the existential a prioris is, in our view, fundamental also in other kinds of schizophrenic experiences and also in other disturbances, like in melancholic and manic delusions, though maybe with changes in detail.

The mentioned 'disturbances of ego' (*Ich-Störungen*) give access to what we mean by a categorial alteration. Disorders of the ego, e.g. bodily experiences of being influenced, thought insertion, thought broadcasting, etc., belonging to the so-called first-rank symptoms, are not only particularly useful from the point of view of diagnosis, but they also show the way to the recognition of the essence of schizophrenia. These 'disturbances of ego', even though they are often combined with delusional contents, are as such not delusional experiences, because, according to Spitzer (1988), they are formally presented as statements about a mental state (e.g. like feeling pain). Therefore, they should not be interpreted as false statements about reality, but as true statements about the patient's own experience.

Phenomenological-anthropological approach and the concept of *Dasein*

An alteration of the self- and world-experience underlying the delusions and the hallucinations of people with schizophrenia and expressed by them, has been explicated particularly by the different approaches, which can be summarized under the title of a so-called phenomenological-anthropological psychiatry (Kunz 1931; Binswanger 1957, 1965; Blankenburg 1980, 1991; Lopez-Ibor 1982; Mundt 1989; Kraus 1991, 1994, 2001; Sass 1992; Schwartz and Wiggins 1992;Bovet and Parnas 1993; Naudin 1997; Parnas 1999). A recent survey of phenomenological-anthropological psychiatry has been given by Kraus (2001) and Schmidt-Degenhard (2000).

These approaches were (at least immanently) strongly inspired by transcendental philosophy. Kant (1998) was the first to bring about a far-reaching revolution in philosophy by supposing that, in contrast to former beliefs, knowledge does not only conform to its objects, but objects also conform to our ways of knowing. This was a big blow to the belief that it could be possible to achieve positive knowledge about reality as it is itself. Kant showed that, without what he called transcendental categories, without the a priori forms of space and time, causality and reality, no kind of experience could emerge. Hundert (1990), Spitzer (1990), and others referred to these Kantian categories in order to understand psychiatric phenomena.

The influence on psychiatry of Husserl, who himself owes very much to Kant, was greater and more manifold than that of Kant. Suffice it to mention his new understanding of consciousness with its reality-constituting, intentional acts. In recent time the phenomenological approach has got a new impetus by possible relationships to cognitivism and neuroscience and thus also to empirical research (see Naudin *et al.* 1997).

An even stronger influence on psychopathology came from Heidegger (1953), particularly through H. Kunz (1931), Blankenburg (1971), Tellenbach (1983), Binswanger (1994), and others. What is new in Heidegger is, as we have already stated, his strict differentiation between a being in the sense of *Vorhandenheit*, the being of objects, and that of *Dasein*, in the sense of being-in-the-world. Let us take an example by Heidegger (1994, p. 94) to make this clear. A pair of shoes standing near the door is different from a man standing there. It is a different kind of 'being-with' the door. Human 'being-with' objects has the basic trait of 'standing open' or openness (*Offenstehen*) to the 'present-being' (*Anwesende*) or to the thing that is there (1994, p. 94). Shoes, however, placed near the door do not allow access to the door. The door is not present to the shoes. 'There' (*Da*) in Heidegger's notion of human *Dasein* therefore signifies this kind of openness, which is fundamental to human beings, in which beings (*Seiendes*), things, the others can be present, indeed the person can be present to him-or herself (1994, p. 157). The German word *Dasein* could be written with a hyphen, that is *Da-sein*. In order to avoid the possiblity that *Dasein* might be misunderstood as referring to location, (here and there), it could be better translated as 'being the there' in analogy to Heidegger's own translation into French: *être le la* (1994, p. 43). *Dasein* in its openness to the present is a letting oneself in for beings, a being taken up with one's action and behaviour (1994, p. 143). As a relation to the being of beings, *Dasein* always already understands being. Openness, understanding being respectively thus characterize the basic condition of humankind. The openness of *Dasein* makes the being-in-the-world of the person possible (ontologically understood), which in this way always already belongs to humankind. Being-in-the-world is a being completely different from that of *Vorhandenheit*, which is thus being only within the world. Being-in-the-world is the essence of humankind and therefore cannot be added to the person. Being-in-the-world is not a quality of a subjectivity, however it may be imagined. It is intrinsic to the existing of humankind (1994, p. 286). Heidegger, thus, goes back behind the differentiation of subject and object; or of ego, or self and world. And in this he differs fundamentally from Kant as well as from Husserl.

The existentials and their clinical application

The fundamental structures of *Dasein* are called existentials (*Existenzialien*) by Heidegger. Because they present the characteristics of the being of *Dasein*, they differ from the entities of a being not of the *Dasein* kind, e.g. beings of nature. Because *Dasein* is the condition of the possibility of being-in-the-world, the existentials can be conceived as different kinds of possible-being (*Sein-können*) (1994, p. 203).

Dasein, ontologically understood, constitutes the being of the world and the self (also ontologically understood) through the endowing of meaning (p. 22). According to Needleman (1969), the existentials function in a manner analogous to the Kantian categories, in that they are the forms through which ontic reality can manifest itself to the *Dasein*. These existentials, for Heidegger, are

In-sein (in-being), *Sein-bei* (be-immersed-in), *Mit-sein* (with-being), *Zeitlichkeit* (temporality), *Räumlichkeit* (spatiality), *Verstehen* (understanding), and so on. All these notions in Heidegger's Daseinsanalytic are to be understood ontologically as characteristics of humankind, taken as *Dasein*, in preparation for inquiry into the fundamental question for the meaning of being. In contrast, Daseinanalysis, which is different to Daseinsanalytic, has an ontic orientation, i.e. it is concerned with factual phenomena of a certain existing *Dasein*. Now, what Binswanger (1958) did in his Daseinsanalyse (existential analysis—a 'phenomenological empirical science' that aimed to make ontic statements) was to take the ontologically determined existentials of Heidegger and bring them into the frame of concrete human existence. The intention governing his Daseinsanalyse was to understand psychiatric symptoms as the expression of an alteration of the structural components of one's basic being-in-the-world, which we have mentioned above.

Needleman (1968), on whom we draw in the following, in his introduction to the *Selected papers of Ludwig Binswanger* described Binswanger's way of applying the ontological a prioris to the concrete individual. Because Binswanger was on the one hand concerned with the transcendentally a priori essential structures and on the other hand with the possibilities of concrete human existence, Needleman labels his approach 'meta-ontic'— since it is neither ontological nor ontic, but rather lying somewhere in between. For the same reason he renamed what Binswanger (1958) calls a 'transcendental category' as an 'existential a priori'. The existentials, or to say it better, the existential a priori, give meaning to and thereby constitute the world of anybody (in the present discussion, the patient). As such they are one's matrix of possible experience. The existential a priori structure, according to Needleman, represents 'the being of this particular man as he exists in his particular world' (p. 67). This extension of Heidegger's ontology to the ontic level is very important for psychiatry. However, much work has still to be done to clarify the relationship between the two kinds of existentials, which should not be identified with each other.

The *existential a priori* structure serves as a clue to the world-design of a patient—what her/his world holds out as potential experience. Binswanger used his Daseinsanalyse as a biographical method for the investigation of the development of psychiatric disturbances as well as for the analysis of psychiatric phenomena such as delusion and hallucination. We use existential analysis here only in the last sense.

As already mentioned, the notion of being-in-the-world goes beyond the separation of subject and object and is related to a pre-conceptual being of the human person. Such a pre-objective, pre-predicative and pre-intentional being has also been thematized by other philosophers, such as Husserl in his notion of life-world, by Merleau-Ponty, by Sartre and others. It has become an increasingly important topic not only for different approaches to phenomenological psychopathology, but in a certain sense also for much empirical research, which attempts to avoid objectifying or isolating the individual from his experiential world. Of interest here is the human being's state of *already being related-to*, i.e. to a life-world in the sense of habits, self-evidence, familiarity, etc., wherein intentional behaviour and experience is based. Thus, for example, intentional trust in somebody presupposes human familiarity. This pre-objective, pre-predicative being is expressed in the already mentioned verbalized nouns of temporalization, spatialization, etc., but also in prepositional determinations, as in Heidegger's notion of being-in, being-with, etc., in Merleau-Ponty's *être-au-monde*, etc., in Sartre's *être-pour-soi*, *être-pour-autrui*. A modification of this pre-objective being can be assumed in many psychiatric disturbances, such as in delusion, which, according to Blankenburg (1967, p. 647), manifests itself in intentional acts, but is not founded in these acts. For psychopathology, it is important that being on this level, as these notions already indicate, is by no means something static, but has to be understood as a process of happening.

Technical delusions and hallucinations

In the following we summarize some of the results of our studies on 21 schizophrenic patients with delusions and hallucinations of technical contents (preliminary study Kraus 1994). These are mainly patients with so-called 'made up' experiences, experiences of being influenced in their will, their thinking, and their feeling in a positive or negative way, as well as being explored by others by technical means. These technical means are, for example, electric streams, different kinds of rays, like X-rays, laser, short-, medium-, and long-waves, ultra-short-waves, UHF- and VHF-rays, infra-red and micro-waves, as well as different kinds of electromagnetic fields (EMF rays), and so on. Not only are their acts, movements, and bodily feelings influenced, but also parts of their body or their whole body may be heated or cooled, numbed, or destroyed, etc., by these technical influences. The same kind of influencing, harming, or supporting by technical means may also originate deliberately or spontaneously in the patients themselves and have effects on others. Both possibilities of experience, being influenced by others and influencing others, may occur in the same patient at the same time.

A case report

In the following we present a crimped-haired, and much younger looking patient of 61 years, who shows an extraordinary self-assertive behaviour, when coming to the clinic. She explains she is out of place in our clinic, because she feels psychologically well. She then tells us that her husband, who separated from her five years ago, for reason of hate and rage, had implanted two little wires and a capsule in her brain. These electrodes were located 2 cm above her left ear. Since then she has been controlled by remote electrodes. The whole neighbourhood has smaller or bigger appliances with buttons by which she is steered; she has even seen these herself. Everybody in her place of residence knows that she has electrodes in her head and everybody talks about it, even making video films of her. The whole experimental project is, apparently, connected to a cable television, so that she can be watched constantly.

At the same time as her husband moved out, a young man moved into the house. This was the beginning of it all; he had made the first installation of this kind. The apparatus would also cause pains in her kidneys, muscles, and in her hand. In the night her consciousness would be switched off, and she could not rule out the possibility that she was then sexually manipulated. Anyway, she would, astonishingly enough, wake up with pains in her lower abdomen. Above all, she would hear in the night how the neighbours would speak about her and laugh spitefully. Once she had heard: 'Tonight I did it eight times' (the patient speaks here in the first person!). The patient tells us that her husband had had affairs with other, younger, married women for 17 years. This, however, was vehemently denied by her husband as well as by her only son. Only after his moving out of the house had he established a relationship with another woman.

Clinically we have here delusions of persecution and observation, delusions of reference and jealousy, acoustical hallucinations as well as bodily sensations in the frame of schizophrenia.

Technical contents indicating an altered being-in-the-world

We think it is not by chance that people with schizophrenia so often use technical metaphors to explain their schizophrenic experiences. There must be some analogy between the characteristics of technical processes of the above mentioned kind and the way patients experience their altered psychotic self and world. In the following we try to explore the altered pre-objective being-in-the-world of our patients by examining their technical delusions, using the phenomenological characteristics of technical processes as guidelines. We deem this alteration to be prior to the appearance of delusion and hallucination.

Classical psychopathology, discriminating between the form and content of psychotic experiences, is for diagnostic reasons mainly interested in the form of the contents, asking, for example, if we are dealing with delusional ideas, delusional perceptions, hallucinations or illusion, and so on. For diagnosis, especially for the diagnosis made by diagnostic manuals, the respective contents of psychotic experiences seem not to be important, because they are seen to be just the material for these symptoms coming from the biography of the patient or her/his actual situation. But, in this way much of the information given by the contents of her/his delusions and hallucinations about the alteration of the pre-objective, pre-predicative formal structures of her/his relationship to her-/himself, to others and to her/his world is lost. In so far as the pre-predicative being of the patient is, as we will show later on, especially important for diagnosis, this information is also lost considering diagnosis. The analysis of these transcendental, or as we would prefer to say, a priori existential structures, is not only important for the understanding of the world in which a patient lives, but they also show how the phenomena that we diagnose clinically as symptoms, e.g. as delusions and hallucination, become possible.

Alteration of temporalization and spatialization, of 'being-in'

The technical processes of the kind mentioned above are in many respects different from non-technical 'natural' processes, especially if we see them from the aspect of temporality and spatiality. This particular relationship to time and space is what makes technical processes so useful for practical purposes. Rays, for instance, bridge space and time and can penetrate solid objects. They have effects at long distance. The apparatus from which they originate, and the people using them, seem to be near and present, but in reality they are not. The 'natural' spatial and temporal discursivity, the 'natural' sequences of events, the environmental coherences and connections, the mutual references of objects and events are interrupted. A technically transmitted talk (like, for instance, a telephone call) is compared to a talk in the presence of the interlocutors, lacking background information about what is told. The partners in a telephone call do not know the present condition or the situation of each other. They may only have suppositions without any certainty. All these characteristics of real technical processes characterize also the delusional experiences of our patients. So one of our patients, hallucinating voices, supposed that her mother was giving her orders, which had been recorded on a tape when the patient was a child.

If we now look at our patients under the aspect of the existential a priori of 'being-in' (*In-sein*), in the context of their being-in-the-world, we have to start with the fact that the being-in, of the kind of being of *Dasein*, has nothing to do with the kind of being in the world of things like wine in a bottle or a tree in its surroundings. 'Being-in-the-world' of humans signifies that one's world is not intended in the sense of Husserl, but is part of the *Dasein*, of one's being itself. That means, time and space are essential features of one's being. *Dasein* as such spatializes and temporalizes itself, and (for example) opens the space for the appearance of things. As we have already shown, 'being there' (*Dasein*) means that this being is open to its world. It lets beings appear as they are, constructs its own world, understands it, and is always already familiar with it. If we now compare this with the *Dasein* of our patients, they have suffered a loss of their 'being there' in their delusions and hallucinations. They have lost the spatial as well as the temporal presence in their real world, which in a certain sense, they are sliding over. They can be contacted and be influenced, wherever they are, from far distances and from anywhere. Their attention is completely absorbed by these occurrences.

So, with the electrodes in her brain, our patient is, because of what she experiences, always anywhere and nowhere, but not where she really is. She has completely lost her position in the real world in which she lives. The natural connections of things and real human relationships are broken down. Also, the quality of delusional human relationship is extraordinarily poor and without any background information. The patients themselves—as well as their partners—are without a certain place in space and time. With their delusional partners they lack the unity of a common world. It is significant that hallucinatory experiences are mostly monomodal, either acoustical or tactile, etc., whereas normal perceptions are usually multimodal, e.g. what we see we can also touch and smell. The private room in which a patient lives has lost its protecting boundaries. For this reason, everything happening in the private space is at the same time made public. Coming back to our patient, in reality she does not inhabit her world. Because she communicates with her husband by electrodes, she hardly realizes that her husband is, on a daily basis, looking after things in her house.

Is the same not also true for somebody who is using real technical media, e.g. a mobile phone? The fundamental difference is that such a person, also operating in another relationship of time and space, is always at the same time related to her/his 'natural' space and time, she/he can change it and is not passively exposed to it.

The loss of the existentiality of our patients is expressed by the fact that their whole being has received features of the being of the *Vorhandenheit* like that material things. In technical delusions and hallucinations the patients feel like being treated as objects, they are available, at hand for everybody at any time. Even their thoughts have received the quality of a material thing that can be extracted from their brains, as one patient told us. Thoughts can directly be transformed into waves or rays and waves into thoughts. A merging of ego and material objects, an inter-penetration of both is taking place. Not only have the boundaries between the ego and its surroundings become permeable, as K. Schneider (1967) showed, but even those of one's subjectivity and the material world, between *res cogitans* and *res extensa*.

Alteration of the bodily being

It is worth noting that the body—more exactly bodily being—belongs to the being-in-the-world. The openness to beings, according to Heidegger, is characterized by the fact that we are immediately *with* the things, which 'catch' us in a bodily way. In the psychotic kinds of experience, however, this openness for real things is restricted. As a body available (*vorhanden*), at hand (*zuhanden*) to the manipulations and attacks of others, this body exists as *Dasein* (as characterized above) only very restrictedly. As an alienated body, this body is no longer a possibility of openness for beings, but only a prison. So Minkowski's (1970) 'loss of vital contact with reality' of people with schizophrenia can be understood in the sense of a loss of bodily openness of being-in-the-world.

Degraded in their personhood to such an excessive degree, deprived of their openness for beings, and insufficiently appealing to beings, these patients have no needs or little interest in doing anything; acting may even become impossible. In our opinion, insufficient attention has been paid to the so-called apathy of people with schizophrenia, which—if it is described at all—is mostly seen merely as an intrapsychic state. Such 'apathy' is based on the particular kind of being-*in* of their being-in-the-world. Their particular kind of relationship to the world is also the reason why their apathy is therapeutically so difficult to influence. The lacking discursivity, the altered spatiality and temporarality, which is expressed in their delusional assumptions, do not allow them to react in any way, e.g. to protect themselves against the delusionary technical influences that they describe. For instance, the patient will very seldom investigate where the technical influence actually comes from and who causes it.

Alteration of 'being-with' others

Let us also have a look at the alteration of the structure of being-with others in connection with the altered experience of the self. Kurt Schneider (1965) found that in technical delusion there is always the assumption that another person, or several others, use the technical means. One could assume that this is only a *post hoc* explanation by the patient for her/his acoustic 'sensory perceptions'. Mostly, however, the patients maintain that they were already conscious of the intention of others at the first appearing of a hallucination. The articulation of the other in the delusion and hallucination of those with schizophrenia suggests a fundamental alteration of the existential a priori of being-with. According to Heidegger (1963), being-with cannot be seen apart from being-in-the-world, but is always a part of it. 'The In-being is always also being-with others'. 'Being-with structures being, even when another person is not there or not perceived' (p. 120). It seems important to us that every instance of knowing each other is founded in a primary understanding of being-with (p. 124), and that consequently empathy is possible only on the basis of the existential a priori of being-with (p. 125).

If we now turn to our patients in their schizophrenic delusional and hallucinatory experiences, there is no direct, immediate communication possible with others, because the technical medium is always in-between, in the way. The patients are not free to communicate with others, but are forced to get into contact, because they are the object of rays or waves sent by these others. They are not only forced to listen to the information they get by their voices, but they are also explored by the technical medium: they have to reveal themselves to the delusionary others. They cannot hide from them or protect themselves. They are commanded by these influences, have lost their freedom and are victims of the other, or of others. We have already pointed to the mono-modality of hallucinatory experiences. The patients hear other persons without seeing them and they have the feeling of being touched without the concomitant presence of the other. Thus, no background information, no meta-communication is possible. This makes it difficult for them to know the motives, the intentions of the others carrying out such manipulations, or fully to understand the meaning of what the voices say. It is also because of the neutrality of the technical medium that they often do not know whether the manipulations should help or harm them. Because everybody can use a tech-nical medium and meta-communication is not possible, they often cannot identify the user. Because nobody is able to participate in what they experience, the patients feel isolated, cut off from the others. By means of technical media like rays and waves it is possible to be near from afar. This can be a particular torture, if, for example, through bodily hallucinations the most intimate near-ness is realized from afar; so one of our patients suffered from genital manipu-lations and touches by radiation. The patient we have mainly been referring to in this chapter had similar experiences. Here, the near–farness of the delusional other is experienced as a particular stress, because the patient has only his or her own bodily feelings, whereas the other stays abstract—only present in the patient's bodily feelings (we refuse here to speak only of an imagination of the other being inferred from his/her bodily feelings). Rays and waves always have one-way effects. The consequence is that the patient usually has no possibility to react to these, there is no reciprocity possible, the patient is the mere object of the wishes, ends, and purposes of others.

Our analysis of the experience of technical delusion and hallucination makes it immediately recognizable which kind of being-in-the-world in the sense of being-with others is still possible for the patient. It shows at the same time to what degree his/her openness for beings, his/her being with things, and his/her being together and with others, and his/her relationship to him-/herself, are restricted. Together with the alteration of his relationships with others and the imaginations the patient has about him-/herself, even the experience of his/herself as a self alters. So he/she perceives from the behaviour of others that he/she has suddenly become the centre of all that is happening, that he/she has got (for example) a messianic mission. The others not only rob him/her of certain possibilities of his/her spontaneity, making him/her move his/her limbs and provoking feelings in him/her, etc., by technical means, but they also sabotage his/her whole being-him-/herself. They put themselves in place of his/her subjectivity, pretending to be his/her subjectivity. Thus, even his/her own subjectivity is felt to be alien.

'What is experienced in the praecox-feeling?'

What patients tell us about their new pre-reflective experiences in their technical delusions and hallucinations, what we see as a consequence of the alteration of basic structures of their existence, their being-in-the-world (their spatialization and temporalization, their being-with, their embodiment), corresponds to what the psychiatrist recognises in the so-called praecox-feeling. Many years ago, Wyrsch (1946) interpreted the praecox-feeling as the recognition of 'a certain mode of being-in-the-world, of taking part in it'. Because what the experienced diagnostician recognizes in the praecox-feeling is a certain mode of being, he is not only confronted with bizarre, not understandable behaviours and ideas, but as Müller-Suur (1958) showed, he/she is faced with a definite non-understandability (*bestimmte Unverständlichkeit*; see also Kraus 1994). He/she realizes in an intuitive way, in the case of patients with schizophrenia, that their reality is constituted in a different way, originating as we saw in an alteration of the existential a prioris.

Delusional mood and delusional ideas

The patient experiences this alteration immediately in the first incident, in the so-called delusional mood (*Wahnstimmung*), which is mostly connected with great anxiety, often of an apocalyptic kind. In the consecutive development of (technical) delusional ideas and hallucinatory experiences, the patient tries not only to translate these original pre-reflective experiences into our common language, but also looks for explanations which best fit the new experiences. In an absolutely creative act, by using the technical 'metaphor' in his/her delusional ideas, the patient performs an adaptive integration of the primordial experiences into quasi-normal experiences of reality. The delusional technical medium, by reconciling schizophrenic experiences with real possibilities, makes the strange new experiences plausible for the patient and for others. By using technical 'metaphors' the person with schizophrenia is able to give words to things not sayable. Methodologically, we have gone just the other way round, and have tried to get access to the primary experiences that are expressed in the technical delusions and hallucinations.

The technical content, is it merely a metaphor?

The experience of delusion and hallucination often seems to be associated with vivid phantasy and imagination. However, we think that this phenomenon must be seen in connection with the lack of openness for being and the lack of response to, and insufficient involvement with being, as we have mentioned above. Consequently those with schizophrenia do not experience the resistance of reality, which, according to Heidegger, characterizes being-in-the-world, which presupposes a disclosed world and constitutes the sense of reality. 'Reality is resistance' (p. 209). The lack of openness for the being of the beings of the out-side world and the resulting lack in the experience of resistance is, in our view, the reason not only for the fact that his/her thoughts can so easily adopt the character of being somehow 'real', but also for the fact that these may gain such power over the patient. Because the contents of delusion emanate from the patient her-/himself, she/he relates everything to her-/himself, she/he has the experience of a *'tua res agitur'*. And, because the contents of delusion contain a concealed, repressed knowledge about him-/herself, his/her most secret wishes and anxieties, the delusion and hallucination are able to stir his/her own being in such an extreme way. This is also the explanation for the character of message and revelation of schizophrenic hallucination, excellently described by Lopez-Ibor (1982).

This leads us to the question of whether the theme of technical processes in delusion and hallucination really has to do merely with a metaphoric representation of a psychotic experience of the patient, which, as such, cannot be described by means of our normal language. The patient would certainly refuse such an explanation. Whereas the non-psychotic person knows that he/she visualizes, for example, an unclear subject by using metaphors, the patient does not. For the patient, the visualized picture of being manipulated by technical means itself for him has the character of reality, even if she/he is able to see the difference to 'normal' reality.

The reason for the quasi-reality of her/his assumptions of technical processes is above all her/his passively experienced. global pre-objective alteration of her/his self and world.

That we here are dealing with a very different kind of being-influenced than that of normal life in someway has also been expressed by the concept of an altered intentionality (see clinical concepts of recent time, among others of Fulford (1989) and Mundt (1991)). Thus Fulford showed that in schizophrenic thought-insertion it is not just the content of thinking but *thinking as such* that is influenced.

To summarize: We saw that the primary, altered experiences are not the classical symptoms of delusion and hallucination, but are related to an alteration of fundamental structures of being-in-the-world, which we called existential a prioris and which only make possible delusion and hallucinations.

To recognize the primordial experiences in the contents of delusional ideas and hallucinatory experiences is not only of great importance for the understanding of schizophrenia, but also for diagnosis and last but not least for therapy.

Summary

Existential a prioris are fundamental elements of the a priori structure of one's being-in-the-world. They relate to Heidegger's existentials, such as being-in and being-with, in the context of *Dasein* as being-in-the-world. Our thesis is that schizophrenic delusions and hallucinations are secondary phenomena, being founded in a primary alteration of the existential a prioris, the very 'categories' that make possible the anchoring and orientation in the life-world.

This is demonstrated by the so-called technical delusions and hallucinations. The alteration of the existential a prioris is what the trained psychiatrist recognizes in his/her so-called praecox feelings, as a certain mode of being different from ours. We have tried to make this diagnostic intuition scientifically accessible. The recognition of the alteration of these basic pre-objective structures, which is not as yet part of the diagnostic manuals, is not only important for diagnosis, but also for the understanding and therapy of people with schizophrenia.

References

Binswanger, L. (1955). *Ausgewählte Vorträge und Aufsätze*. Bern: Francke.

Binswanger, L. (1957). *Schizophrenie*. Pfullingen: Neske.

Binswanger, L. (1958). The existential analysis school of thought. In: *Existence* (ed. R. May, E. Angel, and H.F. Ellenberger). New York.

Binswanger, L. (1965). *Wahn*. Pfullingen: Neske.

Binswanger, L. (1994). Der Mensch in der Psychiatrie. In: *Ludwig Binswanger* (ed. A Holzhey-Kunz), *Ausgewählte Werke*, Bd. 4, pp. 57–72. Heidelberg: Asanger.

Blankenburg, W. (1971). *Der Verlust der natürlichen Selbstverständlichkeit*. Stuttgart: Enke.

Blankenburg, W. (1980). Anthropological and ontoanalytical aspects of delusion. *Journal of Phenomenological Psychology*, **11**: 97–110.

Blankenburg, W. (1991). Perspektivität und Wahn. In: *Wahn und Perspektivität*. Stuttgart: Enke.

Bovet, P. and Parnas, J. (1993). Schizophrenic delusions: a phenomenological approach. *Schizophrenic Bulletin*, **19**: 579–597.

Fulford, K.W.M. (1989). *Moral theory and medical practice*. Cambridge, UK: Cambridge University Press.

Heidegger, M. (1963). *Sein und Zeit*. Tübingen: Niemeyer.

Heidegger, M. (1994). *Zollikoner Seminare*. (ed. M. Boss). Frankfurt: Vittorio Klostermann.

Hundert, E. (1990). *Are psychotic illnesses category disorders?—proposal for a new understanding and classification for the major forms of mental illness*. Berlin: Springer.

Jaspers, K. (1965). *Allgemeine Psychopathologie*. Berlin: Springer.

Kant, I. (1978). *Anthropolgy* (trans. V.L. Dowdell) (ed. H.H. Rudnick). Carbondale: Southern Illinois University Press.

Kraus, A. (1991). Der melancholische Wahn in identitätstheoretischer Sicht. In: *Wahn und Perspektivität* (ed. W. Blankenburg). Stuttgart: Enke.

Kraus, A. (1994). Phenomenological and criteriological diagnosis: different or complementary? In: *Philosophical perspectives on psychiatric diagnosis and classification* (ed. J. Sadler, O.P. Wiggins, and M.A. Schwartz), pp. 148–162. Baltimore: John Hopkins University Press.

Kraus, A. (2001a). Phenomenological-anthropological psychiatry. In: *Contemporary psychiatry* (ed. F. Henn, N. Sartorius, H. Helmchen, and H. Lauter). Berlin: Springer.

Kraus, A. (2001b). Phenomenology of the technical delusion in schizophrenics. *Journal of Phenomenological Psychology*, **25**: 51–69.

Kunz, H. (1931). Die Grenze der psychopathologischen Wahninterpretation. *Zeitschr. f. d. ges. Neur & Psych*, **135**: 671–715.

Lopez-Ibor, J. (1982). Delusional perception and delusional mood: a phenomenological and existential analysis. In: *Phenomenology and psychiatry* (ed. A.J.J. De Koning and F.A. Jenner). London: Academic Press.

Minkowski, E. (1970). *Lived time. Phenomenological and psychopathological studies.* Evanston, Ill: Northwestern University.

Mundt, C. (1984). Der Begriff der Intentionalität und die Defizienzlehre von den Schizophrenien. *Nervenarzt*, **55**: 582–588.

Naudin, J. (1997). *Phenomenology and psychiatry. The voices and the thing.* Toulouse: PUM.

Needleman, J. (1968). *Being-in-the-world. Selected papers of Ludwig Binswanger.* New York: Harper & Row Publishers.

Parnas, J. (1999). On defining schizophrenia. In: *Schizophrenia. WPA series: evidence and experience in psychiatry*, vol. 2 (ed. M. Maj and N. Sartorius) Chichester: John Wiley & Sons Ltd.

Sass, L.A. (1992). 'Ontological difference'. In: *Phenomenology, language and schizophrenia* (ed. M. Spitzer, F. Uehlein, M.A. Schwartz, and C. Mundt). New York: Springer.

Schmidt-Degenhard (2000). Anthropologische Aspekte psychiatrischer Erkrankungen. In: Psychiatrie und Psychotherapie. (Hrsg Möller HJ, Laux G, Kapfhammer HP). Berlin, Springer.

Schneider, K. (1967). *Klinische Psychopathologie*. Stuttgart: Thieme.

Schwartz, M.A. and Wiggins, O.P. (1992). The phenomenology of schizophrenic delusions. In: *Phenomenology, language and schizophrenia* (ed. M. Spitzer, F. Uehlein, M.A. Schwartz, and C. Mundt), pp. 305–318. London: Springer.

Spitzer, M. (1988). Ichstörungen: in search of a theory. In: *Psychopathology and philosophy*. Berlin: Springer.

Spitzer, M. (1990). Kant on schizophrenia. In: *Philosophy and psychopathology*. Berlin: Springer.

Spitzer, M. (1994). The basis of psychiatric diagnosis. In: *Philosophical perspectives on psychiatric diagnostic classification* (ed. J.Z. Sadler, O.P. Wiggins, and M.A. Schwartz). London: John Hopkins University Press.

Tellenbach, H. (1983). *Melancholie. Problemgeschichte, Endogenität, Typologie, Pathogenese, klinik*, 4. erw. Aufl. Berlin: Springer.

Wyrsch, J. (1946). Über die Intuition bei der Erkennung des Schizophrenen. *Schweiz Med Wochenschr*, **46**: 1173–1176.

6 Schizophrenia: a phenomenological-anthropological approach

Osborne P. Wiggins and Michael A. Schwartz

We shall approach schizophrenia from the point of view of phenomenological-anthropological psychiatry. We shall first provide a brief introduction to the phenomenological-anthropological point of view. This introduction will provide the context for explicating the basic phenomenological concepts that we will borrow from Edmund Husserl (1973, 1983) and apply to schizophrenia, namely, intentionality, synthesis, and constitution. We shall then address schizophrenic experience as a whole, insisting that the transformation of human experience that it involves affects even the most basic ontological constituents of the world, namely, space, time, causality, and the nature of objects. It will be necessary at that juncture to distinguish between an early stage of schizophrenia and a later one. We shall then be prepared to focus on the peculiar nature of schizophrenic hallucinations, first through an anthropological description of them and subsequently through a phenomenological one. We conclude by briefly addressing one final puzzle: if schizophrenic hallucinations exhibit the characteristics we attribute to them, why do the people who encounter them experience them with such certainty?

Phenomenological-anthropological psychiatry

Our approach to schizophrenia falls within the multifaceted tradition of phenomenological-anthropological psychiatry (Doerr-Zegers 2000; Kraus 2000). The adjectives 'phenomenological' and 'anthropological' refer to two sources in continental philosophy of the methodological and conceptual components of the approach (Blankenburg 1962). Phenomenological-anthropological psychiatry should therefore be seen as having been inspired by different continental philosophers but as also having been developed much further by a variety of psychiatrists who have themselves been identified as phenomenological, anthropological, or sometimes both (May *et al.* 1958; Spiegelberg 1972; De Koning *et al.* 1982; Doerr-Zegers 2000; Kraus 2000). 'Phenomenological' refers to those components of the approach that were initially derived from Edmund Husserl (1970, 1973, 1983; Doerr-Zegers 2000,

p. 357), although other influences stem from Jean-Paul Sartre (1956), Michel Henry (1975), and Maurice Merleau-Ponty (2000). The methodological components of phenomenological psychiatry were initially delineated by Karl Jaspers (1963; Wiggins *et al.* 1997). 'Anthropological' connotes those elements that originated primarily with Martin Heidegger (1996, 2001). These thinkers, however, represent only points of origin (Binswanger 1963; Boss 1963). The psychiatrists who were influenced by them developed remarkably original and fruitful concepts and theories of their own (Natanson 1969; Blankenburg 1971; Kraus 1977; Ey 1978; Boss 1979; De Koning *et al.* 1982; Straus 1982; Naudin 1997; Tatossian 1997). Therefore, it is important to understand that 'phenomenological-anthropological psychiatry' signifies today an ongoing research programme rather than an achieved theory and set of categories. At this juncture in its development the research programme, we maintain, should incorporate results from empirical neuroscience as well as some concepts from the philosophical anthropologists, Max Scheler (1962), Helmut Plessner (1981), and Arnold Gehlen (1988), and the philosophical biologists, Hans Jonas (1966), Marjorie Grene (1974), and Adolf Portmann (1990a, 1990b).

A fundamental thesis of phenomenological-anthropological psychiatry is that the patient, in order not to be misconceived, must be comprehended as inseparably related to his or her world. Hence in this psychiatry one is always examining a relationship. In phenomenology this relationship is called 'intentionality' (Husserl 1973, 1983; Merleau-Ponty 2000). 'Intentionality' connotes the correlation between the experiencing subject and his or her experienced world. The notion of a correlation means that one cannot understand the human subject without also understanding the world *strictly as this subject experiences it*. From the anthropological point of view this correlation between the human subject and his or her experienced world is called 'being-in-the-world' (Binswanger 1963; Heidegger 1996). Hyphens appear in the phrase 'being-in-the-world' because this phrase designates a single complex reality, a unified whole. Of course, this whole is composed of component parts, but it should always be kept in mind that these parts must ultimately be understood in their relations to the other parts of the whole. Hence one may examine the part, mind, the part, brain, or the part, body; but these parts must ultimately be more fully construed in terms of their world-relatedness in order to comprehend them adequately. Mind, brain, body, and world are interrelated parts of the complex whole, 'being-in-the-world' (Zaner 1981).

In the phenomenological-anthropological tradition it is generally recognized that psychopathology must be conceptually based on psychology (Straus 1958, 1980). Restated phenomenologically, a theory of abnormal mental life presupposes a theory of normal mental life. Restated anthropologically, a theory of abnormal being-in-the-world presupposes a theory of normal being-in-the-world. Hence we shall begin our exposition by outlining some central features of normal human experience. In other words, we shall explicate some concepts of phenomenological-anthropological psychology.

We shall then indicate in what respect these features of normal experience are significantly altered in schizophrenic experience. In other terms, we shall develop some concepts of a phenomenological-anthropological psychopathology of schizophrenia. This characterization of some features of schizophrenia as a whole will permit us to focus on auditory hallucinations.

Some concepts of phenomenological-anthropological psychology: intentionality, synthesis, and constitution

In phenomenology the term 'intentionality' refers to the fact that mental processes are awarenesses of something (Husserl 1973, pp. 31–33, 39–41; 1983, pp. 211–235). Correlated with this feature of mental processes are the 'objects' of which they are aware. The word 'object' in this context is used by the phenomenologist in its broadest possible sense, the sense in which anything whatsoever can qualify as an 'object.' Thus an 'object' of mental life may be a physical thing, an algebraic formula, a divine power, a human being, a mythological creature, a character in a novel, the lost city of Atlantis, and so on. The object is to be considered exclusively as it is meant in the mental process that is aware of it. In other words, nothing is to be attributed to the object except the meaning it has for the mental process under examination.

If we examine individual mental processes in this manner, we note that the same object can be intended by a multiplicity of mental processes (Husserl 1973, pp. 41–44). For example, the same physical thing—indeed, even the same side of a physical thing—can be intended by a multiplicity of perceivings of it. Even the same brief sound can be intended in a multiplicity of awarenesses of it; once I have actually heard the sound, I can always recall the sound in memory again and again. In all of these mental processes their object can be intended as one and the same.

When an object is meant as identically the same by manifold mental processes, the phenomenologist speaks of a 'synthesis' (Husserl 1973, pp. 41–44). The mental processes are synthetically joined together by virtue of the intended sameness of their object. It is in the same sense that the phenomenologist speaks of 'constitution'. Objects are 'constituted' as the objects they are for mental life by virtue of the multiple mental syntheses through which those objects are intended as one and the same across time. For instance, throughout the exploration of a physical object the various features of it that come to be experienced are all intended as features of one and the same object. Hence we can speak of a 'unity' of these features by virtue of the fact that they are experienced as belonging to the same entity.

The word 'constitution' is to be taken here exclusively with regard to what can be found when we reflect on our own mental lives and recognize that objects, along with their various features, are meant as identically the same objects throughout a multiplicity of awarenesses of them. In other words, 'constitution' is not to be understood in a causal or metaphysical sense. Mental life does not 'make' objects in the ordinary sense of 'making', the sense in which a boatwright makes a boat or a baker makes a cake. Through a unified multiplicity of mental processes mental life is aware of objects as identically the same, and this alone is what is signified by 'constitution'.

Active and automatic syntheses

Processes arise in mental life in two basically different ways. Some mental processes arise because they are actively generated by an agency within mental life. Husserl gives a name to this active agency within mental life; he calls it 'the ego' (Husserl 1983, pp. 190–192). For example, the thoughts that are arising in my mental life as I formulate these sentences are being actively generated by my ego. These thoughts would not simply come into being 'on their own', even if I were wide-awake and seated at my computer. *I* must actively *think* them. It is to be noted that the theme of my awareness at any given moment is that to which my ego is attending. The mental acts actively generated by my ego are thematizing, attentive, or focal acts.

There are, by contrast, many processes that occur in my mental life without my ego actively producing them. For instance, the grassy playground of which my mental life is also aware as I focus on my daughter skillfully riding her bicycle appears only in the background of my awareness. This perceiving of the playground occurs automatically. Husserl described these mental processes as 'passive', but we believe that the term 'automatic' better conveys the manner in which such processes occur in mental life (Husserl 1973, pp. 41–46). To return to our example, as I actively thematize my daughter's skilled movements on her bicycle, my mental life 'on its own' sees the playground, just as it 'automatically' perceives the houses across the street. To convey this notion of automatic mental processes, we might also say that perceivings of items in the background arise 'behind the back' of the ego. Of course, my ego could choose to turn to the houses or the playground and focus on them. With this change of focus my awareness of my daughter's bicycle riding would recede into the background; and, as long as she remained in my field of vision, my awareness of her would occur only automatically.

Now it can be seen that some syntheses occur in mental life automatically while others, if they are to arise at all, must occur actively (Husserl 1973, pp. 56–61; 1983, pp. 272–285). Every time my daughter circles around the playground my mental life automatically intends the houses in the background as the same houses she passed before. If, however, I actively attend to the houses, compare them, and as a result judge, 'That brown house has three stories whereas all the others have two', such a judgment must be actively generated by my ego. Making this comparison among several objects and synthesizing the result in a judgment must occur actively.

Among the many automatic processes that occur in mental life, some function in syntheses that constitute the basic ontological components of what we take to be the reality of the world. For example, in some automatic syntheses objects are experienced as having spatial relations to one another; say, one object is intended as 'in front of' another. Moreover, other automatic syntheses intend events as occurring at different moments of time; for instance, one event may be experienced as taking place 'just before' another event occurred. Furthermore, some mental processes synthesize different events as causally related: one event may be experienced as the effect of another event that immediately preceded it. And finally, different features may be automatically meant by mental life as features of the same object: the hardness of the object I hold in my two hands may be intended as a feature of the hammer that I also watch as I, with some effort, lift it to hit a spike. All of these features, although given through different senses, are synthetically intended as features of the same object.

In order to indicate the ways in which the various ontological components of reality are constituted, we have elected to sketch space, time, causality, and objecthood separately. However, for our automatic mental lives, these ontological constituents of reality are not experienced as distinct. They are rather entirely interlaced and mutually implicated in one another. For example, objects that are synthetically intended as composed of multiple features are intended as possessing a typical causal efficacy. The hammer whose visual, tactual, and kinesthetic aspects are synthetically co-given as features of the same object is also intended as (causally) producing a typical sort of sound when it strikes a metal spike; just as the spike, as it is given with its visual and other aspects, is co-intended as (causally) emitting a typical kind of sound when struck by a metal hammer-head. Moreover, the various aspects of the hammer and spike are co-experienced as lying at a familiar spatial distance from one another; that is precisely why my body in its lifting and swinging of the hammer controls the hammer's thrust and movement as it does, guiding it to fall at a particular speed and angle toward the spike's head. Similarly, all of these bodily movements, feelings, and metallic sounds are synthetically intended as temporally related to one another; lifting the hammer is experienced as temporally earlier than the kinesthetic pressure of guiding it forcefully toward its target, and the as-yet-unheard sound of the meeting of the two is intended as just about to occur, in the near future. At the higher mental level of intellectual differentiation and abstraction my ego can actively conceptualize space, time, causality, and objecthood as distinct general categories. But at the level of hammering the spike these ontological aspects of things seamlessly form the fabric of one, unified world. Hence the basic ontological components of the world, space, time, causality, and the object-property relationship, are constituted at a fundamental level of automatic mental life through multiple constantly occurring syntheses.

A phenomenological-anthropological psychopathology of schizophrenia in its beginning: the overwhelming complexity of reality

From the phenomenological-anthropological point of view, much can and has been said about schizophrenic experience (Binswanger 1963; Blankenburg 1971; De Koning *et al.* 1982; Wiggins *et al.* 1990; Schwartz *et al.* 1992; Schwartz *et al.* 2005). The sole component we wish to discuss pertains to the weakening of the synthetic power of mental life in schizophrenia (Wiggins *et al.* 1990; Schwartz *et al.* 2005). This weakening affects syntheses at both the automatic and active levels of experience. Schizophrenic mental life no longer synthetically connects worldly events with one another or unites the features of objects with one another in the ways that normal mental life automatically and reliably does. This accounts for the instability, unforeseeability, and mutability of events and objects in a world disturbed by schizophrenia. Even the most fundamental components of this world fragment and restructure themselves.

Because of the weakening of mental syntheses in schizophrenia, some aspects of objects—that 'normal' subjects experience as clearly and obviously there—may not be synthetically joined with one another. A case reported by James Chapman of a patient in the early stages of schizophrenia illustrates this phenomenon. The patient says, 'Everything I see is split up. It's like a photograph that's torn to bits and put together again. If somebody moves or speaks, everything I see disappears quickly and I have to put it together again' (Chapman 1966, p. 229). Chapman quotes another patient who provides an example of the same kind of experience: 'I have to put things together in my head. If I look at my watch I see the watch, watchstrap, face, hands and so on, then I have got to put them together to get it into one piece' (Chapman 1966, p. 229). Notice that for this patient, as for the immediately preceding one, his automatic mental life does not synthetically unite the various features of the object, his watch. Hence this patient's experience shows that one basic onto-logical component of the world, namely, what we have called 'objecthood' or the fundamental fact that the world consists of individual objects in which various features are united, has crumbled. Because of this fragmenting of the 'objecthood' of the object, the patient's ego must then come to his aid and actively synthesize the constituents together as all features of one object. The objecthood of things must be actively rather than automatically constituted.

The failure of mental life in early schizophrenia to automatically constitute the spatial dimension of reality can be seen in another of Chapman's cases (1966, p. 230):

> I see things flat. Whenever there is a sudden change I see it flat. That's why I'm reluctant to go forward. It's as if there were a wall there and I would walk into it. There's no depth, but if I take time to look at things I can pick out the pieces like a jigsaw puzzle, then I know what the wall is made of. Moving is

like a motion picture. If you move, the picture in front of you changes. The rate of change in the picture depends on the speed of walking. If you run you receive the signals at a faster rate. The picture I see is literally made up of hundreds of pieces. Until I see into things I don't know what distance they are away.

Chapman summarizes the sorts of changes in the experience of lived space that the patient undergoes: ' ... the phenomena experienced by schizophrenic patients include alterations of the size, distance, and shape of objects (metamorphopsia), loss of stereoscopic vision, defective revisualization, and illusory acceleration of moving objects' (Chapman 1966, p. 230).

Max Scheler claimed, in a pioneering work on philosophical anthropology, that human beings are inherently 'world-open' (Scheler 1962, pp. 35–55). A later philosophical anthropologist, Arnold Gehlen, adopted and extended Scheler's term (Gehlen 1988, pp. 24–31, 248–255). In Gehlen's words, 'Human beings are exposed to an excess of stimulation toward which they remain world-open' (Gehlen 1988, p. 181). Gehlen specified that these 'stimuli' may be either internal or external ones; i.e. they may issue from within the individual's body or mind, for example, in inner urges or thoughts, or they may consist of sensory data coming from the external world. Because of this 'barrage of sensation and stimulation to which human beings are exposed' (Gehlen 1988, p. 181), they must develop means for reducing its complexity. The reduction of the complexity of both internal and external stimuli is, from the phenomenological point of view, the achievement of automatic syntheses. Gehlen maintained that if some such reduction of the complexity of stimuli were not automatically achieved, the ego of the person would be overburdened with the constant task of having to reduce this complexity through active thinking and selecting. Fortunately, for the normal person the acquisition of innumerable habits and skills that function automatically suffices to structure the person's world such that an adequate reduction of its complexity is achieved. Thanks to this reduction of complexity through the acquisition of skills and habits, the individual may devote his or her energies to 'higher level' intellectual and cultural accomplishments (Gehlen 1988, pp. 54–64).

With the weakening of its automatic syntheses during the early phases of schizophrenia, mental life loses the normal capacity to structure and organize the internal and external stimuli to which it is subjected. Hence the subject becomes too 'world-open'. Again Chapman furnishes several pertinent examples. These cases illustrate both the weakening of the syntheses and their common result, an overabundance of stimuli. The ego must then assume the daunting task of attempting to actively organize these stimuli. One patient reports (Chapman 1966, p. 231):

It's like a temporary blackout—with my brain not working properly—like being in a vacuum. I just get cut off from outside things and go into another world. This happens when the tension starts to mount until it bursts in my brain. It has to do with what is going on around me—taking in too much of my surroundings—vital not to miss anything. I can't shut things out of my mind and everything closes in on me. It stops me thinking and then the mind goes a blank and everything gets switched off. I can't pick things up to memorize because I am absorbing everything around me and take in too much so that I can't retain anything for any length of time—only a few seconds, and I can't do simple habits like walking or cleaning my teeth. I have to use all my mind to do these things without knowing it and I'm not controlling it. When this starts I find myself having to use tremendous control to direct my feet and force myself round a corner as if I'm on a bicycle. I want to move and the message goes from my brain down to my legs and they will not move in the right way. What I'm worried about is that I might get myself so controlled that I will cease to be a person. I find it difficult to cope with these situations that get out of control and I can't differentiate myself from other people when this comes on. I can't control what's coming in and it stops me thinking with the mind a blank.

Another patient reports the same sort of experience (Chapman 1966, p. 232):

Nothing settles in my mind—not even for a second. It just comes in and then it's out. My mind goes away—too many things come into my head at once and I lose control. I get afraid of walking when this happens. My feet just walk away from me and I've no control over myself. I feel my body breaking up into bits. I get all mixed up so that I don't know myself. I feel like more than one person when this happens. I'm falling apart into bits. My mind is not right if I walk and speak. It's better to stay still and not say a word. I'm frightened to say a word in case everything goes fleeing from me so that there's nothing in my mind. It puts me into a trance that's worse than death. There's a kind of hypnotism going on.

As these examples illustrate, the weakening of the automatic syntheses affects even the ones that constitute the basic ontological components of the world. Space, time, causality, and objecthood undergo vacillation, de-structuration, and reconfiguration. This de-structuring of the ontological components of reality we have in another essay called 'the unbuilding of the world'. And, in a manner that attempts to supplement the insights of R.D. Laing, we sought there to depict the 'ontological insecurity' that overcomes the experiencing self during early stages of schizophrenia when this unbuilding of reality occurs (Wiggins *et al.* 1990).

Schizophrenia as it continues: the reduction of complexity

In the beginning stages of schizophrenia the individual comes to be over-burdened by the complexity of his or her experience. As the disorder continues, however, this complexity must be somehow reduced. With the persistence of the patient's schizophrenia, the reduction does occur in several ways. In a way that we think remains ultimately 'un-understandable'—to appropriate Jaspers' term—new automatic syntheses do emerge in the patient's mental life and the person's world begins to achieve a novel structure. We deem the emergence of these new syntheses 'un-understandable' because we believe, like Jaspers, that it is inexplicable why the person's world comes to be re-constituted in the way it does rather than some other. Nevertheless, new syntheses do come to constitute the world in new ways.

The hitherto weak syntheses are not entirely eliminated by the emergence of new ones, however. The world of the person with schizophrenia still remains 'unbuilt' to some extent; and consequently its space, time, causality, and objects remain relatively unstructured.

Moreover, this novel make-up of reality that begins to take form may only slightly resemble the structure of the world that other people intersubjectively share. In other words, the world that other people take to be the 'real world' because it appears to them as the same for all, will cohere in only limited respects with the newly constituted world of the person with schizophrenia.

Another way in which the complexity of schizophrenic experience is reduced is through the emergence of hallucinations and delusions. Hallucinations and delusions impart an organization to the patient's mental life that at least minimally stabilize his or her world and self. Hallucinations and delusions thus at least partially diminish the extreme 'world-openness' that had strained mental life in the early stages of schizophrenia. Hallucinations and delusions thereby accord a degree of relief to this mental life, albeit a relief that is purchased at the price of severing the individual even further from the realm of experience shared with others. We turn now to hallucinations in schizophrenia.

An anthropological psychopathology of hallucinations in schizophrenia

We shall first advance an anthropological description of hallucinations in schizophrenia. An anthropological account offers two advantages:

1. It employs a less technical terminology than the phenomenological concepts we have sketched above. This, we hope, will provide a description of these highly unusual phenomena, hallucinations in schizophrenia, that will be more readily intelligible and accessible than the more technical phenomenological one we shall offer subsequently.

2. We can more easily survey the wide variety of features of hallucinations from this anthropological perspective precisely because its analyses are

less technical. Hence our account can provide a more comprehensive and well-rounded representation.

We shall follow the description of hallucinations in schizophrenia given by the anthropological psychiatrist, Erwin Straus (1958, 1980), and we shall confine our descriptions to auditory hallucinations since most schizophrenic ones fall within this sensory modality.

The first feature that should be noted is that the entire acoustic sphere in which the 'voices' emerge is distorted and abnormal. Nevertheless they are experienced in a manner that most resembles hearing; they are 'quasi-acoustic' (Straus 1958, p. 166).

Second, the 'voices' hallucinated by the person suffering from schizophrenia may not sound precisely like what we or they perceive ordinary human voices to sound like. 'Voice' may be selected to categorize them because they sound somewhat like a voice and moreover they convey a meaning.

Third, the auditory hallucinations of an individual with schizophrenia are given with a brute immediacy. The voice is simply there, and consequently it is unavoidably heard. Therefore, no one can disprove their existence through argument: the hallucinations themselves refute all logical disproof by their pre-logical, factual givenness (Straus 1958, p. 166; 1980, p. 287).

Fourth, something about this givenness lends to hallucinations a prominence or outstandingness in the person's experiential field that shoves other sensory givens as well as rational thought into the background. Hallucinations, in their brute, immediate givenness, compel the experiencing subject to thematize them and pay attention to them, to hear what they say.

Fifth, in the paradigmatic cases the sound of the voice occurs independently of a reference to the source of the sound (Straus 1958, p. 166). Granted, in some cases the identity of the speaker is co-given along with the voice, but in characteristically schizophrenic cases it is not. The subject may also attribute the voices to a group, for instance, a hidden cell of terrorists (Straus 1980, p. 286). Moreover, the subject may report that some extraordinary machine generates the voice (further evidence, we think, that the sounding voice alone is immediately given).

Sixth, the space in which the voices occur exhibits an abnormal structure. As Straus writes, 'The common order of things, in which each object has its place, with its own limited range and sphere of influence, is no longer valid. There are no boundaries, there is no measure and no standard of measurement, there is no organization of space into danger- and safety-zones' (Straus 1958, p. 166). Within this world, the voices have no definite spatial position. They may sound everywhere. They may call from unusual directions, from above or from below. The voices may penetrate the subject's body, his head or his heart. In various parts of his body he feels them rather than hears them (Straus 1980, p. 286). The occurrence of this experience confirms us in our interpretation of hallucinated 'voices' as only 'voice-like' rather than ordinary human voices.

Because they emerge in this generally uncanny space, the voices may elude all ordinary spatial limitations. They may not be dampened by walls. They may cross enormous distances. They may exert an overwhelming and inescapable power over the individual. The voices may attack and torment him. The patient hears these tormenting voices and is certain that they mean him and no one else. He has been singled out by them. The voices may issue commands to him alone, even very harsh ones (Straus 1966, pp. 166–167; 1980, p. 287).

Eugen Bleuler (1950, pp. 110–111) furnishes examples that illustrate several of the features enumerated above:

> The independence (of hallucinated voices) from real sensations was very emphatically expressed by Koeppe's patient: 'I could be stone deaf and still hear the voices'. Sometimes it appears to the patients 'as if they heard', which does not prevent them from opening the window a hundred times a day in obedience to such commands, or from making a special journey to the Rhine to jump in. The latter patient described the feeling: 'It was as if someone pointed his finger at me and said, "Go and drown yourself"'. It was as if we were speaking to each other. I don't hear it in my ears. I have a feeling in my breast. Yet it seems as if I heard a sound.'

A phenomenological psychopathology of schizophrenic hallucinations

The weakening of the automatic and active syntheses, excessive world-openness, and subsequent reduction in complexity in schizophrenia can be seen in auditory hallucinations. We claimed above that this weakening affects even the constitution of the most fundamental ontological components of reality, space, time, causality, and object. Moreover, what we also explained should be kept in mind: these various ontological components of reality are not experienced as distinct but rather as entirely interwoven with one another. Hence the weakening of the syntheses that connect temporal sequences with one another will *eo ipso* affect the relating of cause and effect to one another. The weakening of the syntheses that normally unite the various features of an object with one another will also weaken the experience of location in space and movement across distances.

Let us take the unbuilding of objects in schizophrenia. Since objects are no longer fully constituted as they are in normal mental life, only particular aspects or features of them may be given, separated from other aspects and features. Hence in the hearing of hallucinated voices, voices are intended without being synthetically joined to the objects and aspects of objects to which they would be automatically joined in normal mental life. For example, the voice is intended without the synthetic co-intending of a person speaking; the voice alone is meant. And since the individual inhabits a world whose ontological structure has been generally unbuilt, he may not even experience this voice without a source as especially unusual.

This awareness of voices without speakers also evinces the unbuilding of causality. The cause, a speaker, is not synthetically co-intended along with its effect, the spoken voice. Hence it is an unexpected and uncaused voice that directly addresses the hearer. The unbuilding of causality and space together is seen in the fact that barriers like brick walls and thick doors do not muffle the force or loudness of the voice. Spatial distances too have no effect on the volume of the voice. Location of the voice in space undergoes destructuration: the voice can be intended as sounding within the person's heart or leg.

Certainty of the reality of the voices

With this disordering of the basic ontological structure of voices, it would seem that the experience of them would progressively move from uncertainty to doubt to disbelief. The person with schizophrenia could be expected to finally conclude that the voices are unreal. On the contrary, however, in schizophrenia the reality of the voices is experienced as certain. We shall now sketch a phenomenological account of this persistent certainty.

The reality of the voices is not doubted, despite the ontological disorder in which they occur, because of three constituents of them. First is the brute facticity of their givenness. There are simply there; they sound forth, even when unexpected, uncaused, unwanted, or even feared. The person with schizophrenia is helpless in the presence of the voices: he/she can do nothing to avoid or escape hearing them. The patient is left entirely unfree and powerless: he/she *must* hear them speak to him/her; he/she *must* endure their pronouncements.

Second, the same voices repeatedly speak to him/her. They may say different things at different times, but the individual experiences the voices as the same ones that spoke to him/her before. Hence his/her mental life automatically identifies them as the same object across time. As we know from Husserl, this identifying of a sound as the same across several temporal phases is the most basic level at which an item is constituted as real. Indeed, their reality can come to be so constituted that the person's mental life automatically protends their recurrence sometime in the future.

Third, the voices usually have a meaning. They are not simply sounds; they are sounds that signify. And their signification carries a personal relevance for the patient. The patient's existence is somehow implicated—whether condemned, insulted, consoled or praised—in what the voices say. This personal involvement in the meaning of the voices makes them inescapable as constituent parts of the patient's life. We might even say that to some extent the voices constitute the patient: his being is connected to their meaning.

Conclusion

We have sought to develop a phenomenological-anthropological psychopathology of schizophrenia and of schizophrenic hallucinations in particular. We have thus assumed that schizophrenic hallucinations are their own specific kind of hallucination; i.e. we have presupposed that they can be adequately understood only when they are conceived in terms of the basic pathological features of schizophrenia in general. This assumption, we believe, is consistent with the traditional thrust of phenomenological-anthropological psychopathology: the main mental disorders manifest a particular kind of human being-in-the-world. The component parts of the disorder, then, must be theoretically situated within the general context of this mode of being-in-the-world. Only within this basic anthropological context can it become intelligible how the experiencing subject construes and deals with itself and with its experienced world.

References

Blankenburg, W. (1962). Aus dem phaenomenologischen erfahrungsfeld innerhalb der psychiatrie (unter beruecksichtigung methodologischer fragen). *Schweizer Archiv fuer Neurologie, Neurochirurgie und Psychiatrie*, Bd **90**, Helft 2.

Blankenburg, W. (1971). *Der verlust der natuerlichen selbstverstaendlichkeit: ein beitrag zure psychopathologie symptomarmer schizophrenien.* Stuttgart: Ferdinand Enke Verlag.

Bleuler, E. (1950). *Dementia praecox or the group of schizophrenias.* New York: International Universities Press.

Binswanger, L. (1963). *Being-in-the-world.* New York: Harper and Row.

Boss, M. (1963). *Psychoanalysis and Daseinanalysis.* New York: Basic Books, Inc.

Boss, M. (1979). *Existential foundations of medicine and psychology.* New York: Jason Aronson.

Chapman, J. (1966). The early symptoms of schizophrenia. *British Journal of Psychiatry,* **112**: 225–251.

De Koning, A.J.J. and Jenner, F.A. (ed.) (1982). *Phenomenology and psychiatry.* New York: Grune and Stratton.

Doerr-Zegers, O. (2000). Existential and phenomenological approach to psychiatry. In: *New Oxford textbook of psychiatry* (ed. M.G. Gelder, J.J. Lopez-Ibor, and N. Andreasen). Oxford: Oxford University Press.

Ey, H. (1978). *Consciousness: a phenomenological study of being conscious and becoming conscious.* Bloomington: Indiana University Press.

Gehlen, A. (1988). *Man: his nature and place in the world.* New York: Columbia University Press.

Grene, M. (1974). *The understanding of nature: essays in the philosophy of biology.* Dordrecht, Holland: D. Reidel Publishing Co.

Heidegger, M. (1996). *Being and time.* Albany: State University of New York Press.

Heidegger, M. (2001). *Zollikon seminars* (ed. M. Boss). Evanston: Northwestern University Press.

Henry, M. (1975). *Philosophy and phenomenology of the body*. The Hague: Martinus Nijhoff.

Husserl, E. (1970). *The crisis of european sciences and transcendental phenomenology*. Evanston: Northwestern University Press.

Husserl, E. (1973). *Cartesian meditations: an introduction to phenomenology*. The Hague: Martinus Nijhoff.

Husserl, E. (1983). *Ideas pertaining to a pure phenomenology and to a phenomenological philosophy, first book*. The Hague: Martinus Nijhoff Publishers.

Jaspers, K. (1963). *General psychopathology*. Chicago: University of Chicago Press.

Jonas, H. (1966). *The phenomenon of life: toward a philosophical biology*. New York: A Delta Book.

Kraus, A. (1977). *Sozialverhalten und psychose manisch-depressiver: eine existenz- und rollenanalytische untersuchung*. Stuttgart: Ferinand Enke Verlag.

Kraus, A. (2000). Phenomenological-anthropological psychiatry. In: *Contemporary psychiatry*, vol. 1, *Foundations of psychiatry* (ed. F.Henn, N.Sartorius, H. Helmchen, and H. Lauter). New York: Springer Verlag.

May, R., Angel, E., and Ellenberger, H.F. (1958). *Existence: a new direction in psychiatry and psychology*. New York: Simon and Schuster.

Merleau-Ponty, M. (2000). *Phenomenology of perception*. New York: Routledge.

Natanson, M. (ed.) (1969). *Psychiatry and philosophy*. New York: Springer Verlag.

Naudin, J. (1997). *Phenomenologie et psychiatrie: les voix et lachose*. Toulouse: Presses Universitaires du Mirail.

Plessner, H. (1981). *Die stufen des organischen und der mensch, gesammelte schriften IV*. Frankfurt am Main: Suhrkamp Verlag.

Portmann, A. (1990a). *Essays in philosophical zoology: the living form and the seeing eye*. Lewiston: The Edwin Mellen Press.

Portmann, A. (1990b). *A zoologist looks at humankind*. New York: Columbia University Press.

Sartre, J.-P. (1956). *Being and nothingness: an essay in phenomenological ontology*. New York: Philosophical Library, Inc.

Scheler, M. (1962). *Man's place in nature*. New York: The Noonday Press.

Schwartz, M.A. and Wiggins, O.P. (1992). The phenomenology of schizophrenic delusions. In: *Phenomenology, language & schizophrenia* (ed. M. Spitzer, F. Uehlein, M.A. Schwartz, and C. Mundt). New York: Springer-Verlag.

Schwartz, M.A., Wiggins, O.P. Naudin, J., and Spitzer, M. (2005). Rebuilding reality: a phenomenology of aspects of chronic schizophrenia. *Phenomenology and Cognitive Science*, **4**: 91–115.

Spiegelberg, H. (1972). *Phenomenology in psychology and psychiatry: a historical introduction*. Evanston: Northwestern University Press.

Stephens, G.L., and Graham, G. (2000). *When self-consciousness breaks: alien voices and inserted thoughts*. Cambridge, MA: The MIT Press.

Straus, E. (1958). Aesthesiology and hallucinations. In: *Existence: a new direction in psychiatry and psychology* (ed. R. May, E. Angel, and H.F. Ellenberger), pp. 139–169. New York: Simon and Schuster.

Straus, E. (1980). *Phenomenological psychology*. New York: Garland Publishing, Inc.

Straus, E. (1982). *Man, time, and world: two contributions to anthropological psychology*. Pittsburgh: Duquesne University Press.

Tatossian, A. (1997). *La phenomenologie des psychoses*. Paris: L'Art du Comprendre.

Wiggins, O. P., Schwartz, M.A., and Northoff, G. (1990). Toward a Husserlian phenomenology of the initial stages of schizophrenia. In: *Philosophy and psychopathology* (ed. M. Spitzer and B.A. Maher). New York: Springer-Verlag.

Wiggins, O. and Schwartz, M.A. (1997). Edmund Husserl's influence on Karl Jaspers' phenomenology. *Philosophy, Psychiatry, Psychology—PPP,* **4**(1).

Zaner, R.M. (1981). *The context of self: a phenomenological inquiry using medicine as a clue*. Athens: Ohio University Press.

7 Schizophrenia and the sixth sense

Giovanni Stanghellini

Understanding and schizophrenia

Listening to a person affected by schizophrenia is a puzzling experience for more than one reason. If I let his/her words actualize in me the experiences he/she reports, instead of merely taking them as symptoms of an illness, the rock of certainties on which my life is based may be shaken in its most fundamental features. The sense of being *me*, the one who is now seeing this sheet, reading these lines, and turning this page; the experience of perceptual unity between my seeing this book, touching its cover, and smelling the scent of freshly printed pages; the feeling that it is me the one who is having this strange growing anxiety; and it is again me the one who agrees or disagrees with what I am reading; the sense of belonging to a community of people, of being attuned to the others, and involved in my own actions and future; the taken-for-grantedness of all these features of everyday life may be put at jeopardy. Although my efforts to understand, by suspending all clinical judgement, allows me to see this person's self-reports as a possible configuration of human consciousness, I must admit that there is something incomprehensible and almost inhuman in these experiences, something that makes me feel radically different from the person I am listening to. What do I share with someone who says that he can perceive his thoughts as quasi-material objects in his head? Or that he experiences the body or some part of it not as his own, but as a mechanism capable of feeling, perceiving, and acting? Or that he feels so disconnected from all the others that he is trying to find out an algorithm suitable for interacting with other people?

This supposed incomprehensibility (Jaspers 1913) has been for decades a cast-iron alibi for many and has been taken by some as a legitimate reason to give up understanding and to look for causes and explanations (see Eilan 2000; Heinimaa 2003). What is challenging and tackling my capacity to understand these experiences is that they reveal a special kind of non-understanding. If I try to understand them, I will also understand some basic features of my own way to experience and to make sense of my experiences, and by doing so I will feel displaced from what holds fast in my life and seems intrinsically obvious and convincing. Schizophrenic 'abnormalities' exhibit usually unnoticed conditions of normal daily experience (Zahavi and Parnas 1999). When I listen to my schizophrenic partner, I may have the opportunity to see in front of me what I cannot be aware of when I am turned to the life-world in the so-called 'natural' attitude. If I try to follow him, I am at risk of seeing that most (if not all) of what I consider 'natural' is indeed not such and can be put in brackets, suspended. If I turn away my gaze, as he does, from the life-world, I will become engaged in perceiving, almost as concrete objects and material processes, what was hidden to me when I was immersed in the life-world, as a part of it. I will nearly see my self, my body, and my world from another place. If I was previously feeling, perceiving, and acting, I will make these feelings, perceptions, and actions into external objects to be explored.

There is not much more incomprehensibility in the schizophrenic existence than in the modern mind (Sass 1992): they are both victims of the same attitude of spatialization and concretization of 'life' in order to make of it an object of knowledge, as philosophers and psychopathologists have shown (Bergson 1927; Gabel 1962; Foucault 1963; Minkowski 1968; Jonas 1994). The following quotation from Minkowski (1929) makes this point, at the criss-cross between philosophy and psychopathology, very clear:

> Intuition and intelligence, the living and the dead, the flowing and the still, becoming and being, lived time and space, these are the diverse expressions of the two fundamental principles that, with Bergson, govern our life and our activity. [...] We came to distinguish two large groups of psychopatho-logical phenomena: the former is characterised by the loss of intuitive elements and a morbid hypertrophy of rational ones; the latter shows a diametrical opposite state of things.

If I bracket the common-sense attitude, I will find myself at the outskirts of life. This move, and only this, allows me to investigate and know theoretically what I previously sensed practically and intuitively. The experiences of a schizophrenic person remind me that practical sense and intellectual know-ledge are antithetical. This feeling of displacement has been, right or wrong, also considered the kernel of the 'encounter' with the schizophrenic: a preco-cious feeling of alterity (*praecox Gefuehl*, Ruemke 1941) that I feel in front of him. Indeed, this displacement hides a much more complex structure. It is not just an intuitive and pre-categorial diagnostic devise. It hides some of the secrets of the alterity of the schizophrenic existence, which the phenomeno-logical gaze helps to reveal. In the first place, I have the sensation that he is not there where I see him. The here-and-now experience is at stake. He seems to look and to listen from another place. I hope that the meaning of this puzzling sensation will become clearer and clearer in this paper. For the moment, let us say that he does not seem to have an immediate perception of what is going on, but that he is having a sensation, elaborating this sensation, and structuring its parts and the context in which it takes place in a meaningful whole: 'I do not taste the soup, but its ingredients', a young schizophrenic person told me, 'Sensing the whole taste of the soup requires a reconstruction'. A schizophrenic person is sometimes like the spectator of the single steps of his perceptive processes—*natura transcendentaliter spectata* (nature watched from elsewhere). This fragmented experience can also be illustrated as what happens to viewers of a movie when the film breaks: instead of watching passively and being absorbed by what goes on in the screen, the viewer first observes the shot with an increasing feeling of unreality concerning what is represented in it, then turns their eyes towards the shaft of light and finally to the room of the cine-projector. The self-reports by schizophrenic persons suggest that the distance between the perceiver and the perceived object becomes somehow manifest—or, if you prefer, the timing and the process of perception becomes spatialized. 'Sometimes it is as if my sensations remained out of my head.' 'I am not sure of what I have seen, or that it was me the one who saw that object.' Sensations may remain out of one's head, or the feeling of myness of the sensations may be missing. A schizophrenic person gave me this representation of such an experience of de-realization, which goes hand in hand with the spatialization of the perceptual process: 'Life is an illusion,' he said, 'because it is seen through a brain'. This person also described his becoming aware of the otherwise implicit process of visual scanning of an object:

> When I watch something, I would like to see it better. While watching, say, a tree, I can but *scan* with my eye its profile and count its sides. For instance, a dog is seven parts. I called this *counting*, because for me everything in this way is reducible to a certain number according to its sides. It started as a sort of game, then it turned into a kind of obsession. I *become aware* of my eye watching an object.

Indeed, he describes himself in this case as a mechanical scanner: he watches himself from a third-person perspective, instead of being embedded in his own experiences as the owner of these experiences. He conceives of himself, and especially of his brain, as a computational device. I feel him displaced from the here-and-now since he is not directly and immediately in touch with worldly objects and persons; he experiences these as objects of a perceptual process and he is more involved in the inspection of the process of perception, than in the phenomena that appear to him. In phenomenological terms, this is called noetic experience, which was described elsewhere in a group of persons oscillating between the obsessive and the schizophrenic conditions (Ballerini and Stanghellini 1989, 1993). A person affected by schizophrenia is also displaced from his perceptual process, and therefore he can become aware (although in a rudimentary way) of them. His gaze is turned inside—he watches, so to say, his eyes watching. The precocious feeling of alterity

I have in front of him may be the outcome of the fact that he is not watching me, at the moment, but he is watching the way he is watching me.

A second layer of displacement concerns the feeling I have that something is lacking while trying to communicate with a schizophrenic person. Phenomen-ologists think that schizophrenic persons show an enhanced aptitude to the bracketing of common-sense experiences and shared meanings (Blankenburg 1969, 1971). This is supposed to be one of the major features of the vulnerability to schizophrenia (Stanghellini 1997). As we have just seen, they can bracket the natural attitude, i.e. being turned to the object of consciousness, and have access to the way their consciousness appropriates the object to itself. This is not, for them, an achievement, but so to say a natural experience. Whereas for non-schizophrenic persons this performance requires an un-natural exercise, for people with schizophrenia it is part of the natural attitude situated in ordinary life. The same happens with the meanings we usually attach to words, so that we often lack a common ground for understanding each other. I may for instance have the impression that we use the same word but we attach different meanings to it. Thus, I have the sensation that he does not share the same horizon of meanings that I take for granted to share with the other persons I usually get in touch with. Not only does he show an hyper-extension of the horizon of meanings, reflecting a flood of free-floating associations (Schwartz *et al.* 1997). The problem here concerns the situational relevance (Schutz 1970) of one meaning that should be (and is not) selected from the multitudes of those that are grammatically correct. As with the learning and the use of everyday language (Bourdieu 1980), the real problem is not the capacity to produce an infinite number of grammatically correct sentences, but the capacity to generate the sentences really adapted to the infinite number of situations that present us. What seems to be missing in schizophrenia is not only the cognitive capacity to select an appropriate verbal behaviour, but the emotional attunement between the person and the situation (Parnas and Bovet 1991).

This feeling of displacement in human relationships shows a further layer of the encounter with a schizophrenic person. He may complain that he needs to study the 'rules of the social game' that all the others know without making any effort to learn them. It is not uncommon that schizophrenics become *naif ethologists* or *naif psychologists* to overcome their separatedness from the human world and to establish a quasi-mathematical system of key-rules to appropriately interact with the others. It is a matter of debate whether this separatedness is just a consequence of the lack of a body of propositional knowledge about the 'language games' played in human societies, as cognitive psychologists hold; or else a problem arising from a disorder of emotional-affective, non-propositional attunement with the others (Stanghellini and Ballerini 2002):

Although an explicit algorithm is what is being looked for by this young person, something else than propositional knowledge about human interaction is what is missing here. What is missing is a pre-conceptual link between this person and the other persons, a pre-cognitive, intuitive experience and direct perception of the others' emotional life.

Schizophrenia in the light of Aristotle

The senses of common sense: *koiné aisthesis* and *sensus communis*

Schizophrenic persons undergo a special kind of depersonalization: the living body becomes a functioning body, a thing-like mechanism in which feelings, perceptions, and actions take place as if they happened in an outer space. They also endure a special kind of de-socialization: the interpersonal scene becomes an empty stage on which the main actor is unaware of the plot, out of touch from the role he is acting and unable to make sense of what the others are doing. Is there a common root for this twofold experience of de-realization? Is the feeling of disconnectedness that takes place in the realm of the experience of oneself somehow related to the experience of disconnectedness taking place in the inter-subjective scene? Do the crises of the self-experience and that of the social self share a common conceptual organizer? These questions are of capital importance if we want to understand schizophrenia not as a contingent agglomeration of disconnected symptoms, but as Parnas (2000) has suggested, as a unitary psychopathological condition organized around the self-disorder autism complex.

What follows is just one way to tell the story of the supposed missing link between self-experience and inter subjectivity, and their disorders. It is nearly like a detective story, one of those hard-boiled plots in which the runaway changes names and identities to shake off the investigators, but does not succeed to cover all his tracks. It is, as in some of the best thrillers, the very first page of this story that puts us on the right track and allows us to catch the culprit red-handed.

To my knowledge, it was Aristotle who wrote the first page of this story. So there is at least a historical interest in Aristotle's ideas for the understanding of schizophrenia. This is the first answer to the question: why look at Aristotle? Obviously, it is not the only one. A more philosophical reason is that concepts like 'self-awareness' and 'common sense' are enjoying a revival in the psychopathological studies on schizophrenia (see Sass 2001) and Aristotle's philosophy of mind provides a deep account of both these concepts with the advantage that he frames both of them inside a single theory based on the notion of *koiné aisthesis* (literally: common sense; *aisthesis* means that perception is the common ground of the internal and the social dimensions of awareness). There is a crucial question for the philosophical understanding of schizophrenia: is the act by which we are aware of ourselves an act of rational thought or an act of sense? Aristotle decided in favour of sense (Kahn 1966). We have seen how sensory (implicit, pre-reflexive) self-awareness is disordered in schizophrenic persons and how noetic (explicit, reflexive) self-awareness may take its place. Aristotle frames sensory self-awareness inside his theory of *koiné aisthesis*. This move allows him to describe this form of self-awareness as an embodied phenomenon: he recognizes such self-awareness as an act of *aisthesis*, hence as an essentially embodied act (Kahn 1992). Last but not least, through the concept of *koiné aisthesis* (as we will see) Aristotle bridges this form of embodied self-awareness to the phenomenon of supramodal perception (sensory integration), which has turned out (in today's developmental psychology) to be the basis of social awareness and in doing so he provides the philosophical background for the joint understanding of the two main roots of schizophrenic psychopathology, i.e. disordered self-awareness and autism. Let us analyse all these points in detail.

In Aristotle's *De Anima*, *koiné aisthesis* (common sense) has two different functions: the first is to combine the different modalities (*koiné dunamis*) of specific senses (*aisthesis idia*) like hearing, touching, seeing, etc.; the second is to accompany each sensation with the *awareness* of the sensation itself.

In this first sense (*De Anima*, III, 1, 425a, 14), *koiné aisthesis* is the common root of the outer senses. Aristotle's argument goes as follows: each sense perceives one class of sensible objects. However, something must happen in virtue of which when different qualities, e.g. colour and smell, happen to meet in one sensible object, we are aware of both contemporaneously. Also, there is not a special sense-organ for the 'common sensibles' (*koiné aistheta*), i.e. for the objects that we perceive incidentally through this or that special sense, like movement, rest, shape, size, number, unity. In the case of the 'common sensibles' there is in us—says Aristotle—a general sensibility, which enables us to perceive them directly; there is therefore no special sense required for their perception. The second function of *koiné aisthesis* is to accompany each sensation with the awareness of the sensation itself (*De Anima* 425b, 427a), since this awareness cannot belong to one specific sense organ (*De Somno*, 2, 455a, 13). Aristotle argues that, since it is through the senses that we are seeing or hearing, it must be either by sight that we are aware of seeing, or by some sense other than sight. But the sense that gives us this new sensation, i.e. awareness of the sensation itself, should perceive both sight and its object: so that either (1) there will be two senses both percipient of the same sensible object; or (2) the sense must be percipient of itself. Further, even if the sense that perceives sight were different from sight, we must either fall into an infinite regress, or we must somewhere assume a sense which is aware of itself.

Aristotle warns us from any reification of this function and clearly states that *there is no need to postulate a sixth sense*. Those above described are all functions of the soul—they are not intellectual functions. They are located in the heart, which is the organ in which the blood carries all the sensations from different modalities to their point of integration (*De Memoria* 450a, 10). The first function of *koiné aisthesis* affords the experience of a perceptual unity, and the perception of those qualities that belong to all sense modalities ('common sensations') and do not belong to one specific sense modality, such as loudness (hearing), brightness (seeing), smoothness (touching), and so on. The second function affords the experience of oneself as the subject of one's own perceptual experiences—it is the source of self-awareness. What we call self-awareness is for Aristotle a direct perception of oneself while perceiving something: 'The common power accompanying all the senses, by which we perceive that we are seeing and hearing' (*De Somno* 455a, 15). Self-awareness is for Aristotle sensory self-awareness, it 'belongs to the animal principle of sentience' (Kahn 1992). It is an embodied act, an immediate act, which happens in the flesh and which Aristotle elsewhere compares with touch (*De Somno* 455a, 22–24), and as such must be distinguished from noetic self-awareness, which is disembodied and intellectual. This is a crucial point both in Aristotle's philosophy of mind (Kahn 1966, 1992), and also, as we will see, in the phenomenology of schizophrenia.

The integration between different sense modalities, and the integration between sensations and awareness are the functions attributed by Aristotle to *koiné aisthesis*. Quite a different meaning is attributed in the Latin world to the corresponding concept of *sensus communis*. *Sensus communis*—the literal translation of *koiné aisthesis* into Latin—in the Roman classics and in the humanist tradition means habit, taste, judgement (Gadamer 1986). There is here an apparent discontinuity between a naturalistic and a humanistic view of common sense, which parallels the seeming discontinuity that we observe in schizophrenia between self-disorders (depersonalization) and autism (de-socialization).

Sensus communis designates self-evident, commonly shared notions and truths—*koiné ennoia* according to the stoic tradition. *Koiné ennoia* is what we would nowadays call 'social knowledge' and as such *sensus communis* is what establishes the connection between individuals and society. After the metamorphosis into *sensus communis*, *koiné aisthesis* has thus become a *social sense*.

Are *koiné aisthesis* and *sensus communis* different facets of the same phenomenon? Is Cicero's, Reid's, and Vico's common sense the same concept that we find in Aristotle? Do they share a common conceptual root? Or is it misleading to look for analogies between them? (See Fig. 7.1.)

Koiné aisthesis and social attunement: the bodily basis of inter-subjectivity

Aristotle was right: from the earliest days of our life, we experience a world of perceptual unity. For the baby, the touched and the smelled breast is the same breast: supramodal perception is a primordial phenomenon (Stern 2000). The

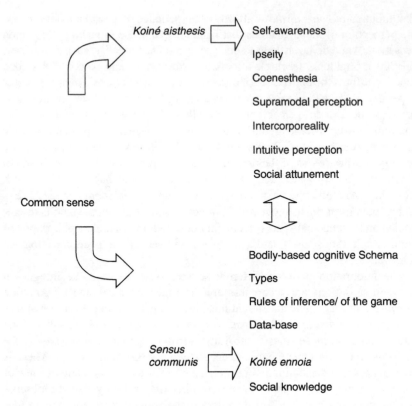

Koiné aisthesis → Self-awareness

Ipseity

Coenesthesia

Supramodal perception

Intercorporeality

Intuitive perception

Social attunement

Common sense

Bodily-based cognitive Schema

Types

Rules of inference/ of the game

Data-base

Sensus communis → Koiné ennoia

Social knowledge

Fig. 7.1 The family-tree of common sense.

breast emerges as an already integrated, global experience, and not from the *post hoc* combination between tactile and olfactory perceptions—as associationism supposed was the case (Hunt 1995; Butterworth 1999; Lagerstee 1999). Infants appear to have an innate capacity to translate the information received from one sensory modality into another sensory modality. Information is supposed to transcend one modality and exist in some supra-modal form. Moreover, infants experience a world whose basic features are akin to Aristotle's 'common sensibles': they do not experience sights, sounds, and touches, but rather shapes, intensities, and temporal patterns (Stern 2000). This kind of perception echoes Aristotle's *koiné aisthesis*. 'Common sensibles' are the bricks with which the interpersonal world of the infant is built. The primary organizers of the emergent sense to be a 'self' in the life of an infant are three, according to Stern (2000):

(1) amodal perception, i.e. the capacity to grasp objects across appearance in different sense modalities;

(2) vitality affects, i.e. the ability to capture the dynamic character of an experience through its qualitative spatio-temporal feature (e.g. a burst of anger or a crescendo of fear); and

(3) physiognomic perception, i.e. the perception of the others' emotions and affects based on perception of the other's physiognomy (e.g. facial expression).

Amodal perception and vitality affects reflect Aristotle's concept of *koiné aisthesis* and *koiné aistheta*, respectively, i.e. sensory-to-sensory integration. Physiognomic perception plays a major role in the constitution of inter-subjectivity. It is a kind of pre-conceptual and pre-reflective supramodal perception based on imitation (Butterworth 2000) or sensory-to-motor integration. This means that the understanding of the others' physiognomy is probably based on a transfer of corporeal schema or inter corporeality (Merleau-Ponty 1945). 'The transfer of corporeal schema, the immediate (that is, reflexive-but-unreflected) perceptual linkage through which we recognize other beings as like unto ourselves [is] the phenomenal ground of syncretic sociability, pathetic identification, or, in a word, inter-subjectivity' (Dillon 1998). When the baby perceives his mother's happy face, tone, actions, etc., he imitates her facial expression, voice, movements, etc., and then feels her happiness himself. It is by reproducing in himself the bodily schema of the happy mother that he recognizes that her behaviour 'means' happiness. Sensory-to-motor integration plays a major role in the phenomenon of inter-subjectivity (Gallese and Goldman 1998; Gallese 2000; Ramachandran and Hubbard 2001). A set of visuo-motor neurons called 'mirror neurons' has been discovered in the monkey's premotor cortex (Di Pellegrino *et al.* 1992; Rizzolati *et al.* 1996). These neurons fire both when a particular action is performed and when the same action, performed by another individual, is observed. It is hypothesized that mirror neurons do an internal simulation of the actions observed and as such are involved in 'action understanding': meaning is assigned to an observed action by matching it on the same neuronal circuits that generate it (Gallese 2000). This is a tempting biological model of the neuronal basis for Merleau-Ponty's intercorporeality, i.e. the intuitive recognition of others' intentions and mental states through the identification with the other's body. According to simulation theory (Gallese and Goldman 1998), sensory-to-motor integration, by tracking or matching other people's mental states with resonant states of one's own, plays a pivotal role in the constitution of inter-subjectivity.

Consequently, Aristotle's *koiné aisthesis* is not only the basis for the integrated perception of the physical world, but also for the meaningful perception of the others' behaviours in the social world. This concept is originally expressing both embodiment and attunement to the social world (Hunt 1995). The bodily and the social selves share the same experiential foundations (Sheets-Johnstone 1999). *Koiné aisthesis* is the basis for the phenomenon of emotional-affective attunement (Stern 2000), which is the prerequisite for the emergence of the social self and of inter-subjectivity. It is the root of the learning of our shared world picture, which we absorb during our psychological and cultural development or *Bildung*. It is the non-propositional, emotional-affective prerequisite for the acquisition of commonsensical propositional knowledge (*koiné ennoia* or *sensus communis*).

The relationship between social attunement and *sensus communis* is of great philosophical and psychopathological interest. Wittgenstein's remarks on this topic are enlightening. He compares common sense to a 'nest of propositions' (Wittgenstein 1969): 'What stands fast does so, not because it is intrinsically obvious or convincing; it is rather held fast by what lies around it'. We may call this the nest-effect: explicit teachings are held fast by what lies around them, i.e. a background (*der ueberkommene Hintergund*) that is not a topic of overt reasoning, or asserting, or doubting. This implicit background for social knowledge, we may argue, is a non-propositional flow of communications and therefore immune from doubts, hence certain. It owes its character of certainty to its being philosophically ungrounded. The taken-for-granted is ungrounded in explicit arguments, therefore it is certain. If the taken-for-granted becomes explicit, *ipso facto* it becomes an object for reflection and doubting. This is the common premise for philosophy and insanity. This kind of non-propositional background, which conveys propositional knowledge, is what we have called social attunement. Social attunement 'permits to convey to the infants what is shareable, that is, which subjective experiences are within and which are beyond the pale of mutual consideration and acceptance [...]. [This is] one of the most potent ways that a parent can shape the development of a child's subjective and interpersonal life' (Stern 2000). Is this function of *koiné aisthesis*, now visible in the light of developmental psychology and neurobiology, the link with the notion of *sensus communis* as we find it in the Latin world and in eighteenth-century philosophy?

Koiné aisthesis, self-awareness, and other-awareness: the mutual constraints of inter-subjectivity and embodiment

The first function attributed by Aristotle to *koiné aisthesis* concerns the bodily basis of inter-subjectivity, the other function is related to self-awareness. We will take into account Aristotle's explanation concerning how these two functions are related in the next section; what we know for certain is that the modifications of these two facets of *koiné aisthesis* are the fundamental domains in the phenomenology of schizophrenic psychoses (Parnas 2000). Self-awareness is not just being conscious of a foreign object, but to be conscious of my experience of that object as well—of my experience of that object as my own. To be self-aware is being aware of things in the world, including my own presence in the world. When I touch this table, I am not only aware of the table, but also of my hand that is touching it. As Zahavi and Parnas (1999) put it:

> To be self-aware is not to apprehend a pure self apart from the experience, but to be acquainted with an experience in its first-personal mode of givenness, that is, from 'within'.

The integration between sensation and awareness is the ground for becoming a self, i.e. to have an immediate experience of oneself. This non-reflexive, non-propositional acquaintance with oneself is called 'ipseity' (Henry 1963) or auto-affection. Ipseity is an experience, not a mediated phenomenon arising from introspection, or reflexivity, or from an eidetic intuition. It is the implicit and tacit presence to oneself, the self-feeling of one's self. Out of ipseity no self is possible. It not only affords the character of *my-ness* of an experience, but also the experience of oneself as the subject having that experience. It is the direct access to oneself as the subject of an experience, the sense of being the centre of one's own experiences, 'the implicit sense of being a centre of consciousness and source of intentionality' (Sass 2000). Ipseity, or as Aristotle would say sensory self-awareness, carries out much of the work that Descartes attributed to the disembodied *cogito*: my perceiving that I think (or have feelings and emotional states) is an act of *aisthesis* and as such an essentially embodied act (Kahn 1992).

Does ipseity grow like a pearl inside an oyster? Or are there mutual constraints between ipseity and the environment, and especially inter-subjectivity? Henry (1963) sees ipseity as a primary emergent phenomenon, prior to anything we are aware of, 'not mediated by anything foreign or external to the self' (Zahavi 2001). However, ipseity can also be seen as a phenomenon that is reinforced by self-perception—the experience of oneself as the subject of one's own perceptual experiences. The shaping of my sense of a core self, the self-feeling of my own self is also based on my perception of myself while perceiving something. As Aristotle put it: to perceive that we are perceiving is to perceive that we exist (*Ethica Nichomachea* 1170a).

The relationship between self-experience and the social self are very tight. It is acknowledge the crucial role of the lived body in this process that grounds attunement. Social attunement is intercorporeality, and as such is based on a 'smooth' perception of my own bodily schema. There is a circular process involving the emergence of a core- and a social self. A crucial point in the psychopathology of schizophrenia is that anomalous self-experiences are associated with disorders of inter-subjectivity. The self is not purely personal. Self-awareness is a social phenomenon having an interactive and linguistic structure. Social attunement is involved in shaping and preserving ipseity and its abnormalities entail disorders of ipseity, as shown by 'strange situation' protocols (Ainsworth *et al.* 1978): when social attunement is disordered, not only the others appear enigmatic and the social environment uncanny, but also my sense of my self and the boundaries between myself and the others may become blurred. Abnormal attunement may de-structure self-perception, but the reverse is also true—attunement may help to re-structure one's own self-experience as in the following self-report:

> I cannot feel my *being* anymore. If I cannot feel myself, I cannot have control over an action. If I cannot feel myself, I cannot feel. I cross the street, and I don't realize it, and I must cross it again. I wash myself, and I am not aware of it. I eat, and I don't perceive what I am doing. I am not aware of the presence of my own person. What I lack is spontaneity. With spontaneity, one realizes that one has done something even without being aware of it. Since I lack spontaneity, then I must use reason in order to be aware of something. And with reason, in order to be aware of something, one must be cognizant of what one is doing. One must think of it. But reason at the end exasperates you! If one thinks of all one is doing, things and actions become more and more unreal. I cannot say 'I' in relation to myself, but only in relation to the others. *But when I am here talking with you all this does not happen.*

In this vignette, lack of self-awareness ('I cannot feel my 'being' anymore... I am not aware of the presence of my person') entails hyper-reflexivity ('One must be cognizant of what one is doing'), establishing a vicious circle ('Reason exasperates you... things and actions become more and more unreal'). Lack of self-awareness also engenders sensory-motor disintegration ('If I cannot feel myself, I cannot have control over an action') and the loss of the capacity to have sensations. There is not an internal sense of ipseity, but only an external one ('I cannot say "I" in relation to myself, but only in relation to the others'). Only empathic attunement mitigates this loop ('When I am talking with you all this does not happen').

There is also strict connection between my self-experience and *sensus communis*, since I apprehend myself through typificatory schemes derived from the data-base of social knowledge, as it appears evident in the case of bodily sensations (Stanghellini 1994). 'The perception of our body constantly needs a metaphor' (Ey 1973): metaphors are needed to make sense of the experience of our own body, to metabolize and normalize bodily perceptions. We derive these metaphors from *sensus communis*, and in this sense the perception of our body is conditioned by social, public symbols. When we cannot find these expressions in *sensus communis*, we find ourselves between the devil and the deep blue sea. Abnormal bodily sensations (i.e. coenesthopathic troubles), which often characterize the prodromal phase of schizophrenic psychoses (Huber 1957; Parnas 2000), reveal a discrepancy between the perceptual level and the level of socially shared linguistic categories. On the one side, the impossibility to find metaphors for normalizing one's bodily experience may entail perceiving one's own body, completely or partially, as an object outside of oneself. On the other side, the urge to form

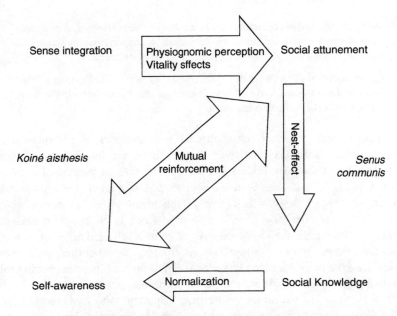

Fig. 7.2 Exploring the relationships within the family-tree of common sense.

new words to explain away uncanny bodily feelings may entail the formation of neologisms, leading to concretism and somatic delusions—as Schnell (1852) 150 years ago had already noticed—which are typical phenomena in chronic schizophrenic psychoses (Agresti and Ballerini 1965). (See Fig. 7.2.)

Aristotle in the light of schizophrenia

The stream of consciousness

Schizophrenia has long been considered as a disorder of 'common sense' (Stanghellini 2004). There are two main interpretations of this:

(1) schizophrenia is a disorder of coenesthesia, an impairment of the 'functional symphony' (Guiraud 1950) in which all the single sensations are synthesized;

(2) schizophrenia is an impairment of practical knowledge, a disorder to appreciate the 'rules of the human game' (Blankenburg 1969).

In the following vignette, these two domains of schizophrenic psychopathology co-occur, although enigmatically for the person who experiences them:

> I feel lifeless. I have this 'feeling of vagueness' especially at sunset hours. I see colours as brighter. All sensations seem to be different from usual and to

fall apart. My body is changing, my face too. *I feel disconnected from myself*, from my muscles, my emotions, my sensations. It happens that my sensations become 'malleable', as if they cropped up in an outer space.

It also occurs that in this state I get lost when I stay with the others. *What I lack is the common thought*. I have nothing to share with them. In this way, the others become incomprehensible and scaring.

The first interpretation of schizophrenia as a disorder of common sense focuses on coenesthesia—the 'deep but more or less indefinite awareness that we have of our own bodies and the general tone of functional activity' (Dupré 1913). Coenesthesia—a concept shaped in French early twentieth-century psychopathology, which largely duplicates Aristotle's theory of *koiné aisthesis*—is the *carréfour* of all sensibility, which is the basis for personal identity including the feeling of existing, of being a self, and of being separate from the external world. Coenesthopathic troubles, i.e. abnormal bodily sensations, are the epiphenomena of a global disturbance of the synthesizing role played by coenesthesia. Abnormalities in coenesthesia are supposed to be the core dysfunction in psychotic syndromes: 'A patient who finds himself gay, full of energies or who declares to feel hopeless or even dead is affected by coenesthopathic troubles' (Guiraud 1950). Especially hebephrenia 'is characterised by the specific impairment of those cellular nervous systems which govern the coenesthetic and kynesthetic synthesis and instinctual vital activity' (Dide and Guiraud 1929).

The second interpretation focuses on the schizophrenic persons' difficulty to share with the others the 'axioms of everyday life' (Straus 1949). They are affected by a 'global crisis of common sense' (Blankenburg 1971) and by a deficit in social cognitions (Bellack *et al.* 1999; Hogarty *et al.* 1999). This interpretation is twofold: on the one hand there are those who emphasize the schizophrenic persons' lack of *sensus communis,* i.e. of the propositional knowledge consisting in a set of rules of inference, shared by their social group, through which its members conceptualize objects, situations, and other persons' behaviours. On the other hand, the schizophrenic dis-sociality is considered the effect of a disorder of social attunement, i.e. of a kind of non-propositional knowledge consisting in the affective-conative-cognitive ability to perceive the existence of others as similar to one's own, make emotional contact with them and intuitively access their mental life (Parnas and Bovet 1991; Hobson 1994; Stern 2000; Stanghellini and Ballerini 2002).

What is surprising is that Aristotle's conception of *koiné aistheisis* reflects both interpretations of schizophrenic psychopathology (although he does not explicitly relate sensory integration to social attunement). Aristotle's explanation of this may sound odd today, nonetheless it is intriguing: the setting of *koiné aisthesis* is the heart, i.e. the organ in which the blood carries the stream of sensation from different sense modalities 'to their point of integration and coalescence' (Hunt 1995). Aristotle argued that sensory integration and self-awareness are indissoluble since both are produced by the flowing and blending together of all the senses (*syn-aisthesis, con-scientia*). The heart, in Aristotle's physiology, is also responsible for perceiving time and is the seat for imagination (Kahn 1966). Hunt (1995) comments that this is 'an accurate, if tacit, phenomenology buried within all this erroneous anatomy'. The kernel of Aristotle's proto-phenomenology is that the self originates from a stream, a current amalgamating different sensations; that self-awareness coalesces at the edge between an inner and an outer flow; that it is linked in the heart to the sense of time and to the power of image-formation.

De-animated bodies and disembodied spirits

Aristotle's theory of *koiné aisthesis* provides a solid philosophical ground from which the phenomenological understanding of the schizophrenic modifications of self- and social awareness can depart. The question is now: can the phenomenological understanding of persons affected by schizophrenia enhance Aristotle's theory of mind?

Schizophrenic persons experience a world in which sensory self-awareness is disrupted. The sense of aliveness, the feeling of being embedded in oneself, the unity of self-experience are disrupted. This involves the experiencing of a dualistic Cartesian form of existence in which embodied sensory self-awareness is substituted, as I will argue, by incorporeal noetic self-awareness. Schizophrenic persons experience a world similar to that portrayed in modern objective psychology, as described by Erwin Straus (1935) in his timely criticism of early objectifying psychological approaches and polemically epitomized in the sentence, 'Persons think, not the brain'. Both in the experience of schizophrenic persons and in cognitive theories of the mind, the immediate sensory awareness of one's perceptions, actions, and thinking as one's own is replaced by a second-order noetic awareness of something that perceives that one is perceiving, acting, or thinking. Literally: life is seen through a brain.

Schizophrenic persons often describe their condition as that of a de-animated body or a disembodied spirit. Lack of sensory self-awareness entails the feeling of being a lifeless body (*Koerper*, i.e. the body I have, as opposed to *Leib*, i.e. the body I am). This state is often mis-diagnosed as melancholic de-personalization, but whereas melancholic patients complain about their feeling of the loss of feelings (e.g. 'I feel that I don't feel'), schizophrenic ones report two apparently contrasting experiences: loss of self-awareness (e.g. 'I don't feel that I feel') and a special kind of objectified awareness (e.g. 'It is not me who feels—*It* feels'). This existence as a zombie or de-animated body comes to its apotheosis in the state of a scanner or dis-embodied spirit, which lives as a mere spectator of one's own perceptions, actions, and thoughts. This pathological condition not only is an argument confirming Aristotle's theory of (normal) self-awareness as based on *koiné aisthesis* ('the common power accompanying all the senses, by which we perceive that we are seeing and hearing'), but it reinforces his fundamental distinction between sensory and noetic self-awareness, and in addition may shed new light on it.

> If the mind is empty it works like a *plotter* or a photo-camera, and retains the objects' contour. If it is full, it must be much more controlled to obtain the same result. Therefore one must keep in a good balance the emptiness of the mind and the fullness of ideas.

In these sentences there is, in my view, much more than a sheer reproduction of the obsolete praise of the optimal state of the mind as a *tabula rasa* in order to mirror the world in the most accurate way. If we want to understand exactly what is meant here, we must also question the assumption that 'plotter' and 'photo-camera' are used here like mere metaphors or like 'as-if' similes to represent the activity of the sentient mind. If we do so, then we can speculate that what is described is a kind of awareness of the act of perception (the same holds not only for perceptions, but also for motor actions and thinking). If sensory self-awareness—i.e. the unity of perception and self-perception—breaks down, then the 'I' breaks down into an experiencing I-subject contemplating an experienced I-object, while the latter is performing the act of perception. The act of perception itself is no more experience from within, but from without ('through a brain'). It becomes an object of noetic awareness. The phenomenality of this experience is no more implicitly embedded in itself; the act of perception turns out to be an explicit intelligible object. Can we say then that schizophrenic persons, in virtue of the abnormality of the structure of their self-awareness, can thus become aware of usually unnoticed conditions of normal daily experience? If with 'usually unnoticed conditions' we refer to the normal structure of self-awareness the answer must be 'No', since what they become aware of—*ex hypothesi*—are not normal experiences embedded in normal self-awareness, but experiences set in an abnormal state of self-awareness, i.e. in the position of a disembodied spirit: a state characterized by the shift from sensing one's own experiences as one's own to examining their constitution after the subject-object split has occurred. Schizophrenic persons are not in this respect like *Uebermenschen*, as Cutting (2002) seems to suggest, who have a privileged knowledge on the enigma of self-awareness: they certainly have a privileged insight into the problem, but not into the solution of such enigma.

Does this experience of disconnectedness that takes place in the realm of self-awareness share a common root with the experience of disconnectedness taking place in the realm of the social life of schizophrenic persons? This was the *Leitmotiv* of this paper and I will try to sum up my ideas here. In short, these are the two roots of schizophrenic psychopathology:

(1) disorders in self-awareness, implying morbid objectification of sensations and emotions and of bodily and mental functions, and

(2) disorders in sense integration, more precisely in sensory-to-sensory and sensory-to-motor integration, implying disorders of attunement (which is based on simulation routines, i.e. the coupling between action perception, simulation of action, and understanding of intentions), and consequently autism.

What we need now is a panoramic view on these two phenomena—anomalous self-experience and autism.

In the section devoted to *koiné aisthesis* and social attunement I tried to demonstrate, in the light of recent developmental psychology and neurobiology, that Aristotle's *koiné aisthesis* is not only the basis for the integrated perception of the physical world, but also for the meaningful perception of the others' behaviours in the social world, since it is the basis for the phenomenon of emotional-affective attunement, which is the prerequisite for the emergence of the social self and of inter-subjectivity.

In the following section, the mutual constraints between sensory self-awareness and inter-subjectivity were outlined, i.e. circular process of the emergence of a core- and a social self: abnormal attunement may de-structure self-perception (but the reverse is also true: attunement may help to re-structure one's own self-experience). It was also suggested that abnormal bodily sensations (coenesthopathies), a very common phenomenon in early phases of schizophrenia, may affect the inter-corporeal resonance on which attunement is based.

Developmental psychology and psychopathological data legitimate to consider that disordered *koiné aisthesis* is the common ground for schizophrenic anomalous phenomena in self- and social experience. What I would like to suggest in these concluding remarks is that the mode schizophrenic persons relate to the others shares with the mode they relate to themselves the same objectifying attitude. In a nutshell, the social world of schizophrenic persons is a lifeless land. If one feels one's self as a de-animated body, then the others' bodies are lifeless too. The disintegration of one's own sensory self-awareness implies the impossibility of attunement and without attunement the others are meaningless things—*Koerper*. Also, if one conceives of oneself as a disembodied spirit, an entity who is split into a spirit watching one's body as an operating mechanism, then the others are pictured as mechanisms too. Social interactions are also mechanical and their performance requires the knowledge of abstract algorithms. If empathic attunement fails, the search for propositional knowledge appropriate to social interactions takes its place. As it happens in self-experience, also in social experience; there is a shift from first-person to third-person perspective: the social world is conceived of as an impersonal game regulated by impersonal norms. The social experience of schizophrenic persons is penetrated through and through by conceptual elements. In such a world, the comment that Walter Benjamin addressed to Paul Valéry in occasion of his sixxty-fifth birthday looks appropriate:

> 'He bends himself on facts as if they were nautical charts, and, without being pleased by the sight of 'depths', he is just happy to be able to follow a not dangerous route.

References

Agresti, E. and Ballerini, A. (1965). Aspetti del vissuto corporeo nella schizofrenia. *Rassegna di studi psichiatrici*, **54**(6): 679–683.

Ainsworth, M., Blehar, M., Waters, E., and Wall, S. (1978). *Patterns of attachment: a psychological study of the strange situation*. Hillsdale: Erlbaum.

Aristotle De Anima, De somno, de memoria, ethica nichomachea. Loeb Classical Library, St Edmundsbury Press Ltd.

Ballerini, A. and Stanghellini, G. (1989). Phenomenological questions about obsessions and delusions. *Psychopathology*, **22**: 315–319.

Ballerini, A. and Stanghellini G. (1993). Obsession et révélation. *L'Evolution psychiatrique*, **58**(4): 743–756.

Bellack, A.S., Gold, J.M. and Buchanan, R.W. (1999). Cognitive rehabilitation for schizophrenia: Problems, prospects, and strategies. *Schizophrenia Bulletin*, **25**(2): 257–274.

Bergson, H. (1927). *Essai sur les données immédiates de la conscience*. Paris: Presses Universitaire de France.

Blankenburg, W. (1969). Ansaetze zu einer psychopathologie des 'common sense'. *Confinia Psychiatrica*, **12**: 144–163.

Blankenburg, W. (1971). *Der verlust der natuerlichen selbstvertaendlichkeit. Ein beitrag zur psychopathologie symptomarmer schizophrenien*. Stuttgart: Enke.

Bourdieu, P. (1980). *Le sens pratique*. Paris: Editions de Minuit.

Butterworth, G. (1999). A developmental-ecological perspective on Strawson's 'the self'. In: *Models of the self* (ed. S. Gallagher and J. Shear), pp. 203–211. Thorverton: Imprint Academic.

Butterworth, G. (2000). An ecological perspective on the self and its development. In: *Exploring the self. Philosophical and psychopathological perspectives on self-experience* (ed. D. Zahavi), pp. 19–38. Amsterdam: Benjamins.

Cutting, J. (2002). *The living, the dead, and the never-alive: schizophrenia and depression as fundamental variants of these*. Mill Wood: The Forest Publishing Company.

Di Pellegrino, G., Fadiga, L., Fogassi, L., Gallese, V., and Rizzolati, G. (1992). Understanding motor events: a neurophysiological study. *Experimental Brain Research*, **91**(1): 176–180.

Dide, M. and Guiraud, P. (1956). *Psychiatrie clinique* (3rd edn). Paris: Le Francois.

Dillon, M.C. (1997). *Merleau-Ponty's ontology*. Evanston: Northwestern University Press.

Dupré, E. (1913). Les cénesthopathies. In: *Themes and variations in European psychiatry* (ed. S.R. Hirsch and M. Shepherd). Bristol: John Wright (1974).

Eilan, N. (2000). On understanding schizophrenia. In: *Exploring the self. Philosophical and psychopathological perspectives on self-experience* (ed. D. Zahavi), pp. 97–114. Amsterdam: Benjamins.

Ey. H. (1973). *Traité des hallucinations*. Paris: Masson.

Foucault, M. (1963). *Naissance de la clinique. Une archéologie du regard médical*. Paris: Presses Universitaire de France.

Gabel, J. (1962). *La fausse Conscience*. Paris: Editions de Minuit.

Gadamer, H.G. (1986). *Warheit und methode*. Gesammelte Werke, vol. 1. Tuebingen: Mohr.

Gallese, V. (2000). The acting subject: toward the neural basis of social cognition. In: *Neural correlates of consciousness* (ed. T. Metzinger), pp. 325–334. MIT Press.

Gallese, V. and Goldman, A. (1998). Mirror neurons and the simulation theory of mind-reading. *Trends in Cognitive Sciences*, **2**(12): 493–501.

Guiraud, P. (1950). *Psychiatrie générale*. Paris: Le Francois.

Heinimaa, M. (2003). Incomprehensibility. In: *Nature and narrative. International perspectives in philosophy and psychiatry* (ed. K.W.M. Fulford, K. Morris, J.Z. Sadler, and G. Stanghellini). Oxford: Oxford University Press.

Henry, M. (1963). *L'essence de la manifestation*. Paris: Presses Universitaire de France.

Hobson, R.P. (1994). Understanding persons: the role of affect. In: *Understanding other minds: perspectives from autism* (ed. S. Baron-Cohen, H. Tager-Flushberg, and D.J. Cohen), pp. 204–227. Oxford, UK: Oxford Medical Publications.

Hogarty G.E. and Fleischer S. (1999). Developmental theory for a cognitive enhancement therapy of schizophrenia. *Schizophrenia Bulletin*, **25**(4): 677–692.

Huber, G. (1957). Die coenaesthetische schizophrenie. *Forstschritte der Neurologie und Psychiatrie*, **25**: 491–520.

Hunt, H.T. (1995). *On the nature of consciousness*. London: Yale University Press.

Jaspers, K. (1913). *Allgemeine psychopathologie*. Baltimore: The Johns Hopkins University Press (1997).

Jonas, H. (1994). *Das prinzip leben. Ansaetze zu einer philosophischen biologie*. Frankfurt am Main: Insel.

Kahn, C.H. (1966). Sensation and consciousness in Aristotle's psychology. *Archiv fuer Geschichte der Philosophie*, **48**: 41–82.

Kahn, C.H. (1992). Aristotle on thinking. In: *Essays on Aristotle's de anima* (ed. M.C. Nussbaum and A.O. Rorty), pp. 343–379. Oxford: Clarendon Press.

Lagerstee, M. (1999). Mental and bodily awareness in infancy: Consciousness and self-existence. In: *Models of the self* (ed. S. Gallagher and J. Shear), pp. 213–230. Thorverton: Imprint Academic.

Merleau- Ponty, M. (1945). *Phénoménologie de la perception*. Paris: Gallimard.

Minkowski, E. (1926). *La notion de perte de contact vital avec la réalité et ses applications en psychopathologie*. Paris: Jouve & Cie.

Minkowski, E. (1927). *La schizophrénie. Psychopathologie des schizoides et des schizophrènes* (2nd edn, 1953). Paris: Payot.

Minkowski, E. (1929). Les idées de Bergson en psychopathologie. *Annales Médico-Psychologique*, **88**(1): 235-

Minkowski E. (1968). *Le temps vécu*. Paris: Presse Universitaire de France.

Parnas J. (2000). The self and intentionality in the pre-psychotic stages of schizophrenia: a phenomenological study. In: *Exploring the self. Philosophical and psychopathological perspectives on self-experience* (ed. D. Zahavi), pp. 115–148. Amsterdam: Benjamins.

Parnas, J. and Bovet, P. (1991). Autism in schizophrenia revisited. *Comprehensive Psychiatry*, **32**: 7–21.

Ramachandran, V.S. and Hubbard, A.M. (2001). Synaesthesia—a window into perception, thought and language. *Journal of Consciousness Studies*, **8**(12): 3–34.

Ricoeur, P. (1990). *Soi-meme comme un autre*. Paris: Editions du Seuil.

Rizzolati, G., Fadiga, L., Gallese, V., and Fogassi, L. (1996). Premotor cortex and the recognition of motor actions. *Cognitive Brain Research*, **3**: 131–141.

Ruemke, H.C. (1941). The nuclear symptoms of schizophrenia and the praecoxfeeling. *History of Psychiatry* (1990), **1**: 331–341.

Sass, L.A. (1992). *Madness and modernism. insanity in the light of modern art, literature, and thought.* Cambridge/London: Harvard University Press.

Sass, L.A. (2000). Schizophrenia, self-experience, and so-called 'negative symptoms'. In: *Exploring the self. Philosophical and psychopathological perspectives on self-experience* (ed. D. Zahavi), pp. 149–182. Amsterdam: Benjamins.

Sass, L.A. (2001). Self and world in schizophrenia: three classic approaches. *Philosophy, Psychiatry, and Psychology*, **8**(4): 251–270.

Scheler, M. (1973). *Wesen und formen der sympathie*. Bern: Franke.

Schnell, B. (1852). Ueber die veraenderte sprechweise und die bieldung neuer worte und ausdruecke im wahnsinn. *Allgemeine Zeitschrift fuer Psychiatrie*, **9**: 11.

Schutz, A. (1970). *Reflections on the problem of relevance*. New York: Yale University Press.

Schwartz, M.A., Wiggins, O.P., and Spitzer, M. (1997). Psychotic experience and disordered thinking: a reappraisal from new perspectives. *Journal of Nervous and Mental Disease*, **185**(3): 176–187.

Sheets-Johnstone, M. (1999). Phenomenology and agency: methodological and theoretical issues in Strawson's 'the self'. In: *Models of the self* (ed. S. Gallagher and J. Shear), pp. 231–252. Thorverton: Imprint Academic.

Stanghellini, G. (1994). Body, language and schizophrenia. *Comprendre*, **7**: 107–122.

Stanghellini, G. (1997). For an anthropology of vulnerability. *Psychopathology*, **30**: 1–11.

Stanghellini, G. (2004). *Disembodied spirits and deanimated bodies. The psychopathology of commnon sense*. Oxford, UK: Oxford University Press.

Stanghellini, G. and Ballerini, M. (2002). Dis-sociality: the phenomenological approach to social dysfunction in schizophrenia. *World Psychiatry*, **1**(2): 102–106.

Stern, D.N. (2000). *The interpersonal world of the infant*. New York: Basic Books.

Straus, E. (1935). *Vom sinn der sinne*. Berlin: Springer.

Straus, E. (1949). Die aesthesiologie und ihre bedeutung fuer das verstaendnis der halluzinationen. In: *Existence* (ed. R. May, E. Angel, and H.F. Ellenberger), pp.139–169. New York: Basic Books.

Wittgenstein, L. (1969). *On certainty*. Oxford: Basil Blackwell.

Zahavi, D. (2001). Schizophrenia and self-awareness. *Philosophy, Psychiatry and Psychology* (Special Issue: The phenomenology of Schizophrenia: Three Classic Approaches; guest editor L.A. Sass), **8**(4): 339–341.

Zahavi, D. and Parnas, J. (1999) Phenomenal consciousness and self awareness: a phenomenological critique of representational theory. In: *Models of the self* (ed. S. Gallagher and J. Shear), pp. 253–270. Thorverton: Imprint Academic.

8   The paralogisms of psychosis

Grant Gillett

If today we try to relate the syndromes of insanity to particular developmental stages of personality, we have few hypotheses on which to base
our arguments. If these attempts are to be more than tentative gropings,
we must trace the phenomena of our inner life back to their roots in the
psyche of the child, of primitive man, and of animals.

(Emil Kraepelin 1920)

Psychotic paranoia is a type of unreason. However, when we consider the
contents of paranoid thought we find that, rather than being irrational or
disorganized, they are often hyper-rational. This chapter will argue that this
variety of reason is an aberration; although in logical form, it seems to be
consistent and carefully structured. The puzzle presented by paranoid reasoning is closely linked to the problems encountered in attempts to define
delusions. Both spring from a philosophical view of mind and epistemology
in which reason and the apprehension of the true nature of reality are seen as
individual attainments by a Cartesian thinker. However, the unreason of
psychosis looks very abnormal when we adopt the discursive naturalism
of post-Wittgensteinian philosophy of mind and epistemology.

Discursive naturalism relates psychotic thinking to the kind of informed rule-following and practised habits of reason that are useful in
human language games and cultural evolution. When language games and
human forms of life are seen as the true home of reason (with logic and
deductive consistency as an abstraction from idealized forms of those natural
activities) the aberrations in psychotic thinking become readily apparent. For
instance, we begin to see that psychotic thought represents a departure from
what is taken for granted in human engagement with others in a real world
where one strives for agreement in judgements. We can also see that an initial
causal unhinging of reason from the regularities of everyday discourse paves
the way for paranoia, such that the elaboration of paranoid thought arises
through the exaggeration of an adaptive tendency in our cognitive response to
the world. One would normally weave a coherent narrative out of the events of
life in the light of common sense, as revealed by the checks and balances
conveyed through communication and interaction with others. In psychotic
unreason that source of correction is lost (Gillett 1999a). Thus the individual

cognitive system must make sense of the world unaided by discursive engagement with others and the drive for experiential coherence can become exaggerated to a pathological extent. An evolutionary account of human rationality and its role in paranoid thought, which takes account of the nature of cultural evolution, coheres well with Wittgenstein's approach to understanding and meaning. The resulting philosophical discussion has a bearing on three key topics in devising a naturalistic approach to the philosophy of mind:

(1) the unconscious (Ucs) and the nature of the conscious mind;
(2) the normative drive to reason as an evolutionary good trick;
(3) the discursive modulation of reason as a further cognitive adaptation.

I well recall an evening when a young friend of our family came around to our home obviously quite agitated. He liked discussing philosophy and was talking excitedly in our hallway. My wife and daughter were upset because they had heard that he was to be taken back in to the acute psychiatric unit for treatment. My wife kept saying to me, 'Just try to understand him because I am sure he is making sense but we are not getting it'. This is a common intuition that arises in folk who are conversationally engaged with a person suffering a psychotic episode. I will try, in exploring the three themes I have identified, to illuminate that intuition.

The unconscious and consciousness

The mind is grounded in our engagement with the world. That engagement results in a stream of activity in the brain and some of that activity is transformed in such a way that a human being consciously lives out an unfolding autobiography (Gillett 2001). In attempting to account for the transformation from brain activity to conscious mental life, Dennett (1991) has devised a multiple drafts theory of consciousness that can be elaborated to yield a narrative theory of the conscious self. The elaboration proceeds by taking account of strands in the cognitive neuroscience, the philosophy of mind, and the relation between culture and rule-following.

From cognitive science we learn that the brain is organized like a massive neural network with areas of local specialization and holism of function (Spitzer 1999). This neural network is in constant dynamic interchange with the world in such a way that it provides a substrate for the operation of processes that yield a stream of conscious thought. The joint operation of top-down and bottom-up influences in that network enable the constraints governing linguistic content to help shape intentional content in general (in human beings). Thus language and language games are the vehicle for the negotiation of the content that will appear in consciousness (Gillett 2001).

The written and spoken signs and their associated information structures and categorical boundaries serve as foci (or nodes of excitation) for the neural network to use when collecting and organizing packages of information from the world. Those packages include stimulus conditions, patterns of human activity, collective responses and rituals, and so on. Taken together, these diverse influences, operating through the interconnected nodes in our neural networks, clothe our lives with meaning so that we can live and move among others, exchanging information with them, benefiting from their experiences, and forging relationships. Notice that these activities form a milieu in which brain activity is itself shaped and configured according to what is happening to and in the world around the person whose brain it is.

From philosophy of mind we derive an account of consciousness and thought, which incorporates the ability of the subject, considered as a whole subject, to find meanings in or confer meanings on segments of a stream of neural activity. This follows from the twin facts that the best account of conscious thought is based on the idea that we read into the activity passing continuously and seamlessly between the brain and the world, a range of contents that obey rules governing our concepts. The forming of contentful mental states and acts, on the basis of ongoing experience and according to the conceptual structure produced in and used by a thinker, allows that thinker to make use of the 'good tricks' of the human group to which the thinker belongs (Dennett 1995, p. 78). The result is a stream of conscious experience, thoughts that make the happenings of life available to the thinker in ways that mesh with the cognitive skills of that thinker. I have argued that these cognitive skills (or 'good tricks') can only usefully be explained by appeal to the culture in which the individual has been shaped as a subject of experience (Gillett 1999b).

The relevant argument basing content in culture and discourse goes through a conception of rule following in which the rules we follow in applying concepts to experience are a product of the socio-cultural group to which we belong and therefore importantly dependent on historical and discursive forces operating on and within that group to shape their practices.

From the importance of rule-following in the articulation of conscious content we are led to Winch's work on culture and rules (1958). The role of culture emerges when we notice that the specification of any function requires us to take account, not only of the way the function was selected for at the time of its emergence, but also the structures that preserve it in a given form (Millikan 1993, p. 86). It is clear that many of our mental structures, which condition what we do and the ways in which we articulate our thought, are produced by training in a particular historico-cultural setting and then maintained by the same milieu. In this milieu there are multiple connections between the meanings of different signs and there are multiple connections between events and situations, the knowledge of which is much more fully owned by our caregivers and other adults than it is by our young selves. Thus we extend our understanding or consciousness of the world around us by catching on to the validated links that pervade experience and language, and by continually revising our own constructions of the world in the light of corrections and communication by others. We are creatures of whom it is true to say that we are each biologically designed to function in the context of a human group and then further designed (even intentionally crafted) by that group to operate with a cultural endowment that can expand and enrich our cognitive systems.

From the cultural milieu I pick up not only the categories that help me understand what is happening around me but also stories or scripts for episodes and situations in which I am involved, and also for more extended tracts of my lived experience (Taylor 1989). Thus the events of my life take on a significance based on these resources. In effect I come to a negotiated compromise or 'best fit' arising from an accommodation between what actually happened and the way that I understand what is going on between my brain and the world around me within the context of the narrative that I create by living it. Like all narrators I try to make sense of what is happening but I do not always succeed. I realize, in part from the reality checks of others, that some things just happen and that some things have a significance and connectedness that goes beyond my own experience. One can understand why I do this when we look at our narrative ability as an adaptation that helps human beings to deal with their normal ecological domain.

Having laid out certain initial theses about consciousness and the resources that I use to render conscious what happens to me, I can now deepen the discussion of the shaping influences that play on my conception of reality.

Kant and the nature of reason

Kant followed Descartes and the early empiricists in accepting that our knowledge of the world is constructed out of intuitions or the apprehension of appearances, which presented themselves to the mind of a subject (1787/1929). He argued that these intuitions or presentations are only combined into representations apt for thinking (which comprises discursive or logical operations) by being subsumed under concepts which function to pull together otherwise isolated moments of experience in terms of a feature or features which they have in common (functions of unity) according to the judgement of a competent thinker (B130ff). The application of concepts that inform our representations by articulating their content, is rule-governed and imparted from one human being to another by training (B172). The use of judgement to organize experience so that it yields knowledge of the world around one is, in its practical or everyday operation, therefore a disciplined skill and it is constantly evaluated according to its coherence with the hypothetical judgements of suitably placed others (B848). The ability to correct one's own thinking by relativizing it to the judgements that would commend themselves to any competent observer or thinker is what distinguishes mere subjective persuasion about how things are with the world and oneself from objective conviction satisfying the rules governing well-grounded human judgement (B850; B172). By refining my ability to eliminate the subjective biases that can cloud judgement and thereby tending to increase the likelihood of my arriving at judgements that would be converged upon by all suitably placed thinkers, I enhance my ability to think what is true (B849). It is this ability (and the implicit correction that resides in the convergent judgements of others) that gives me knowledge about what is actually going on in the world around me and at large. In this I am dependent on my own fallible cognitive faculties but also upon the ability trained in me to judge as others would judge, to converge with common sense (the *sensus communis* (Kant 1800/1978).

In Kant's *Anthropology,* the active nature of thought is clearly set out in relation to the abstraction that underlies general ideas or universal concepts; he portrays this as an act of the faculty of cognition'(Kant 1800/1978, p. 14) or 'a power of the mind which can only be acquired by exercising it'(Kant 1800/1978, p. 15). He confirms the account he outlined in the *First Critique* and portrays this active cognitive skill as a pervasive feature of human thought (Kant 1800/1978, p. 29):

> Only the understanding, which joins perceptions and combines them under the rule of thought, by introducing order into the manifold. establishes them as empirical cognition, that is, experience.

It is through the ability to ascertain what is actually happening in the world with clarity and accurate use of our cognitive skills that we achieve 'common sense'(which is not common or vulgar but is more like *nous* or informed and critical opinion). Through the exercise of these faculties, we come to relatively objective knowledge of what is going on (or a conscious story based on my experience at the time in question that does justice to what I have perceived and concluded in the light of a reality principle). The reality principle is best understood as informed knowledge of what normally happens around here as judged by competent thinkers (Spitzer 1990, p. 53).

This coheres very well with Kant's discussion of the practical constraints on knowledge that are applied when we use perception and reason to discover the truth about the real world by working towards genuine knowledge: knowledge that would be inter-subjectively validated and which sets aside any subjective biases that might otherwise mislead one (B849). However, this works together with a tendency within myself that is so ingrained it seems innate and indispensable: the tendency to make a rationally coherent story out of the events that I experience.

The rational compulsion

In the antinomies, Kant explores a series of conflicts that are inherent in rationality itself and based on certain ideals of reason (B434). Reason ideally aims for completeness in our understanding of the world and therefore strives for a sense of natural necessity, whereby everything is connected to everything else. We find this set out, for instance, in Kant's third antinomy where he claims that we are inclined to believe that every event is caused or intelligibly connected with every other event. This is clearly a useful tendency for our species to have because it leads us to investigate the origins of phenomena and thus attain the knowledge that allows us to intervene in nature to bring about the aims we devise for ourselves. A degenerate or exaggerated form of this tendency gives rise to the view that everything that happens to me has an explanation and that nothing happens by chance (or through the chaotic configuration of the great chain of being).

Absolute completeness of the system of ideas to provide one with a world concept or 'the absolute totality of the synthesis of the condition of all possible things'(B434) is for Kant 'a natural and unavoidable illusion'(B449). One could say that a sign of maturity is that sometimes, when faced by inexplicable events, one learns to say, 'It happens'. But where do we learn the judgement required to distinguish the occasions when one should pursue a complete and complex explanation and those when one should discount the need for a coherent and rationally structured story about what is happening to me now in the light of 'life, the universe, and everything?' Arguably we learn when to stop seeking an explanation as we learn common sense.

Constraints on reason

Thus it is plausible that what corrects the tendency to seek over-rational completion of the system of ideas is exactly the *sensus communis* that arises through communication and inter-subjectivity. Kant suggests as much when he speaks of common sense and sound human understanding (*bon sens* or 'horse sense'), which looks at life from many angles and comes to reasonable judgements about what is going on by benefiting from the perspectives and opinions of others (Kant 1800/1978, p. 23)

One of the characteristics of mental disorder, according to Kant, is that one lives in a 'stream of thoughts which follows its own (subjective) law (Kant 1800/1978, p. 97) and does not obey the constraints of shared knowledge or common sense. Kant offers a classification of cognitive disorders, whereby individuals are unable to participate in the common, rationally constrained discourse that allows each to attain an adequate knowledge of the objective world. In so doing, he provides the reader with a brief description of the kind of cognitive derangement seen in paranoid schizophrenia (Kant 1800/1978, p. 112):

> Insanity is that disturbance of the mind wherein everything which the insane
> person relates is in accord with the possibility of an experience, and indeed
> with the formal laws of thought; but because of falsely inventive imagination,
> self concocted ideas are treated as if they were perceptions. Those who
> believe that they are everywhere surrounded by enemies, and those who
> regard all glances, words and otherwise indifferent actions of others as
> directed at them personally and as traps set for them belong to this category.

Kant also suggests a hereditary basis for most mental disorder and dismisses
many of the popular explanations by overwork, studying too many difficult
texts, and so on, arguing that a normal mind will cope with these challenges
perfectly well. But he does explain that the loss of cognitive congruence with
others, and thereby the touchstone of objectively valid judgements, can
worsen the situation produced through an inherited defect. He notes the
idiosyncrasy of psychotic ideation concluding as follows (Kant 1800/1978,
p. 117):

> The only general characteristic of insanity is the loss of a sense for ideas that
> are common to all (*sensus communis*) and its replacement with a sense for
> ideas peculiar to oneself (*sensus privatus*).

We can now explore the development of paranoid psychosis and what it
tells us about mind and epistemology in relation to this broadly naturalistic
framework.

The narrative drive and rational explanation

In one's development as a human being, one takes the experiences, events,
contexts, and relationships that arise as life unfolds and weaves them together
so that one lives out a more or less coherent life story. This project becomes
more developed as life progresses, so that in middle life we might find those
with mental disorder showing rich delusional phenomena that are not transient
and disjointed but held together by a strong linking narrative thread to form
systems of paranoid belief and so on (Kraepelin 1920/1974, p. 13) The fact
that a human being does weave a life narrative together recalls the rational
drive to explain and connect events that serves our species so well. One might
expect that such a drive would tend toward the ideal that all life events fell into
a coherent pattern, where the significance of every event was related in some
intelligible way to all others.

I have noted that in constructing an identity for oneself (or a personal
identity), one confers significance on the things that happen and that significance draws on the narrative context that one weaves for it. It is, we could say,
only in the context of a story that any episode has an appreciable, and possibly
deeply connected, meaning. And there is an expectation that one's story is

unifiable as a personal trajectory through the world but it is a matter of judgement to decide what is reasonable as a meaning-giving act and what goes beyond the bounds of common sense. Many delusional systems unify the events of life beyond the point to which any normal person would look for meaning. Thus the paranoid psychotic might say things like, 'But the fact that he is wearing that tie today rather than yesterday or tomorrow must mean something' or, of a passer by, 'I know that her look means something, but I can't quite figure it out'. In order to supply these linking explanations, a person may be driven to invoke conspiracies or patterns of connectedness, which are highly idiosyncratic but which trade on occasional perspicuous moments outside the experience of normal people and therefore need not be explained. Kant remarks of the insane person that (Kant 1800/ 1978, p. 112):

> In their unfortunate madness, [they] are often so acute at interpreting as directed against them what others do inadvertently, that, if the data were only true, we would be obliged to pay the highest respect to their understanding.

Thus a paranoid system of beliefs may become the central and only rationally coherent organizing framework within which a person can make sense of their possibly idiosyncratic perceptions and convictions.

Hundert revealingly interprets some of the paranoid symptoms of a patient he calls Timothy G. in this manner and comments on its evolutionary significance (1992, p. 348):

> Meaning was returned to his life, however. This meaning arises from his delusion because, like so many psychotic patients, his 'symptomatology' is an organising feature of his continued existence. To end his life would be to end the world's only hope for bringing justice to the perpetrator of the Nazi Holocaust. Since the time his brain figured this out his continued survival has not been in jeopardy.

One might quibble with the idea that Timothy's brain figured this out rather than Timothy figured it out as a person whose brain was throwing up very strange connections and associations, but the main point is that paranoia does involve a meaningful narrative, albeit one that a normal person would neither compose nor believe. However, each of us is the centre of our own narrative and therefore is under some pressure to provide an account of the personal trajectory that grounds that narrative. Thus the narrative perspective is, by its very nature, self–interested. As a result, where it has parted company with the narratives of co-travellers because of a dislocation of the cognitive congruence we all tend to take for granted (with good reason), it is apt to personalize all events either as threats to one's well-being or as testimony to one's uniqueness. If we, as a species, are adaptively suited to live in a supportive and co-operative environment (which has, *inter alia*, imparted and affirmed that set of cognitive skills upon which each human being depends), then one might expect that the isolation of insanity would magnify the threats that would otherwise be mitigated by the familiarity of that customary, shared, domain of activity.

The co-operative nature of human adaptation is overlooked by many of the earlier, post-Darwinian, writers. Kraepelin, for instance, expresses the 'red in tooth and claw' version of Darwinism prevalent at the time he was writing (Kraepelin 1974, p. 19):

> Every human being, if he is to survive, needs to have confidence in himself and at the same time a mistrust of the possibly hostile world around him. From this comes his natural tendency... to interpret external events always in terms of their effect on his own well-being or otherwise.

This orientation is also found in the Freudianism that became fashionable in the early twentieth century. However, when we recall Kant's account, the need to balance this bestial view of human cognition with an enlightened discursive naturalism more in tune with the forms of life of a communicative and co-operative species becomes clear. It is against that background that the disordered nature of paranoid thought becomes fully apparent and its persecutory, self-referential features are understandable (DSM IV Casebook, p. 101):

> Mr Simpson maintains that his apartment is the centre of a large communication system that involves all three major television networks, his neighbours, and apparently hundreds of 'actors' in his neighbourhood. There are secret cameras in his apartment that carefully monitor all his activities. When he is watching TV, many of his minor actions (e.g., going to the bathroom) are soon directly commented on by the announcer. Whenever he goes outside, the 'actors' have all been warned to keep him under surveillance....
> His neighbours operate two different 'machines'; one is responsible for all of his voices,... the other machine he calls 'the dream machine'. This machine puts erotic dreams into his head, usually of 'black women'.

Mr Simpson has a story about his life and situation that hangs together and explains everything that happens to him such that it all means something and is connected in intelligible ways to everything else. It is just that the whole story is crazy. There is such an admixture of real events and unreal or impossible interpretations that no-one of sound mind (who shares Kant's *sensus communis*) would ever believe it. This is therefore a glimpse into a mind out of touch with others but for which everything has to connect or mean something in relation to the narrative perspective of the central character. The result is that the drive to rational connectedness has eclipsed realistic thinking about oneself and the world.

We see this tendency vividly evident in the Capgras delusion. In this delusion, the illusion of doubles, 'the patient believes that a person closely related to him has been replaced by a double'(Gelder *et al.* 1983, p. 287). A plausible explanation for this delusion is that the schizophrenic patient does not experience the normal emotional responses to familiar people and seeks an explanation for this odd fact. The explanation—that they are not the people he or she cares for and responds to but duplicates of them— makes sense only in a private or idiosyncratic way and would not be countenanced by a normal thinker guided by common sense. Interpreted this way, it exemplifies what Cutting refers to as 'an increased reliance on a logical, rational, self-conscious mind'(1999, p. 30). Cutting argues that the psychotic patient overlooks the possibility of a subjective change and that there is a disturbance in the 'process of objectivization'. I have argued that our ability to correctly objectify and not to overstep the bounds of common sense in explaining a subjective change by appeal to a strange objective state of affairs is an achievement we make in company with others who impart to us standards of judgement and an understanding of the world which discipline the innate tendency to try and connect everything into a grand objective world scheme.

This tendency is astutely identified by Kant as lying at the root of many overblown metaphysical schemes or theories and is writ large in the delusional systems of paranoid schizophrenia. But how is the tendency to rationally explain everything that happens moderated so that it does not mislead a subject given its obvious adaptive advantages for human beings in general?

Moderating the norms of reason

The difficult task of composing or editing a good-enough narrative of one's experience in the light of common sense and what actually happens to one as an embodied subject (or subjective body) poses interesting problems for human beings, which are illuminated by psychotic thought. This task involves weighing multiple constraints all arising from 'complex types of causal interplay that raise vexing questions concerning the boundaries between mind and brain, and between mind, brain, body, and world (Graham 1999, p. 225). I have argued that there are no fixed boundaries separating the determinants of the lived narrative that is an individual consciousness, there is only a set of negotiable constraints arising from language, the world, the brain, and the social context. These constraints can be understood quite well from an informed understanding of the relationship between the influences of language and signification, and the input to the brain from the individual's causal interaction with the environment; but each of these terms is itself merely a way of indicating a complex and deeply interwoven set of factors, which inscribe us as historical beings (Gillett 2001). The end result of this 'internal negotiation', carried out with the aid of a range of cognitive and discursive skills, is a lived autobiography that more or less hangs together.

This makes *both* my knowledge of my own agency *and* the narrative coherence to be found in my conscious life into achievements of the active subject as narrative subject and intentional agent. Those achievements depend on a normally functioning cognitive system and can disintegrate under certain challenges. What is more the possible types of disintegration reveal the complexity of self-knowledge.

The most basic constraint on the unity of consciousness arises from Kant's appreciation of the need for a unified subject to do the work required to render experience contentful. But Chadwick (1994) notices, when faced with aberrations of thought such as thought insertion, and alien voices, that this Kantian requirement (that all mental states have an experiencing subject who imparts to them the formal unity required for the constitution of mental content) is a different requirement from the sense of one's being the author (and owner in that sense) of one's first-person thoughts and experiences. Indeed neither of these requirements, by itself, suffices to explain phenomena such as thought insertion. Clearly these two things normally go together but in a disordered state of mind, and therefore a state where there is disordered narrative and integrational ability, something else is needed to account for normal function as highlighted by the abnormality of these psychotic phenomena (such as thought insertion, alien voices, and passivity).

Gibbs develops the strands of an account of thought insertion, which identifies agency or authorship of a thought and the subjectivity associated with first-person mental content as crucial aspects of a thought but aspects that may come apart (Gibbs 2000, p. 200). He also notices the responsibility that comes with ownership and the alienness of some of the inserted thoughts complained about by schizophrenics. But one gets a sense that there is something more to it than these momentary phenomenological characteristics and that the notion of authorship has more to it than what is usually displayed. Stephens and Graham pursue the difficult issue of ownership of thoughts and suggest that not only a failure to align agency with subjectivity but also an alienness with respect to the (more or less coherent) owned conscious autobiography of a person may play a role in the disorders of self-attribution. This narrative flavour to self-consciousness is highly congenial to a view in which the conscious lived narrative is both a first-person construction (involving subjectivity and agency) and imposes its own narrative (and therefore evaluative) constraints and coherence on the thoughts one has (Gillett 1999a). The skilled nature of the implicit narrative task draws heavily on an intact cognitive system and is clearly threatened by a major psychotic illness.

The key role played by the subject in constructing a first-person, lived, conscious narrative normally results in a congruence between authorship, first-person experience, and coherence within an unfolding life story, but states of disordered self-consciousness vividly illustrate what happen when this bedrock of first-person cognitive discursive skills is undermined and collapses (Stephens and Graham 2000). In fact the idea of nesting one's experiences in a coherent narrative (in accordance with a common sense view of what is going on in one's life) and thus discerning their significance for oneself, has evident appeal for psychology and psychiatry. Reflective equilibrium about the contents and tendencies of one's own mind, on this model, is seen as an individual and collective enterprise in which we fashion liveable life stories from the resources shared with us by others and on the basis of a set of narrative choices one makes for oneself.

On the view I am recommending, the world nurtures me practically and cognitively so that I grasp and correctly apply the techniques of conscious articulation of experience as employed by other human beings around here. To succeed in mastering these techniques, I need my brain to be working well in terms of the attentional and other cognitive skills that others use, but also I must be able to attune my networks of association and inhibition or constraint of information flow so that they are 'in synch' with those of others. If I were out of synch with others I would also be poorly attuned to the world and likely to be subject to disturbances of perception and action (as indeed we see in schizophrenia). A biochemical anomaly in my brain, distorting my internal and highly structured patterns of information flow, would be expected to contribute to thought patterns that were fragmented and aberrant, so that I would be prone to disruptions in many aspects of my thought. This would plausibly affect features of thought (such as subjectivity and ownership) that would normally be automatically linked and also make me prone to misinterpret the thoughts and experiences that do occur to me. However, my rational drive towards coherence, faced with distorted and misinterpreted experiences, might force them into a coherent but idiosyncratic world picture, even where it is a picture that, in my right mind and able to engage in fruitful interchange with others, I would not be inclined to accept.

We might therefore see schizophrenia as a breakdown in *con*-sciousness (from com- or *con*-together with, or jointly and *scio*—I know). Our brains are designed to work con-sciously and we are shaped and refined as thinkers so that the principle of con-scious knowledge pervades our thoughts about the world and ourselves. This is a radical departure from the view that each cognitive individual is somehow programmed to formulate his or her own 'internal picture' of reality, which is structured by logical rules and based on Cartesian sensations and ideas. The paranoid schizophrenic has logic aplenty; what is missing is a commonsensical ability to adjust one's thought and experience to what goes on around here—which is validated by shared experience and discourse.

Inter-subjectivity, knowledge, and action

In *On Certainty*, Wittgenstein advances a theory of knowledge that is deeply informed by a kind of pragmatism. Certainty arises from the sharing of knowledge among individuals who have mastered a common set of epistemic and practical techniques, which are used to engage them with the world in sophisticated and complex ways. We induct children into these techniques as we share our lives with them and we teach them to distinguish those occasions when they know things from those when they only believe them, and how to anchor their thoughts in their dealings with the environment around them (both egocentric and extended). The result of the integration of epistemic and practical techniques is certainty and assured action in a shared or public environment that they come to understand and negotiate.

Wittgenstein's analysis of knowledge casts considerable light on the reasons why thinkers such as Fulford are inclined to identify mental illness with action failure (1989). Action, evaluation, and knowledge form a seamless whole in which one benefits by the suggestions and corrections of others and thereby becomes increasingly adept at forging a life trajectory for oneself. Even in something as cognitive as an understanding of one's nature as a human being and one's place in the world, the seamless (but tripartite) endeavour is evident. When I depart from the trajectory that a normal brain is capable of negotiating, and fall prey to such afflictions as delusional thinking, my engagement with the world goes seriously awry. Things do not work for me; my information-gathering techniques let me down; and the connections I make between experiences leave me adrift in a bewildering world because they seem to provide me with no structured framework for action and no shared experience with others.

I am therefore alienated: from others, from the world, and increasingly from myself as a being among others. This is frightening and strange, and it means that I have to make my own sense of the world—armed only with my own rational drive to connect things into a coherent story or picture of life, the universe, and everything. It is natural that, in a world where I have been deserted and am therefore trapped in a lonely journey that I am struggling to understand and cannot get any reliable clues about, I should move to a more defensive position (Hundert 1992, p. 350). Kraepelin's image of the mistrust that each individual must have for the possibly hostile world around him springs into stark clarity with a different productive origin (1920/1974, p. 19). Reason by itself cannot resolve the problem that one is then faced with as a creature designed by nature to seek *con-sciousness*, fellow feeling, and conjoint solutions to problems. Thus the world of the psychotic is a lonely and threatening world, and it is only the insight that reason gives into the intricate structure that explains all the phenomena that he encounters, that assures the psychotic of any kind of stability. Mr Simpson's world is threatening and hostile but he understands the conspiracy behind it all and therefore he can protect himself against it, even though there is no one else who understands and can help him.

The schizoid break

Schizophrenia, particularly of the paranoid type, is a break with reality and as such is highly significant for philosophy. It exposes the fragility of the human brain as an organ that takes a cacophony of stimuli and moulds them, according to cognitive techniques honed in a shared discursive environment, so that they form a coherent lived experience. At its base level this organ causally interacts with that environment but the information it takes in does not organize itself, it is powerfully structured by a set of influences arising in a context of nurture and conjoint adaptation and out of those influences it moulds consciousness.

One of the most important shaping influences on lived conscious life is the rational connections between events that have been discerned by human beings acting collectively and sharing their knowledge. All are individually moved by a tendency to make connections in experience and this tendency is reinforced by shared systems of meaning making or signification. The cohesion this adds to experience, along with the techniques we shape in each other for tracking what happens in the world, yields a conscious narrative or lived autobiography for each of us to inhabit.

The psychotic loses the coherence of thought through losing control of the associations that have been painstakingly shaped by the natural and social environment. Some psychotics retain an impressive ability to connect things together into a coherent story and this story, disconnected from the sense of reality that is common sense (or the *sensus communis*) serves as a foundation for a *sensus privatus*. The psychotic thus replaces syllogisms and sound argumentation and reason, with paralogisms—delusory rational trains of thought leading to empty and unfounded conclusions. Having lost the fundamental cognitive ability to walk in step with others, and therefore to use the fine-grained tuning mechanism that we have developed as a collective and shared tool, the psychotic experiences a break with reality. This break with reality is also a break with the shared reality that constantly strengthens and affirms one's own well-grounded assessments of self and one's place in the world. The lonely, disjointed, and uncaring world that the psychotic finds himself in is, understandably, not a place that any normal human being could live in.

References

Cutting, J. (1999). Morbid objectivization in psychopathology. *Acta Psychiatrica Scandinavica,* **99** (Supp): 30–33.

Dennett, D. (1991). *Consciousness explained*. London: Penguin Press.

Dennett, D. (1995). *Darwin's dangerous idea*. London: Penguin Press.

DSM IV casebook. American Psychiatric Association (1994b) *Diagnostic and statistical manual IV: case book*. Washington: APA.

Fulford, W.K.M. (1989). *Moral theory and medical practice*. Oxford, UK: Oxford University Press.

Gelder, M., Gath, D., and Mayou, R. (1983). *Oxford textbook of psychiatry*. Oxford, UK: Oxford University Press.

Gillett, G. (1999a). *The mind and its discontents*. Oxford, UK: Oxford University Press.

Gillett G. (1999b). Dennett, Foucault, and the selection of memes. *Inquiry,* **42:** 3–24.

Gillett,G. (2000). *Moral authenticity and the unconscious in the analytic Freud* (ed. M. Devine). London: Routledge.

Gillett G. (2001). Signification and the unconscious. *Philosophical Psychology* **14**(4): 477–498.

Graham, G. (1999). Mind, brain, world. *Philosophy, Psychiatry and Psychology* **6**(3): 223–226.

Hundert, E. (1992). The brain's capacity to form delusions as an evolutionary strategy for survival. In: *Phenomenology, language and schizophrenia* (ed. Spitzer, Uehlein, Schwartz and Mundt). New York: Springer Verlag.

Kant, I. (1787/1929). *The critique of pure reason* (trans. N. Kemp Smith). London: Macmillan.

Kant, I. (1800/1978). *Anthropology from a pragmatic point of view* (trans. V.L. Dowdell). Carbondale: Southern Illinois University Press.

Kraepelin E. (1920/1974). Patterns of mental disorder. In: *Themes and variations in European psychiatry* (ed. S. Hirsch and M. Shepherd). Bristol: John Wright and Sons.

Millikan, R. (1993). *White queen psychology and other essays for Alice*. Cambridge, Mass: MIT Press.

Spitzer, M. (1999). *The mind in the net*. Cambridge, Mass: MIT Press.

Stephens, G.L. and Graham, G.(2000). *When self consciousness breaks*. Cambridge, Mass: MIT Press.

Winch, P. (1958). *The idea of a social science and its relation to philosophy*. London: Routledge.

Wittgenstein, I.. (1969). *On certainty* (ed. G.E.M. Anscombe and G.H. von Wrigh). New York: Harper.

9 How to move beyond the concept of schizophrenia

Jeffrey Poland

The causes of dementia praecox are at the present time still wrapped in impenetrable darkness.

Emil Kraepelin

Introduction

The concept of schizophrenia (and its predecessor, *dementia praecox*) has played a major role in conceptualizing certain forms of severe mental illness for a century.[1]

Such conceptualization impacts how individuals suffering from mental illness are viewed and treated, how relevant research is conducted, and how mental healthcare policy and reimbursement practices are set. The concept has its origins in a clinical psychiatric tradition that includes such figures as Kraepelin, Bleuler, and Schneider, and it has found a secure home in major contemporary diagnostic systems, such as DSM-IV (American Psychiatric Association 1994), that purport to underwrite scientifically based classification, research, and clinical practice concerning mental illness.

Numerous claims have been made buttressing the place of schizophrenia in contemporary clinical and research practice: e.g. that schizophrenia is a mental disorder having a characteristic clinical manifestation and course; that the diagnostic criteria for the disorder have adequate levels of reliability; that it is well-established that schizophrenia has a genetic component in its aetiology; that there are promising leads for identifying the pathophysiological basis of the disorder; and that there have been significant improvements in psychopharmacological treatments for schizophrenia. In addition, it is claimed that epidemiological studies have established stable prevalence rates across cultures and over time, and that schizophrenia represents a major public health problem for which aggressive scientific research programmes are required. These claims ('the received view'), along with the lengthy clinical tradition of employing the concept, have led to the firm entrenchment of schizophrenia in clinical and research practices and in the public imagination.

Critics of the received view of schizophrenia have not been in short supply, however, and it is useful to distinguish two general sorts: socio-political and scientific. The socio-political critics, such as Szasz, Laing, Scheff, and Foucault, have criticized the concept of schizophrenia, as well as psychiatric concepts and labels more generally, in terms of their social and cultural significance: e.g. the role they play in managing deviance, the social, economic, and guild interests they serve, their rhetorical power, their impact on personal and inter-personal processes. Such critics have been concerned to unmask the non-scientific and non-clinical interests, forces, ideas, and processes that lead to the introduction of mental illness concepts like schizophrenia and to the maintenance of social practices organized in terms of them. More broadly, the socio-political critics have attempted to demonstrate the cultural and historical contingency of psychiatric practices employing mental illness concepts, to undermine their credibility, and to identify the moral, social, economic, and political issues they raise.

In contrast, the scientific critics pursue a less radical line. Taking schizophrenia researchers at their word when they articulate their commitment to science as the avenue to theoretical understanding of, and effective intervention concerning, mental illness, these critics (e.g. Cromwell 1983; Bentall 1990; Boyle 1990; Sarbin 1990) argue that the concept of schizophrenia lacks the features of a sound scientific concept and that it ought not to occupy the central role it does in either clinical practice, scientific research, or mental health policy. Unlike the radical critics, the scientific critics locate themselves squarely within the research community concerned to understand 'mental illness' from a scientific point of view, and they argue that the concept of schizophrenia, as well as the claims formulated in terms of it, fail to satisfy the standards of that community. Such critics challenge the significance of research practices and results centred around the concept of schizophrenia, and they deny both that schizophrenia, as conceived by the received view, exists and that it is now an appropriate object of ongoing clinical concern and scientific investigation. Rather, such critics see the concept of schizophrenia as being an impediment to sound and productive scientific and clinical practice.

Today, despite decades of criticism of both sorts, the entrenchment of the concept of schizophrenia and associated practices appears to be as deep as ever. Schizophrenia is fully expected to reappear in DSM-V as one of the official diagnostic categories of mental disorder, journals are replete with articles reporting on research concerning schizophrenia, mental health policy and practice continue to be widely conceptualized in terms of a brain disease called 'schizophrenia', and the public is being aggressively 'educated' about the nature of this disease, partly in an attempt to offset widespread stigma associated with the label and partly to reinforce the existing practices centred around the concept. Advocacy groups like the National Alliance for the Mentally Ill (NAMI) are especially outspoken regarding the disease status of schizophrenia for reasons having to do with mental health policy, research funding practices, and access to health care. Thus, it would appear that neither the advancement of arguments designed to undermine the scientific credibility of the schizophrenia concept, nor the advancement of deep socio-political analyses and critiques of its cultural role, have been sufficient to undermine its entrenchment in contemporary mental health practice. How could this be?

There are, at least, three possible explanations to explore. The first, predictably articulated by those of a more socio-political bent, is that the powerful vested interests served by the schizophrenia concept, the inertia of well-entrenched practices, and perhaps the contemporary *Zeitgeist* (e.g. concerns about efficiency and technological control, tendencies toward pathologizing problems and deviance) all have combined to overpower any purely academic considerations concerning the scientific merits of the concept or the role it plays in cultural practices. With respect to making significant social changes, considerations of money, power, prestige, political interests, and the like tend to be more effective than good arguments.

A second explanation is that, even if the concept of schizophrenia and the claims and practices based upon it are in some ways flawed, the concept still plays a useful role in contemporary culture (e.g. a role in providing access to healthcare or in distributing research funds and organizing scientific research programmes) and there is no alternative ready to take its place while maintaining comparable levels of efficiency. Hence, short of the emergence of a viable alternative for serving a wide range of pragmatic functions, the status quo is maintained.

A third explanation is that the arguments just are not as strong as the critics think: there are flaws and loopholes that make it possible for the defenders of the schizophrenia concept to argue that, although the critics may make some good points, they are not nearly good enough to justify the abandonment of the concept or the practices it supports.

There is some plausibility in each of these explanations, especially the third. Although there are core truths in both the scientific and the socio-political criticisms of the schizophrenia concept, the specific arguments advanced by the critics have serious limitations that have made it easy for the concept to persist, particularly given the powerful interests it serves and the apparent absence of a viable alternative approach. At a minimum, more effective arguments are required; although even good arguments will probably not be enough to effect the serious reform that is required.

My goals in this paper are:

(1) to clarify some serious limitations of the arguments of the scientific critics;

(2) to outline a strategy for strengthening the scientific case against schizophrenia; and

(3) to clarify some issues and strategies involved in moving beyond the concept of schizophrenia.

In doing (1)–(3), I hope to show how the arguments and insights of the socio-political and the scientific critics can fruitfully work in concert with each other.

The master argument of the scientific critics

The scientific case against the concept of schizophrenia is well exemplified in the work of Mary Boyle (1990) and Richard Bentall (1990). Their key claims are: that the concept of schizophrenia fails to satisfy appropriate standards of scientific validity; that schizophrenia, conceived of as either a medical syndrome or a brain disease, does not exist; and, that the concept of schizophrenia ought not to play the role it currently does in research and other mental health related practices.

Although the case for these claims is complex, there is a 'master' argument at the core that will be the focus of my attention. This master argument is signalled in the following summary statement made by Boyle (1990, p. 193):

> The major argument which has been presented here is that the concept of schizophrenia was introduced and has been developed and used in a way which bears little resemblance to the methods of construct formation used in medical and other empirical sciences. It has also been argued that any attempt to transform the concept to a scientific one is futile and is based on a serious misunderstanding of the methods used to develop concepts whose claim to scientific status is less equivocal.

The argument signalled here is one based upon claims about how concepts are legitimately introduced and developed within empirical science. In a nutshell, and simplifying her presentation somewhat, Boyle builds upon a version of logical empiricist philosophy of science and proposes two key conditions for the legitimate introduction and use of a scientific concept. The first is a necessary condition that there must be a well-established empirical pattern among observable features, which justifies inferring the existence of an underlying causal structure ('a hypothetical construct'); the second is a sufficient condition (which therefore implies the first) that the inferred construct be embedded in a system of empirically established relationships to other constructs or observable features. The two conditions can be codified in the following principle for defining construct validity in science:

> (CV1)—A scientific concept, SC, is construct valid if and only if: (a) there exists a pattern of inter-correlated observable features from which the

existence of an associated hypothetical construct, HC, has been inferred; and
(b) SC has predictive power, i.e. the associated construct, HC, is empirically
related to other constructs or observable events.

The significance of this definition of construct validity (CV1) is supposed to
be that justified belief in the existence of entities or conditions picked out by a
scientific concept and justified employment of such a concept for scientific
purposes (e.g. designing experiments and interpreting their results) require
that the concept satisfy conditions (a) and (b). As a consequence, CV1
functions as a standard by which scientific practices can be assessed for
their scientific legitimacy and by which specific concepts, along with claims
framed in terms of them, can be assessed for their scientific credibility.

Given the standard, the argument against the scientific credibility of
the concept of schizophrenia, the claims made in terms of it, and the
practices based upon it focuses attention upon the character of the empirical
research record with the aim of demonstrating that the schizophrenia concept
(henceforth, SZ) fails to satisfy the requirements of scientific legitimacy
specified by the standard.[2]

The 'master argument' then goes like this:

1. A scientific concept, SC, is construct valid if and only if:

   (a) there exists a pattern of inter-correlated observable features from which
   the existence of an associated hypothetical construct, HC, has been
   inferred; and

   (b) SC has predictive power, i.e. the associated construct, HC, is empirically related to other constructs or observable events (CV1).

2. Neither condition (a) nor condition (b) is satisfied by SZ.

3. Thus, SZ is not a construct valid scientific concept.

4. We are justified in thinking that schizophrenia exists and in using SZ in
   research only if SZ is a construct-valid scientific concept.

5. Thus, we are not justified in thinking that schizophrenia exists or in using
   SZ in research.

Within the framework of this argument, the case advanced by the scientific
critics against the validity of SZ has been focused largely on establishing
premise two by showing: first, that at no time has scientific evidence ever been
amassed to reveal the existence of a pattern of relationship among signs and
symptoms that would justify inferring the existence of a hypothetical construct
associated with SZ, and, hence, the existence of a well-defined disease
condition (to wit, schizophrenia); and second, that, to date, no credible scientific evidence establishes any substantial empirical relationships between the
construct associated with SZ (i.e. schizophrenia viewed as a well-defined

disease condition) and other empirically definable variables of interest (e.g. aspects of aetiology, pathology, clinical presentation, and clinical dynamics).

Boyle (1990) advances the case for premise two in two steps. The first, aimed at establishing that condition (a) has not been satisfied, involves examining the historical basis for the introduction and refinement of the concept of schizophrenia (and its precursor, *dementia praecox*) by Kraepelin, Bleuler, Schneider, and ultimately the architects of recent forms of the concept found in DSM-III (American Psychiatric Association 1980) and DSM-III-R (American Psychiatric Association 1987). She argues powerfully that none of the discoverers and developers of the schizophrenia concept have ever been in possession of the kind of evidence (e.g. data based on clinical observations, data gleaned from clinical records, data from experimental studies) sufficient for establishing the existence of empirical patterns among observable features that would justify an inference to the existence of a hypothetical construct.

The second step in her case targets the predictive power of SZ and is focused upon the research record bearing on the alleged genetic component of the aetiology of schizophrenia. She discusses both the existing research frequently cited to support claims about a genetic aetiology and the many criticisms of that research, drawing the conclusion that the research is too flawed and inconclusive to warrant any such aetiological claims. Several of the authors in Bentall (1990) extend the case with more comprehensive coverage of the research record focusing on, in addition to the genetic research, research concerning biological pathology, clinical phenomenology, and clinical dynamics. The conclusion of these critics is that the massive research record concerning schizophrenia does not provide adequate scientific justification for claims about empirical relationships between a hypothetical construct associated with SZ and these other variables of interest (i.e. the research record does not support the predictive power of SZ; see also Sarbin 1990 and Heinrichs 1993). Thus, the critics contend that the scientific case for the construct validity of SZ, and hence the existence of schizophrenia, is virtually non-existent. And yet, the concept of schizophrenia remains in the official diagnostic classification system and it is widely employed in research and clinical practice.

The loophole in the argument

Although there is much that is right about this scientific criticism, it has some limitations that create a loophole for the defenders of the schizophrenia concept. There are two key problems to consider: the first concerns the evidence adduced to support the key empirical premise; the second concerns the scientific standard invoked by the critics.

The problem with the evidence is that there has been an enormous amount of research on schizophrenia between the development of the argument just cited and now. Even if premise two is supported by the research record up to the late1980s and early 1990s, perhaps more recent research has vindicated the concept of schizophrenia in ways that prior research did not. Thus, assuming the correctness of the critics' claims regarding the research record to which they had access, it is possible that more recent research either has identified a pattern of inter-related features from which the existence of a hypothetical construct associated with SZ can be inferred or has demonstrated the predictive power of SZ.

The second problem concerns the critics' understanding of the concept of 'construct validity' and the relevant standard for establishing legitimate scientific concepts (i.e. CV1). The problem is that this standard is a remnant of somewhat dated philosophy of science and does not adequately express current understanding of the requirements on usable concepts in science. Specifically, it is not the case that all legitimate scientific concepts must be associated with patterns of observable features from which the existence of a construct is inferred, even if this is one way of introducing a concept for scientific use. Rather, some concepts can be legitimately introduced and employed on the basis of their occurring within a theoretical framework. So long as the concept is well defined within the theoretical framework, the framework has a substantial level of empirical support, and there are procedures for fixing the extension of the concept as theoretically defined, no barriers will exist to the legitimate employment of the concept in experimental or theoretical scientific work. The clearest examples of such concepts occur in elementary particle physics (e.g. in theories concerning quarks), although there is no reason why such concepts cannot be employed in other sciences as well. As a consequence, a revised standard should be considered:

> (CV2)—A scientific concept, SC, is construct valid if and only if: (1) (a) there exists a pattern of inter-correlated features from which the existence of an associated hypothetical construct, HC, has been inferred, and (b) SC has predictive power, i.e. the associated construct, HC, is empirically related to other constructs or observable events; or (2) SC is well-defined in a theoretical framework for which, as a whole, there is substantial evidential support.

This revised standard suggests that SZ could be a legitimate scientific concept that picks out a real disease condition and plays a justifiable role in scientific inquiry even if CV1 is not satisfied. This is possible so long as the concept is appropriately located in a theoretical framework that, as a whole, has substantial evidential support.

The significance of this second problem for the critics' case is that, because of the latter's reliance on an incorrect articulation of the relevant scientific standard, the critics have not adequately conceptualized and dealt with the possibility that schizophrenia is a complex disease condition that can be defined in the terms of an evolving theoretical framework within the relevant sciences. As a consequence, the critics have failed to appreciate that the defenders of the concept of schizophrenia can take refuge in the possibility that schizophrenia is a disease condition embedded in a highly complex biological system, even though it does not have any well-defined clinical manifestations (e.g. a sharply defined clinical syndrome, a characteristic clinical onset, course, outcome) or bear any clearly identifiable and simple relationships to readily defined variables like specific causal agents, specific pathologies, and response to specific treatments. On this view of the situation, it is only with the march of science that enough theoretical clarification will be gained to allow an understanding of the nature of the disease process and how it interacts with other conditions and processes to produce its highly hetero-geneous clinical appearance and dynamics. In a deep sense, the history of research described and utilized by the critics is just what should be expected of a disease process of this sort given the relative immaturity of the relevant sciences. Thus, rather than bowing to the critics, the defenders can claim that what needs to be done is to step up the research, both in the relevant background sciences (e.g. cognitive science and neuroscience) and in increas-ingly sophisticated scientific research programs aimed at understanding the underlying causal structure (i.e. aetiology, pathology, and dynamics) of schizophrenia and its associated clinical phenomenology.

The two problems just described (i.e. the problem with the evidence and the problem with the standard) imply that there is a loophole in the argument of the scientific critics: viz., the critics have failed to establish that research up to the present does not vindicate the concept of schizophrenia in the light of CV2 by establishing either condition 1 or condition 2.

Now, it is pretty much granted on all sides that the scientific research record has not established the existence of a well-confirmed pattern of inter-correlated features from which the schizophrenia construct can be inferred. Perhaps the most visible expression of this is found in the history of the development of recent DSMs (i.e. DSM-III, III-R, IV): nowhere in the development of the criteria found in these documents is evidence provided that empirically isolates a set of inter-correlated signs and symptoms. What is found is a series of 'consensus' judgements and committee decisions about optimal diagnostic criteria punctuated by limited and questionable empirical data (cf., Boyle 1990; Kirk and Kutchins 1992; Caplan 1995; Poland 2001, 2002). More recent research has not improved on this dismal record (cf., Heinrichs 2001).

Further, it is pretty much granted on all sides that the scientific research record does not provide strong evidence for the predictive power of the concept of schizophrenia: direct-validation research aimed at relating schizo-phrenia to specific aetiology, pathology, response to treatment, or clinical onset, course, and outcome has not produced evidence confirming the existence of substantial empirical relationships involving the schizophrenia construct. In what is, perhaps, one of the more serious understatements made by defenders of the concept of schizophrenia, Frances *et al.* (1996) write as follows (p. 166):

> Schizophrenia is a clinical syndrome of unknown aetiology and pathophysiology. No symptoms are pathognomonic to Schizophrenia, and there are no clinically useful laboratory or imaging markers. The characteristic features of Schizophrenia are heterogeneous, and the boundaries with other disorders can be difficult to delineate. All of this makes for quite a diagnostic challenge, as well as creating problems for research. The clinical diagnosis of Schizophrenia is currently based on the pattern of characteristic signs, symptoms, and course of illness.

The pattern mentioned in the last sentence of this passage can only refer to the currently legislated diagnostic criteria found in the DSM, criteria that have not been empirically validated. And, again, more recent research does not appear to have improved the situation (cf., Heinrichs 2001). It is somewhat poignant, if not instructive, to be reminded of Kraepelin's famous statement made early in the twentieth century: 'The causes of dementia praecox are at the present time still wrapped in impenetrable darkness'. So, it would seem that almost 100 years of research based upon the concept of schizophrenia has led to little change with respect to the scientific validation project (viz., no empirically established inter-correlated features and no predictive power). In the eyes of the scientific critics, this apparent scientific failure means that the clinical conceptualization, initiated by Kraepelin, perpetuated by Bleuler, Schneider, and others, and continued in its current form in the DSM, is a bankrupt conceptualization from the point of view of science. But, given the loophole in the argument of these critics, defenders can continue to believe that there is hope nonetheless.

Consider the following passages from Nancy Andreasen's recent book, *Brave new brain* (Andreasen 2001):

> Schizophrenia is a brain/mind disease.

> (Andreasen 2001, p. 197.)

> Most clinical neuroscientists now suspect that schizophrenia is a 'neurodevelopmental disorder.' Something—and probably several different things—has gone wrong in the orderly process of brain development that begins at the time of conception and continues on into young adult life.

> (Andreasen 2001, p. 201.)

> The scientific evidence suggesting that schizophrenia is a neurodevelopmental disorder affecting multiple stages of brain development is substantial and steadily increasing. This evidence indicates that many different kinds of influences may be involved, and that they may be both genetic and environmental.

> (Andreasen 2001, p. 203.)

These quotes reflect a growing consensus in some quarters that the disease that Kraepelin is supposed to have discovered is a highly complex neurodevelopmental brain disease, which only the advance of neuroscience can help us to fathom, and that there is a substantial and ever-increasing body of evidence in support of this hypothesis. If this view is right, then, in the light of CV2, the concept of schizophrenia is vindicated, schizophrenia research is in fact justifiable, and the argument of the scientific critics is disarmed.

In the next two sections, I shall briefly outline the main features of the neurodevelopmental model of schizophrenia and describe a critical strategy for closing the loophole in the scientific case against the concept of schizophrenia. That strategy will depend heavily on the notion of scientific evidence and will be designed to clarify whether the existing research base does, in fact, warrant the continued aggressive pursuit of schizophrenia research. Since this 'meta-analytic' strategy is still far from being fully articulated and carried out and because of limitations of space, I will only be able to describe the framework of analysis in broad strokes, briefly describe one example, and then, in the last section of the paper, further locate the strategy in the larger framework of critical discussion.

The neurodevelopmental model

According to the Neurodevelopmental Model of Schizophrenia (NDMS),[3] schizophrenia exists and is a brain disease for which, at present, there are only diagnostic criteria focusing upon clinical manifestations (i.e. there are no laboratory tests): that is, clinical inference to the presence of the disease in individual patients involves a diagnostic process of assessing symptomatology based upon DSM criteria and of using sound clinical judgment in the light of auxiliary information (e.g. individual and family medical history.) According to the model, there is a genetic vulnerability for the disease, although currently it is hypothesized that additional non-genetic 'hits' are required to cause the disease process to be initiated during pre-natal stages of neural development (possibly during the first or second trimester, depending upon the type of non-genetic events involved.) In any case, some combination of genetic vulnerability and non-genetic events is thought to initiate a pathogenic neurodevelopmental process, which continues over the course of approximately two decades and leads to a complex neuropathology involving a core abnormality. This neuropathology, in turn, underlies complex and heterogeneous psychopathology, which, in its turn, gives rise to disruptions of social functioning and heterogeneous clinical manifestations and dynamics. The following are the essential features of the model:

- genetic vulnerability plus non-genetic hits;
- disruption of pre-natal neural-development;
- initiation of a developmental pathogenic cascade;

- neuropathology (neural misconnection);
- information processing deficits (neural miscommunication);
- psychopathology (cognitive, perceptual, affective dysfunction);
- clinical phenomenology and dynamics (psychotic episodes, symptoms);
- disruption of social and adaptive functioning.

More specifically, the hypothesized genetic vulnerability and epigenetic hits (e.g. viral infection, malnutrition, mechanical injury, stress, presence of toxins) are thought to lead to neurodevelopmental abnormalities involving failures to complete cell migration processes, ineffective synaptic pruning, and, ultimately, sub-optimal neural connectivity between brain regions and systems. Such abnormalities initiate a developmental pathogenic cascade involving pervasive and variable disruption of normal neurodevelopmental processes the effects of which become manifest over time, as affected regions and connections are called upon to function in the developmental process. At such critical junctures, significant brain systems may not be available to perform their functions properly because of poor connectivity or because they are not adequately developed. For example, relatively subtle 'early signs' (e.g. mixed handedness, lack of co-ordination, social ineptness in childhood), as well as increasingly more manifest clinical signs and symptoms (e.g. psychotic symptoms during late adolescence) are thought to be manifestations of the developmental unfolding of the hypothesized disease process.

According to NDMS, the core abnormality in schizophrenia is one of inefficient neural connectivity resulting from structural abnormalities emerging from the neurodevelopmental process just described. Abnormal neural connectivity, in its turn, underlies abnormal information processing and miscommunication among affected brain systems. And, these more or less pervasive abnormalities are hypothesized to underlie the various biochemical, neurocognitive, and higher level cognitive and affective dysfunctions present in the schizophrenic clinical picture and to be ultimately responsible for the various personal and social consequences of the disease. As noted above, current diagnostic criteria key on the higher level consequences of the disease process.

Given the fundamental character of the core deficit (viz., neural misconnection), as well as its apparent pervasiveness and variability across individuals, it is expected that higher level abnormalities and deficits will be similarly pervasive and variable; and it is also expected that clinical manifestations and dynamics (early signs, onset, course, outcome, response to treatment) will be heterogeneous across individuals with the disease. Because the core defect involves connectivity among neural regions and systems, there are no hypothesized focal lesions (e.g. as in Alzheimer's disease), although neural markers of the disease process are not unexpected (e.g. signs of abnormal cell migration, reduced brain volume). Because the problems of connectivity do not involve disconnection, but rather misconnection, resulting deficits and dysfunctions are expected to be (relatively) mild compared to those characteristic of disconnection syndromes (e.g. ALS, MS). Finally, recent discussions of this disease process have debated the question of whether the disease is progressive or one that involves an early, static defect. According to some, the evidence is tending to suggest that schizophrenia is a progressive brain disease (cf., Woods 1998).

Defenders and developers of NDMS have claimed that there is 'a critical mass of evidence conveying support for the model', evidence that comes from numerous research domains (epidemiological, genetic, neuropathological, neurocognitive, clinical.) Genetic studies (e.g. family, twin, and adoption studies), for example, are frequently cited as providing perhaps the strongest evidence in support of a component hypotheses of the NDMS: viz., that schizophrenia is caused, in part, by a genetic vulnerability (cf., Gottesman 1991; Mouldin and Gottesman 1997). Another cornerstone of the evidential case for the NDMS involves data from epidemiological studies purporting to establish empirical associations between schizophrenia and malnutrition, viral infection, stress, and mechanical injury during the first or second trimester of pregnancy or during the birth process itself. Such associations are supposed to provide support for the hypothesis that schizophrenia is caused, in part, by one or more epigenetic hits that disrupt early stage neurodevelopmental processes. Further, the case for NDMS rests heavily on a number of purportedly well-established findings with respect to structural and functional abnormalities associated with schizophrenia: e.g. reductions in both gross and regional brain volume, ventriculomegaly, functional abnormalities in key brain regions (e.g. frontal hypoactivity, temporal hyperactivity). Structural abnormalities are viewed as markers for the operation of the disease process over time, whereas the functional abnormalities are taken to be expressions of the ongoing neuropathology that is present in schizophrenia and is the consequence of abnormal neural development. Finally, evidence supporting NDMS is obtained from studies concerning both abnormal neurocognitive functioning associated with schizophrenia (e.g. abnormal attentional, sensory-perceptual, and executive processes), and a variety of findings concerning clinical appearance and dynamics (early signs, onset, course, outcome, response to treatment) of the disease (e.g. mixed handedness, typical late adolescent onset, phenomenological reports of patients). Indeed, it has been claimed that various 'predictions' of the model (e.g. presence of information-processing deficits, pervasiveness of the deficits, their relatively mild severity, and their relatively early appearance) have received confirmation (cf., Green 1998, chap. 1).

In short, the proponents of NDMS are claiming substantial evidential support for the model, support that is supposed to be sufficient to justify stepped-up research and development efforts focused upon it. Hence, as pointed out above, this model and the associated research programme provide a potentially powerful response to the scientific critics of the concept of schizophrenia who have not yet fleshed out their arguments adequately to undercut the impact of this bold disease hypothesis. Two questions that now emerge are:

1. Just how strong is the evidential support for NDMS?
2. Is its evidential support sufficient to justify continued employment of the concept of schizophrenia in scientific research concerning mental illness?

I think that a close examination of the research record brought to bear in support of NDMS will reveal that the model has very little evidential support, largely because the data is either irrelevant, weak, or uninterpretable and because neither the model nor its component hypotheses has ever been subjected to anything like a serious scientific test. As a consequence, given the failure of the research record to provide other sorts of validation of SZ (i.e. 1a and 1b in CV2) and given that NDMS is arguably the only serious theoretical framework concerning SZ currently available, there is at present no good basis for continuing to employ the concept of schizophrenia in scientific research. The case in support of these claims, of course, requires a massive undertaking and, in what follows, I shall only outline a strategy for assessing the evidential support for NDMS and indicate the directions in which I expect such an evidential analysis will lead.

Shoring up the case of the scientific critics

To systematically address the question of the strength of the evidential support for NDMS, a map of the evidence bearing on the model needs to be constructed that clarifies how the vast bodies of empirical data, which have been collected over the past several decades, is supposed to provide support for the various component hypotheses of NDMS, and hence the model itself. To this end, the following steps should be pursued:

(1) identify the component hypotheses of NDMS;
(2) for each, identify a class of 'evidential statements', which are intermediate hypotheses and which, if true, provide support for the given component hypothesis;
(3) for each evidential statement, identify a class of studies that, individually or collectively, bear upon its level of evidential support; and
(4) identify various evidentially relevant systemic features (e.g. simplicity, explanatory power) and relationships to background theories and findings that must be taken into account in assessing both the components of this structure (studies, evidential statements, component hypotheses) and the model as a whole.[4]

Given such an 'evidential map', the basic strategy of assessment is to determine the evidential strength provided to evidential statements by individual studies (and groups of studies), to determine the evidential strength provided to component hypotheses of the model by the evidential statements, and to determine the evidential strength provided to the model as a whole given all relevant evidential considerations.

As an example, consider the following component hypothesis of NDMS:

EP1—Schizophrenia is partially caused by one or more epigenetic influences that contribute to early disruption of neuro-developmental processes.

According to defenders of NDMS, this hypothesis receives support from, at least, the following evidential statements:

ES1—Schizophrenia is associated with the occurrence of famine during pregnancy.

ES2—Schizophrenia is associated with the occurrence of mechanical injury during or near birth.

ES3—Schizophrenia is associated with the occurrence of viral infection during the second trimester of pregnancy.

ES1–3, in their turn, are supposed to each receive support from a class of empirical studies that purport to provide data relevant to establishing the empirical associations mentioned in the evidential statements. Each of these studies, drawn from the epidemiological research of the past several decades, makes a specific contribution to the body of data relevant to one or another of ES1–3. Thus, the following list provides a small sampling of the various studies typically cited as bearing on these evidential statements:

ES1—Susser and Lin 1992; Susser *et al.* 1996.

ES2—Done *et al.* 1991; McNeil 1991; McCreadie *et al.* 1992.

ES3—Mednick *et al.* 1988; Barr *et al.* 1990; O'Callaghan *et al.* 1991; Crow 1994.

A complete map of the evidential structure of NDMS will repeat this process for each of the component hypotheses of the model, along with an identification of additional evidential considerations.

With such an evidential map in place, assessment of the strength of the support for NDMS proceeds in a series of steps that focus, in turn, on the individual studies bearing on a particular evidential statement, the classes of such studies, the evidential statements themselves, the component hypotheses of NDMS, and finally NDMS itself. The ultimate goal of the analysis is to provide an assessment of the strength of the evidential support for NDMS, something which resolves into an assessment of the force and relevance[5] of the empirical studies brought individually and collectively to bear on the evidential statements, an assessment of the force and relevance of the various evidential statements bearing on components of the model, and assessment of any other evidential considerations bearing on the status of NDMS (e.g. systemic features, relationships to background science).

There are a number of problems with the evidential case for NDMS that can be preliminarily identified as indicative of the directions the analysis of the evidence for NDMS will take. For example, with respect to the analysis of empirical studies, the following problems are not uncommon (see Heinrichs 2001 for a selective meta-analytic review of several areas of schizophrenia research):

- negative findings;
- weak effect sizes;
- inconsistent or unreplicated findings;
- non-comparable findings (e.g. due to varying conceptions of schizophrenia);
- uninterpretable findings (e.g. due to methodological flaws);
- findings of questionable relevance;
- free rider effects;[6]
- P.T. Barnum effects;[7]
- over-interpretation of findings.

Such problems with the empirical base undermine both the force and relevance of the findings and they contribute to problems higher up in the evidential framework, although new problems can emerge at higher levels as well. Thus, with respect to the evidential statements, they may suffer from lack of support due to problems with the force or relevance of the empirical studies, while the component hypotheses of the model may lack support due to limitations of the force or relevance of the evidential statements alleged to have an evidential bearing on them, or from problems with other sorts of evidential consideration (e.g. coherence with background scientific theories). Finally, the model as a whole, in addition to problems with support for its component hypotheses, might suffer from problems of simplicity, internal coherence, explanatory power, and coherence with background scientific theories and findings.

The main purpose of the sort of evidential assessment just outlined is to clarify the evidential status of the main prop supporting the continued use of the concept of schizophrenia in scientific research concerning severe mental illness. The anticipated outcome of the analysis is negative: namely, that the NDMS fails to have adequate evidential support to justify continued employment of the concept of schizophrenia in scientific research. Consequently, such an outcome will effectively close the loophole in the case of the scientific critics. However, the conclusion of all this will not be that there are no neurodevelopmental disorders or that the research being evaluated is of no value. Rather, it will be that such research and the development and assessment of hypotheses and models concerning severe and disabling mental illness are obstructed by the use of the schizophrenia concept. Schizophrenia is arguably an artificial and scientifically ungrounded imposition on research that leads to misdirection of valuable resources and misinterpretation of potentially important findings.

There are three stock rejoinders to the scientific criticism of NDMS that it is useful to articulate and to show why they are ineffective. The first is that the scientific criticism being developed constitutes harassment of an immature science that is attempting to comprehend and gain control over a highly complex disease entity. The idea is that researchers are doing the best they can, given the immaturity of the relevant basic sciences (e.g. neuroscience, cognitive science) and given the complex nature and heterogeneous forms of the target disease.

Now, although harassment of an immature science is a bad thing, it is not what is going on here. The sort of criticism under discussion is a perfectly legitimate form of critical activity in science, especially when, as in this case, the stakes are high. The argument of the scientific critics implies that the claim that schizophrenia exists and is a disease process worthy of intense scientific investigation has not been vindicated after a century of trying to do so (i.e. the concept of schizophrenia has no demonstrated construct validity). Thus, the concept of schizophrenia simply does not occupy the central role that it does in scientific and clinical practice because there exists a body of scientific evidence supporting it. As a result, it may well not play a justifiable role in such practices. In addition, the critics point out that there are indeed alternative approaches to the conceptualization and study of psychopathology. Critics such as Boyle and Bentall advocate a symptom focus grounded in the basic sciences; the alternative I favour represents a broader, more systematic and integrated extension of that basic idea (cf., Spaulding et al. 2003, Poland and Spaulding forthcoming). Thus, rather than engaging in harassment, the critics are concerned that there is a harmful over-commitment to a hypothesis with no serious evidential support and to which there are viable alternatives. This is a matter of scientific judgement and decision making in the face of the available evidence, and it is a matter of prudence concerning the relevant purposes of the scientific research in this area, not harassment.

The second stock rejoinder to the critics' case is that the concept of schizophrenia is a fruitful heuristic that, although imperfect, is a useful bridge to future scientific and clinical practice (cf., Frances et al. 1996). Again, the problem is with the evidence: it simply does not support the scientific and clinical utility of either the schizophrenia concept or the associated existential hypothesis. The research programme spawned by the concept has not proven to be productive, and it is becoming increasingly clear that diagnostic categories like schizophrenia (and, especially schizophrenia) do not play a useful role in either clinical assessment or the design and implementation of effective treatment plans for people with severe and disabling mental illness (e.g. drug responsiveness is not specific to schizophrenia; a clinical diagnosis of schizophrenia contributes nothing to managing patient heterogeneity and associated clinical uncertainty.) Comparable to the claim that there is no good evidence for the hypothesis that schizophrenia exists, there is no good evidence that the concept and hypothesis are pragmatically useful in clinical and research contexts, not to mention legal, educational, and healthcare policy contexts. Again, this is not to say that people do not have serious problems or that there are not serious needs that must be served and heuristic roles that must be occupied so that clinical practice and scientific research can proceed. But these needs and roles should not be served and occupied by the concept of schizophrenia and related hypotheses. For not only are these not useful, they are also harmful impediments to sound clinical and research practice (cf., Poland et al. 1994).[8]

The final stock rejoinder to consider here is essentially the challenge 'to put up or shut up'. Here the emphasis is on the lack of visible alternatives to current clinical and research practices, and hence on the burden of the critics to produce a viable alternative which, so the challenge goes, they have not done. The underlying assumption of the reply is that, if the critics cannot produce a viable alternative, they ought to cease making criticisms of current practices.

Although there is much that is wrong with this sort of rejoinder to the scientific critics, it is correct in one respect: viz., the critics do indeed have a burden to carry that involves the development of viable alternatives to current research, clinical, and other practices. The work of the sciences, the clinic, the law, education, and social policy concerning mental illness is not optional, and contributing to the constructive task of developing approaches to effectively doing this work is the burden of all participants in the process. But that is where conciliation ends.

This rejoinder (viz., 'put up or shut up') is a regressive, rearguard manoeuvre that fails to acknowledge the serious problems with the research record centred on 'schizophrenia'. It further fails to acknowledge the serious risks we are running of too aggressively pursuing a dead-end research programme and in shaping clinical and other practices around such a research programme. And, it fails to acknowledge the importance of critical activity to the constructive task of developing viable alternatives: to the extent that if we fail to recognize when a research programme is failing and to the extent that if we fail to understand why a programme fails, then we will lack both the will and the understanding to effectively pursue alternatives. As a consequence, 'Put up or shut up' is a potentially very destructive rejoinder if we take it seriously.

Enter the socio-political critics

To this point, I have focused on a major loophole in the master argument of the scientific critics, a loophole created by too close adherence to antiquated philosophy of science and by the limited scope of the evidence surveyed. I have further outlined a strategy for closing the loophole and, thereby, shoring up the scientific critics' case: viz., a tentative revision of the relevant scientific standard and a systematic assessment of the evidential status of NDMS, the dominant contemporary view of schizophrenia and the only available serious hope for successful theoretical validation of SZ. The anticipated outcome of pursuing this strategy is that it will become clear that NDMS lacks significant evidential support and that there is no scientific justification for continued employment of the concept of schizophrenia in research (as well as in clinical and other social practices). I have also surveyed three stock rejoinders to the scientific criticism and argued that each lacks significant force. And finally, I have acknowledged the importance of the critics' recognizing and carrying the burden of developing viable alternatives to the existing framework.

Now, assuming the strength of the scientific case against the employment of the concept of schizophrenia, it is fair to say that we are facing a serious crisis in research, clinical, and other cultural practices concerning severe and disabling mental illness (SDMI) (cf., Poland and Spaulding forthcoming). However, the deep entrenchment of the schizophrenia concept (i.e. the fact that it occupies essential roles in contemporary practices, that it is sustained by ideology, interests, and other cultural forces, and that it remains in place due to inertia and possibly some form of a 'sunk cost' effect) means that recognition of the problems and the need for radical changes will be slow, and that effecting meaningful change will be slower still. This is to say that the first and the second explanations of the ongoing entrenchment of the schizophrenia concept (i.e. the socio-political and the pragmatic explanations) have some merit. And, it is at this point that the insights and strategies of the socio-political critics may be of considerable value.

I have argued elsewhere (Poland and Spaulding forthcoming) that the only plausible course to pursue is a gradual revolution from the current crisis situation to a more stable and more defensible future framework within which scientific, clinical, and other social practices concerning SDMI are pursued. Neither ironic nor uncritical acceptance of the status quo are defensible, nor are vigorous attempts to vindicate the current framework, given its lack of scientific credibility. On the other hand, neither outright revolt nor passive-aggressive resistance are likely to be successful strategies, the former because the entrenchment is too severe at present, the latter because a more concerted and active response is required. Many practitioners have for years engaged in a form of passive-aggressive resistance without seriously shifting practices on a broad scale. Thus, only a gradual revolution pursued actively along a number of fronts is left.[9]

So, how might the insights and strategies of the socio-political critics be useful in pursuing this revolution? I shall mention just a few key ideas, each of which requires extensive development. First, a study of the socio-political critics will help to deepen our understanding of how scientific research and clinical activities are embedded in a matrix of cultural forces, institutions, and practices that influence, and are influenced by, those activities. Such understanding will lead to deeper appreciation of the ways and the extent to which, for better or worse, the science bearing on mental illness is shaped by culture (e.g. due to the social importance of healthcare issues and to the commercial interests of drug and insurance companies.) And, such appreciation will aid the revolution by revealing the grounds of the deep entrenchment of the schizophrenia concept, by helping to identify appropriate targets for change, and by helping to identify processes and strategies by which change can be accomplished.

A concrete example of this can be seen in the ways in which decisions are currently made about the official manual of diagnostic categories concerning mental disorder (i.e. the DSM).[10]

The process is firmly in the grip of a single professional guild that has made decisions that are visibly influenced more by guild interests than by scientific argument. A thorough critical examination of the sociological characteristics of this process will likely reveal that it fails to satisfy basic standards for scientific decision making (e.g. that the process is neither open, nor adequately informed, nor grounded in scientifically appropriate considerations; that it does not conform to appropriate scientific standards; that it is not free from the influence of inappropriate guild or commercial interests; that the relevant community fails to exhibit an authority structure appropriate to scientific communities.) This sort of analysis leads to ideas for how to effect meaningful change; but the ideas are of an essentially socio-political character: e.g. wrest the process away from the firm control of a single professional guild, create the conditions of a scientific community, introduce an appropriate authority structure.

A second example concerns the recognition that entrenchment of the concept of schizophrenia is maintained by the shaping of perception, thought, and action of the public, policy makers, other scientists, and (most importantly) future generations. Such shaping is accomplished by promulgating entrenched ways of thinking through public relations and advertisement campaigns (e.g. drug advertisements), formal education (e.g. textbooks), the informal 'education' of the public and patients about the disease called 'schizophrenia' (e.g. the recent US Surgeon General's report on mental illness (USSG 1999), other sorts of public service announcements, cinematic and literary portrayals of mental illness), and the linking of access to healthcare to a certain understanding of clinical problems (e.g. parity issues regarding reimbursement for healthcare are being linked to conceiving of schizophrenia as a brain disease.) Each of these modes of influence perpetuates a certain way of framing the phenomena, the questions, the evidence, and so on; and, such framing shapes how we perceive, think about, and respond to the phenomena in scientific, clinical, and everyday contexts.

Such forms of influence are exacerbated by the inevitable authority structure within scientific communities, a structure that makes us all dependent on whomever are the identified 'experts' in a given area. We are thus vulnerable to being co-opted into a certain agenda by making specific assumptions about who occupies the role of 'expert' and by accepting how those 'experts' frame the problems, activities, and products in their domain of expertise. This risk is especially severe when a crisis exists in a scientific sub-community, and it is made worse when scientists in adjacent sub-communities become co-opted (e.g. as when neuroscientists and cognitive scientists innocently assume that schizophrenia is a well-defined disease condition because it is recognized as such by the 'experts').[11]

The critics are suggesting that, with respect to severe and disabling mental illness and the crisis outlined above, the questions of what constitutes expertise in this area and who are the real 'experts' are key components of what is under dispute. And, how we answer these questions will directly affect how we conceive the phenomenon of interest and how we approach scientific, clinical, and social issues focused upon it.

In the light of this sort of understanding, a variety of targets and ideas for action are suggested: e.g. counter-advertisement, alternative textbooks (cf., Spaulding *et al.* 2003), policy reform, novel approaches to the training of clinicians and scientific researchers. And, with respect to the training of researchers, in light of the issues of scientific expertise described above, improvements should reach not just those who are directly involved in research concerning mental illness, but also researchers in adjacent or embedding fields as well (e.g. neuroscience, cognitive science), since it is important to protect against the larger scientific community becoming unwitting partners in maintaining entrenched but flawed concepts and practices. This line of thought clearly requires more systematic development, but the thrust is clear: strategies for protecting against this sort of co-opting of the larger scientific community (as well as the general public) should be developed.

The various points discussed in this paper suggest what I shall call a 'recipe for revolution' that combines the ideas of both the scientific and the sociopolitical critics and includes at least the following elements: pursuit of the scientific criticism of the concept of schizophrenia as outlined above; aggressive pursuit of the development of alternative scientific and clinical frameworks; unmasking of the vested interests, sources of bias, and rhetorical strategies of the defenders of the entrenched concept; pursuit of widespread educational reform through a variety of means (e.g. consciousness raising about the crisis, textbooks, professional training); and pursuit of policy reform in a variety of domains (e.g. research funding, access to health care, clinical evaluation standards, mental health legislation.).

Some general morals to be drawn from this discussion are as follows. First, the ideas of the scientific and socio-political critics concerning the concept of schizophrenia and related practices should be refined and integrated to produce more effective arguments and more effective frameworks within which to pursue change in all areas of mental health practice. Second, when critical scrutiny of both sorts is aggressively pursued, the scientific and pragmatic arguments for change become overwhelming and the targets for effective revolutionary action come into view.[12]

And, finally, it is not possible to disentangle the 'purely scientific' issues from the others,[13] since much of contemporary science concerning mental illness is shaped by concepts like schizophrenia, that have a non-scientific origin, are deeply value-laden, and are maintained by powerful non-scientific forces that, at a minimum, need to be closely scrutinized and better understood.[14]

Endnotes

1. The term 'mental illness' is being used here in a colloquial and non-technical way to pick out the various forms of psychological suffering, disability, deviance, and maladaption to the demands of life that lead people to seek help or lead others to seek help for them. This usage does not carry with it any implication regarding disease, disorder, or dysfunction in any of the technical senses advanced in the literature.

2. I shall employ the following conventions in attempting to manage the potential for confusion raised by the various linguistic forms in play: 'schizophrenia' and 'SZ' will both be used to mention the concept of schizophrenia; 'schizophrenia' will be used to mention the hypothetical construct (the putative condition) associated with the concept. I will be assuming for present purposes that a demonstration of the lack of construct validity of SZ (schizophrenia) will be sufficient for establishing the lack of scientific justification for believing that schizophrenia exists.

3. The following description of the NDMS and the evidence advanced in its support is based upon materials found in Weinberger (1995), Green (1998, 2001), Johnstone et al. (1999), Andreasen (2001), and Heinrichs (2001).

4. The structure of such an evidential map can, to some extent, be understood in terms of Bogen and Woodward's (1988) distinction between data, phenomena, and theories. The purpose of constructing such a map is to clarify and make salient the various elements and relations that become the object of an evidential assessment, as roughly outlined in the text and the next footnote. Space limitations prohibit more systematic presentation of the assessment strategy alluded to here.

5. The 'force' and 'relevance' of a study or statement are concepts designed to capture dimensions for evaluating evidential strength. Intuitively, a given study or group of studies that support an empirical finding (e.g. a statistically significant association of a certain size between being classified as schizophrenic and exposure to influenza during the second trimester of pregnancy) provide support of a certain strength for an evidential statement (e.g. schizophrenia is associated with the occurrence of viral

infection during the second trimester of pregnancy), depending upon such factors as inferential connections between the empirical finding and the evidential statement, the support for assumptions made in such inferences, the methodological soundness of the studies (e.g. considerations of internal and external validity), replication and convergence of the studies, and so on. Those factors concerning how much bearing an empirical finding has on a certain target statement is a matter of relevance, whereas those factors concerning how much evidential support a finding provides, assuming that it bears on the target, is a matter of force. In short, the evidential strength provided depends on the extent to which a finding bears on a target statement and the degree of support the finding provides.

6. Roughly, a 'free-rider' effect arises when an inclusively defined hypothetical construct (e.g. schizophrenia) is shown to be correlated to some other variable, but the correlation is due exclusively to the presence of a feature that is included under the definition of the construct (e.g. hallucinations). In such a case, the construct, is a free rider contributing nothing beyond the contribution of the included feature.

7. Roughly, a 'P.T. Barnum' effect is the establishment of a correlation between some vaguely and disjunctively defined hypothetical construct (e.g. schizophrenia) and some other feature: in such cases the vagueness and the disjunctive character of the definition make possible the inclusion of either a single feature sufficient to create the effect (i.e. a free-rider effect) or the inclusion of enough smaller, independent correlations that in aggregate create a significant association that gives rise to the appearance that the construct is significantly associated to some other feature. In both sorts of case, it is an overinterpretation of the findings to say that the identified construct is correlated with some other variable, and hence is 'validated' to some extent.

8. These points are consistent with the fact that many clinicians and researchers use the concept in their various practices to make decisions, and, indeed, with the fact that many clinicians and researchers have a strong sense that the concept is useful. Such psychological and sociological facts do not entail that the clinical work is getting done effectively or that the research is productive. Further, the claims made in the text are also consistent with the observation that some people who are labelled with 'schizophrenia' do respond to certain interventions. A treatment to which some people respond positively is not necessarily a treatment of the putative disease expressed by the diagnostic label, 'schizophrenia', any more than it would be a treatment of demonic possession in an earlier period. The same people who are labelled as schizophrenic today might well have been labelled as demonically possessed a few centuries ago, and some of those people might well have experienced a reduction of 'symptoms' in response to drug therapies. Presumably, we would not be inclined to say either that this validates the category of demonic possession or that the label is therefore justifiably employed in clinical practice. The reason is that responsiveness of specific features in some members of a class is consistent with the class being artificial and problematic. This point is reinforced by the nonspecificity to schizophrenia of response to drug therapies and by the significant number of 'treatment non-responders' among those carrying the label 'schizophrenia'.

9. This way of framing the issues and the argument for revolution has been heavily influenced by the work of Hacking (1999).

10. Information regarding the character of this process is more available than it had been in the past due to the publication of the DSM sourcebook and related development documents. The process of developing recent versions of the DSM has been subjected to critical scrutiny by Kirk and Kutchins (1992, 1997) and Caplan (1995), among others. See Poland (2001, 2002) for reviews of the first and second volumes of the sourcebook.

11. Under such conditions (i.e. the co-option of adjacent scientific sub-communities) the full weight of authority of the scientific community is brought to bear, not because a consensus has been reached on the basis of broadly agreed upon evaluation processes, but because of specious authority relations and unfounded trust. This, at least, is the risk to which we are currently vulnerable. See Poland and Spaulding (forthcoming) for discussion, and see Kitcher (1993, 2001) and Longino (1990, 2002) for more general discussions of authority in science.

12. Space prohibits a discussion of the powerful 'moral' arguments for change in this area.

13. Recent work in the philosophy of science suggests that such a distinction is bogus, that attempts at demarcation are fruitless, and that deeper analysis reveals that the social (the moral, the political) is an essential dimension of the scientific. Neither of these points means that there is no such thing as scientific objectivity; they mean that we need a more sophisticated understanding of what such objectivity consists. See Kitcher (1993, 2001), Longino (1990, 2002), and Lacey (1999) for important, but somewhat different, approaches to these ideas.

14. Thanks to Jonathan Cohen, George Graham, Casey Haskins, Aaron Meskin, Shaun Nichols, and Barbara Von Eckardt for helpful discussion, comments, and suggestions. A version of this paper was presented to the Philosophy Department at Washington University during the Fall of 2001.

References

American Psychiatric Association (1980). *Diagnostic and statistical manual of mental disorders* (3rd edn) (DSM-III). Washington: American Psychiatric Association Press.

American Psychiatric Association (1987). *Diagnostic and statistical manual of mental disorders* (3rd edn-revised) (DSM-III-R). Washington: American Psychiatric Association Press.

American Psychiatric Association (1994). *Diagnostic and statistical manual of mental disorders* (4th edn) (DSM-IV). Washington: American Psychiatric Association Press.

Andreasen, N. (2001). *Brave new brain*. New York: Oxford University Press.

Barr, C., Mednick, S., and Munk-Jorgensen, P. (1990). Exposure to influenza epidemics during gestation and adult schizophrenia: a 40 year study. *Archives of General Psychiatry*, **47**: 869–874.

Bentall, R. (ed.) (1990). *Reconstructing schizophrenia*. New York: Routledge.

Bogen, J. and Woodward, J. (1988). Saving the phenomena. *Philosophical Review*, **97**: 303–352.

Boyle, M. (1990). *Schizophrenia: a scientific delusion?* London: Routledge.

Caplan, P. (1995). *They say you're crazy*. Reading: Addison-Wesley.

Cromwell, R. (1983). Preemptive thinking and schizophrenia research. In: *Nebraska symposium on motivation*, vol. 31 (ed. W. Spaulding), pp. 1–46. Lincoln: University of Nebraska Press.

Crow, T. (1994). Prenatal exposure to influenza as a cause of schizophrenia: There are inconsistencies and contradictions in the evidence. *British Journal of Psychiatry*, **164**: 588–592.

Done, J., Johnstone, E., and Frith, C. *et al.* (1991). Complications of pregnancy and delivery in relation to psychosis in adult life: data from the British Perinatal Mortality Survey Sample. *British Medical Journal*, **302**: 1576–1586.

Frances, A., First, M., and Pincus, H. (1996). *DSM-IV guidebook*. Washington: American Psychiatric Association Press.

Gottesman, I. (1991). *Schizophrenia genesis: the origins of madness*. New York: Freeman.

Green, M. (1998). *Schizophrenia from a neurocognitive perspective*. Boston: Allyn Bacon.

Green, M. (2001). *Schizophrenia revealed*. New York: Norton.

Hacking, I. (1999). *The social construction of what?* Cambridge: Harvard University Press.

Heinrichs, R.W. (1993). Schizophrenia and the brain: conditions for a neuropsychology of madness. *American Psychologist*, **48**: 221–233.

Heinrichs, R.W. (2001). *In search of madness*. New York: Oxford University Press.

Johnstone, E., Humphreys, M., Lang, F., Lawrie, S., and Sandler, R. (1999). *Schizophrenia*. Cambridge: Cambridge University Press.

Kirk, S. and Kutchins, H. (1992). *The selling of the dsm: the rhetoric of science in psychiatry*. New York: Aldine De Gruyter.

Kitcher, P. (1993). *The advancement of science*. New York: Oxford University Press.

Kitcher, P. (2001). *Science, truth, and democracy*. New York: Oxford University Press.

Kutchins, H. and Kirk, S. (1997). *Making us crazy*. New York: Free Press.

Lacey, H. (1999). *Is science value free?* New York: Routledge.

Longino, H. (1990). *Science as social knowledge*. Princeton: Princeton University Press.

Longino, H. (2002). *The fate of knowledge*. Princeton: Princeton University Press.

McCreadie, R., Berry, I., and Robertson, L. (1992). The Nithsdale schizophrenia surveys: X. Obstetric complications, family history, and abnormal movements. *British Journal of Psychiatry*, **160**: 799–805.

McNeil, T. (1991). Obstetric complications in schizophrenic parents. *Schizophrenia Research*, **5**: 89–101.

Mednick, S., Machon, R., Huttunen, M., and Bonnett, E. (1988). Adult schizophrenia following prenatal exposure to an influenza epidemic. *Archives of General Psychiatry*, **45**: 189–192.

Mouldin, S. and Gottesman, I. (1997). Genes, experience, and chance in schizophrenia: positioning for the 21st century. *Schizophrenia Bulletin*, **23**: 547–561.

O'Callaghan, E., Gibson, T, and Colohan, H, *et al.* (1991). Season of birth in schizophrenia: evidence for confinement of an excess of winter births to patients without a family history of mental disorder. *British Journal of Psychiatry*, **158**: 764–769.

Poland, J. (2001). Review of the DSM Sourcebook, vol.1. Metapsychology, http://mentalhelp.net/books/books.php?type=de&id=557.

Poland, J. (2002). Review of the *DSM Sourcebook, Volume 2. Metapsychology*, http://mentalhelp.net/books/books.php?type=de&id=996.

Poland, J. and Spaulding, W. (forthcoming). *Crisis and revolution: toward a reconceptualization of psychopathology*. Cambridge: MIT Press.

Poland, J., Von Eckardt, B., and Spaulding, W. (1994). Problems with the DSM approach to classifying psychopathology. In: *Philosophical psychopathology* (ed. G. Graham and L. Stephens), pp. 235–260. Cambridge: The MIT Press.

Sarbin, T. (1990). Toward the obsolescence of the schizophrenia hypothesis. *The Journal of Mind and Behaviour*, **11**: 259–284.

Spaulding, W., Sullivan, M., and Poland, J. (2003). *Treatment and rehabilitation of severe mental illness*. New York: Guilford.

Susser, E. and Lin, S. (1992). Schizophrenia after exposure to the Dutch hunger winter of 1944–1945. *Archives of General Psychiatry*, **49**: 983–988.

Susser, E., Hoek, H., Brown, A., and Lin, S. (1996). Schizophrenia after prenatal famine: further evidence. *Archives of General Psychiatry*, **53**: 25–31.

USSG (1999). *Mental health: a report of the surgeon general*. National Institute of Mental Health, Washington.

Weinberger, D. (1995). Schizophrenia as a neurodevelopmental disorder. In: *Schizophrenia* (ed. R. Hirsch and D. Weinberger), pp. 293–323. Oxford: Blackwell Science.

Woods, B. (1998). Is schizophrenia a progressive neurodevelopmental disorder? Toward a unitary pathogenetic mechanism. *American Journal of Psychiatry* **155**: 1661–1670.

10 The delusional stance

G. Lynn Stephens and George Graham[1]

Introduction

Delusions are elements in a number of mental illnesses, and clinical descriptions, in particular, of schizophrenia abound in delusion attribution.

Laura, a young woman suffering from schizophrenia and the subject of a case study by McKay *et al.* (1996), exhibited, among other symptoms of this illness, several different sorts of delusions.[2]

She reported that members of the hospital staff were plotting against her (persecutory delusions). She found comments that she said were directed to her or about her in popular magazines and claimed that characters in television programmes were flirting with her boyfriend (delusions of reference). She complained that external agents compelled her to pace the ward and urinate on herself (delusions of control). Though admitting that the agents were not visible to others, she insisted that they spoke to her, commenting on her behaviour and issuing commands (voices).[3]

Indeed, Laura maintained that they sometimes invaded her mind, banishing her own thoughts (thought withdrawal), and projecting their thoughts into her stream of consciousness (thought insertion). She also claimed that other people were directly aware of her thoughts as soon as they occurred to her (thought broadcasting).

Delusions are not peculiar to schizophrenia (see Young and Leafblood (1996) for a case of non-schizophrenic delusions after brain injury). They occur in a variety of functional and organic mental disorders, although some of Laura's delusions, such as thought insertion, are significant for differential diagnosis of schizophrenia (Mellor 1970). Delusions are, moreover, a common feature of schizophrenia. Sartorius *et al.* (1986, p. 922) found that 73% of schizophrenics in a large cross-cultural sample exhibited delusional misinterpretations such as Laura's persecutory delusions; 63% showed delusions of reference; 50% showed delusions of control. Thought broadcasting was found in 22%; 57% experienced verbal hallucinations, often with associated delusions. It seems reasonable to hope, therefore, that understanding delusions would help us to understand the pathological processes at work in schizophrenia. Unfortunately, however, as Young (1999) observes, 'although a common clinical phenomenon, delusions are difficult to explain and have a problematic conceptual status' (p. 571). Students of delusion have long recognized part of the conceptual problem.

According to the traditional account, delusions are 'pathological beliefs' (Marshall and Halligan 1996, p. 8; also Chen and Berrios 1998, p. 167). This is supposed to mean that they are (in part) false beliefs (APA 1994, p. 275). However to err is human, so mere falsity alone does not distinguish them from non-pathological beliefs. Other factors, including bizarreness of content, incomprehensibility, cultural idiosyncrasy, incorrigibility, and so on, have been cited as additional characteristics.[4]

Worse, the recent literature on delusions suggests that even the most basic and heretofore uncontroversial element of the traditional account has become problematic. Are delusions really beliefs? Authors such as Fulford (1989, 1993, 1994), Berrios (1991, 1996), Sass (1994), Garety and Hemsley (1995), Chen and Berrios (1998), Young (1999), and Currie (2000), among others, raise serious challenges to the conception of delusions as beliefs. This challenge is particularly unsettling since, although there is something like a new consensus for rejecting the proposition that delusions are beliefs, there is no comparable agreement regarding the sort of account of delusions that should be put in its place.

In this chapter we want specifically to do two things. First, we shall propose a theory of the nature of delusions that addresses the objections to the traditional belief-based account and resolves its conceptual problems. Second, we shall explore some implications of our theory of delusions for understanding the pathological processes underlying schizophrenia.

To preview our discussion: We shall begin by reviewing the considerations that have led researchers to question the idea that delusions are beliefs. Then we shall explain why objections to the belief-centred understanding of delusions have, so far, failed to coalesce into a satisfactory alternative account. We shall then present a conception of delusions that we call the Delusional Stance Thesis ('DST', for short), which will (we hope) provide the desired alternative account.

Our Delusional Stance Thesis has two parts or component theses. The first part is the thesis of the higher order stance (hereafter 'DST-1'):

> **DST-1:** All delusions are higher order attitudes that constitute a kind of stance taken towards lower order mental contents or intentional states which may be of a variety of different sorts (including, but not restricted to, beliefs).[5]

The second is the thesis of delusional stance characteristics (hereafter 'DST-2'):

> **DST-2:** The higher order or delusional stance involves the deluded person's identifying himself or herself with the relevant first-order contents, so much

so that he or she persistently maintains those contents, incorrigibly, in the face of strong counter-considerations and with a disturbing lack of diagnostic or first-person insight.

We argue that DST does justice to the objections to the traditional account and provides a way of organizing various suggestions, available in the recent literature, for revising that account into a satisfactory alternative theory of delusions.

Finally, we shall suggest that the DST account of delusions connects in a fruitful way with current views on various other phenomena associated with schizophrenia. These include verbal hallucinations (voices) and so-called passivity experiences, such as thought insertion. Various authors argue that the pathological significance of verbal hallucinations, for example, does not lie in the hallucinating subject's primary perceptual experience or first-order representation of the world. It lies in his/her attitudes toward such representations and in his/her attempts (or failures) to integrate them into his/her understanding of her own mental life (see Stephens and Graham (2000) for discussion and references). We shall argue, similarly, that the deluded person's problem does not lie in the content or nature of his/her first-order intentional states, but in his/her failure to appreciate the role that these states play in his/her psychological economy. It is not *what* is thought, but *how* it is thought that explains the pathological character of delusions.

We should add, however, that although what is thought—the lower order content of delusion—does not account for the pathological character of delusions, reference to what is thought may be germane to categorizing types of delusions (Gelder *et al.* 1996, pp. 12–14). The difference, for example, between amorous delusions, whose thematic content is that another person is in love with the deluded subject, and persecutory delusions that the subject him-/herself is being conspired against or cheated, is a difference in lower order content—in what is thought. However, if we allow that victims of delusions are deluded by virtue of the patently false, bizarre, or otherwise problematic lower order content of their delusions, we are bound to wonder how these contents differ from many non-delusional contents which, from certain points of view, can seem equally bizarre. As DSM-IV (APA 1994, p. 296) notes: 'bizarreness' may be difficult to judge, especially across different cultures'. Sedler (1995, p. 259) remarks that, although the content of delusion 'superficially engages one's attention, and indeed has dominated clinical theory', content alone is 'insufficient to understand what makes a delusion'.[6]

Our view is that the hallmark of delusion is not the unusual quality or character of the lower order content of a delusion—its bizarreness, falsity, incomprehensibility, whatever—but the type of overall stance that the victim takes towards relevant lower order thoughts or contents. The delusional stance may include bizarre, false, and incomprehensible lower order attitudes, as often is the case with delusions, and these features of lower order attitudes may be among the foci of therapy for delusions in an effort to disabuse a victim of the delusional stance. But it is the stance that makes for delusion, not the bizarreness. Aspects or relevant characteristics of this delusional stance include those mentioned in DST-2, each of which will be discussed later in the paper.

Delusion and belief

What understanding of delusion is expressed by the claim that delusions are beliefs? We propose (without detailed defence in this context) that the following are the four main prototypical constituents of the very idea of delusions as beliefs.

1. If delusions are beliefs, delusions have content. They express propositions and are a paradigmatic propositional attitude. The believer has in mind a certain way that things are or might be. Suppose I believe that the sky is falling. It is, primarily, this propositional content that distinguishes one belief from another: my belief that the sky is falling from my belief that the sky is cloudy. Just as I can adopt the same attitude toward different propositions, I can adopt different attitudes toward the same proposition. I believe that the sky is falling; I fear that the sky is falling; I imagine that the sky is falling. It is characteristics of the attitude that distinguish believing from fearing, hoping, and imagining.

2. If delusions are beliefs, one is deluded that the sky is falling only if one is convinced that it is true that the sky is falling. I might imagine that the sky is falling, i.e. entertain the thought that the sky is falling, though I know perfectly well that it is not so. I might fear that the sky is falling, but be uncertain that the sky is really falling. Conviction or confidence in the truth of a proposition is one of the essential characteristics that distinguish believing a proposition from other attitudes one might take toward it.

3. If delusions are beliefs, one who has the delusion that the sky is falling will take account of his/her conviction of the truth of that proposition in his/her reasoning and his/her actions. Beliefs are supposed to guide reasoning and action. A person who believes the sky is falling will accept obvious logical implications of their belief, for example, that the sky is the sort of thing that can fall. They will take it for granted that the sky is falling when they reason about other things, for instance, if they try to predict what they will see when they look overhead tomorrow. This is particularly true of what philosophers call 'practical' reasoning, i.e. the reasoning in which a person engages when they try to figure out what to do or how to behave. Changing your beliefs will change your ideas about what actions are possible or

appropriate, about which of your desires can be satisfied and about what you need to do in order to satisfy them.

4. Finally, if delusions are beliefs, delusions will have 'appropriate' effects on one's emotions. Beliefs tend to call up suitable affective states, given one's values and desires. If you have always enjoyed gazing up at the sky, the belief that it is falling will occasion sorrow or regret. If one anticipates some harm to one's self should the sky fall, the belief that it is falling will produce anxiety, distress, or perhaps panic.

Critics of the traditional belief centred account argue that delusions are not, or are not in general, beliefs because delusions fail to exhibit one or more of (1) through (4).

Contrary to (4), Sass (1994, pp. 23–24) observes that victims of schizophrenic delusions may report that others are trying to kill or harm them while apparently remaining completely indifferent to this prospect. Patients claiming to have achieved unique and remarkable insight into the secrets of the universe or to have been selected for some exalted destiny do not seem excited or exhilarated. Sass suggests that, if they genuinely believed what they say, they should exhibit the affective responses appropriate to their imagined situation. Delusions often do not have the emotional impact of the corresponding beliefs.

Contrary to (3), Currie (2000, p. 174) reports that delusions often 'fail to engage behavior'. Patients suffering from the delusion that their nurses are trying to poison them do not act like they believe that their nurses want to poison them. They uncomplainingly eat food served by their nurses, calmly submit to injections, and readily swallow pills (Sass 1994, p. 21). Young (1999, p. 581) observes that, even patients who exhibit some behaviour appropriate to their delusions do not act consistently. A Capgras patient, who claims that his closest relatives have been replaced by imposters, may refuse to carry on natural domestic interactions with the 'imposter' whom he claims has been substituted for his wife. But he does not file a missing person's report or undertake any investigation to determine what has become of his 'real' wife.

Sass (1994, p. 21) remarks that deluded patients often seem to engage in a kind of 'double book-keeping'. They make statements indicating a serious lack of contact with reality but otherwise seem to maintain an accurate appreciation of their situation. The patient who stoutly denies that he is in the hospital may also inquire when he will be discharged. The patient who reports that she has no children will, when asked, provide an accurate list of their names. Young (1999, p. 581) says that delusions are 'highly circumscribed'. Coming to have the delusion that you are dead does not produce the kind of changes in your other beliefs and intentions that would be produced by acquiring the belief that you are dead.

Contrary to (2), Sass (1994, pp. 20–21) suggests that deluded patients do not seem all that convinced of their delusions. Rather they maintain a distant 'ironic' attitude towards them, very different from the typical believer's commitment to the truth of his beliefs. Indeed, the patient frequently gives indications that he/she does not regard the statements expressing his/her delusions as 'literally' or 'objectively' true (p. 8). Young (1999, p. 579) finds that expressions of contents of delusion do not seem to be 'assertoric', but are offered in a sort of 'as if' spirit.

Finally, against (1), Berrios (1996) urges that despite the patient's verbal output, he/she often seems to have nothing definite in mind. On close examination, the patient's speech production doesn't seem to express any specifiable, coherent propositional content. The patient repeats a form of words but cannot say what those words mean or what they imply. This leads Berrios to maintain that verbal expressions of delusions are 'empty speech acts', not backed by any content intelligible to the bearer or to the speaker. Berrios (1996, pp. 115, 126) writes as follows:

> Properly described, delusions are empty speech-acts that disguise themselves as beliefs. Although delusions purport to . . . convey information, they turn out to be epitemologically manque. Their so-called content refers . . . neither to world nor self. They are not symbolic expressions of anything.

In light of frequent failure to exhibit appropriate connections with both affect and action, the patient's failure to integrate the content of delusions appropriately into his/her web of beliefs and other intentional states, lack of genuine conviction on the part of the subject, and the speaker's inability to express any intelligible content, critics charge that 'delusions are so unlike normal beliefs that it must be asked why we persist in calling them beliefs at all' (Berrios 1996, pp.114–115).

On the other hand, even critics of the traditional account acknowledge that the belief picture seems to properly describe *some* instances of delusion. Sass (1994) admits: 'It cannot be denied that . . . patients do at times make claims that give every appearance of being delusional in the traditional sense' (p. 51). Jones and Watson (1997, p. 11), in a study in which they compared schizophrenic delusions with so-called 'overvalued ideas' (associated with anorexia) and conventional religious beliefs, found that their schizophrenic subjects 'were in general certain that their delusions were factually truthful'. They also note that these subjects claim that their delusions (which of course subjects themselves do not classify as delusions) strongly influence their beliefs and actions. Such self-reports do not establish, of course, that the subjects do generally think and act in ways guided by their delusion, but they reinforce the finding that these subjects are convinced of the truth of their delusion. Their delusions may not be beliefs, but certain patients believe that they are.

The above possibility fits nicely with a thesis of Currie (2000) that delusions involve 'cognitive hallucinations'. Although the deluded subject who says that the sky is falling may not believe that the sky is falling, she does believe that she has that belief. However, Currie himself admits 'it would be unwise to suppose that everything commonly described as a delusion in schizophrenia could be adequately re-described in this way. . . . People with schizophrenia do sometimes act on their thoughts [for] perhaps at this point their thoughts have arrived at the status of beliefs' (p. 176).

Young (1999) also recognizes that some patients act on their delusions, which 'shows that [the delusions] are not invariably metaphors, empty speech acts or solipsistic reflections' (pp.580–581). That people may act on their delusions is clear if we turn to erotomania, Othello syndrome, and other such non-psychotic delusions. These cases generally come to the attention of medical and legal professionals precisely because the patient behaves as one would who believes that he is loved from afar by some celebrity or is being cuckolded by his wife. Likewise, patients suffering from non-psychotic paranoid delusions are notorious for their tendency to carefully integrate their delusions into the structure of their beliefs about the world.

Jones and Wilson (1997) found no significant difference between the affective impact of schizophrenic delusions and religious beliefs on the subjects in their study. Similarly, those with Othello syndrome or paranoid delusions give every appearance of experiencing jealousy, suspicion, anxiety, and so forth.

As Young (1999) concludes: 'The issues involved in determining the conceptual status of delusions are tricky—one can draw attention to delusions which seem pretty convincing false beliefs, or one can draw attention to delusions which seem like solipsistic empty speech acts' (p. 581).

The issues as to whether delusions are beliefs or non-beliefs are made trickier by the fact, also emphasized by Young (1999, pp. 582–583), that belief attribution in ordinary, non-psychiatric contexts is beset by the same issues that arise for delusions. As Bayne and Pacherie (2005) remark, 'the category "belief" is far from homogeneous' (p. 179). People often show less commitment to what they claim to believe than a favoured philosophical account of belief would lead one to expect. People frequently fail to accept logical consequences of propositions they endorse, and act in ways that seem inconsistent with what they avow. And, as everyone experienced in undergraduate instruction knows, they are sometimes unable to go beyond mere repetition of verbal formulas when asked what it is they believe. Perhaps the problem is less that many delusions do not conform well to the traditional account of delusions in the psychiatric literature, than that many alleged beliefs do not conform to a prototypical or favoured conception of belief (see, for example, Bayne and Pacherie 2005).

Critical assessment of the problem of delusions

On a superficial level, the problem we have been discussing is that the clinical use of the term 'delusion' is not captured by the traditional concept of delusion. The traditional concept applies only to beliefs; yet, in clinical practice, the term is applied to states of the patient that, for various reasons, cannot be understood or readily described as beliefs. However, the term is also applied clinically to states that are 'pretty convincing beliefs'. So, as regards the clinical use of the term, we can say neither that:

> delusions are beliefs;

nor that:

> delusions are not beliefs.

At any rate, it does not do justice to clinical practice to endorse either of these slogans and let it go at that.

Moreover there is deeper problem here than the need for linguistic caution or for a good semantic model of the category 'belief'. Sass (1994) criticizes the traditional view not so much because he thinks that it is appropriate to call certain states 'delusions' even though they are not beliefs, but because the account focuses our attention on the wrong features of beliefs—features that do not express delusional pathology. In the traditional view, he says: 'One supposes that, whereas there is a disturbance in the content of the patients' worlds (*what* they believe ... is unrealistic or illogical), the form of these worlds (the overall 'structure' or 'feel', the *way* they believe what they believe) is essentially normal' (p. 2). Whereas for Sass, it is not what the patient believes, or even that he believes it, which makes the patient delusional. It is the way the patient believes or relates to the content of the delusion. Sass (1994, p. 4) notes that Jaspers claimed that being deluded involved being in a special 'delusional mood' and that even true beliefs should be considered delusions, if they occur in the grip of such a mood.

Fulford (1993) suggests similar reservations about the traditional concept. He writes, 'It is not the content but the form of the belief which is crucial to its status as a psychotic symptom' (p. 14). Thinking of delusions as 'irrational beliefs' suggests that the patient's problem should be understood 'in terms of impaired cognitive functioning'. Instead, Fulford urges that 'the irrationality of delusions should be understood in terms not of defective cognitive functioning but rather of impaired reasons for action' (p. 14). That is, it is not understanding how the patient gathers, processes, stores information that represents the problem in delusions, rather it is the way the patient uses this information in decision-making. The patient's irrationality is practical (related to choice and action) rather than theoretical (relating to his representation of reality).

Underlying the problematic issue of delusions-as-beliefs is the perplexing question of how to understand the nature of the disturbance of the patient's psychological functioning represented by delusions. Is delusion fundamentally a cognitive deficit (a matter of embracing an erroneous or evidentially unsupported picture of reality) or is it some other sort of defect—a matter of how the patient uses or relates to a given picture of reality? Merely adjusting the traditional concept of delusions as beliefs to handle clinical non-belief counterexamples will not resolve this more basic question.

DST-1 and delusions as higher order attitudes

In this section we address what we called above the 'superficial problem': that in clinical usage 'delusion' refers both to states that are beliefs and states that are not. We reserve the deeper problem of the nature of the delusional impairment for the next section.

Recall Currie's (2000, p. 175) suggestion that 'what we normally describe as the delusional belief that p ought sometimes to be described as the delusional belief that I believe that p'. In our judgement there is an important insight in this approach. Currie's idea is that delusions are 'second-order beliefs': beliefs that take as their content or object, not a proposition about the way things are in the (external) world, but a proposition to the effect that one has a certain (first-order) belief about the way the world is. This reference to higher orders within delusional experience allows Currie to explain why the patient endorses the proposition that the sky is falling, or affirms that she believes that proposition, and yet fails to act on it, reason according to it, or show the appropriate affective response to it. She answers 'Yes' to the question, 'Do you believe that the sky is falling?' because she second-order believes that she (first-order) believes that the sky is falling. She is, as it were, of the conviction or attitude that she has the belief that the sky is falling. However she does not exhibit the full range of behavioural and affective responses appropriate to a person who believes that the sky is falling, because she does not in fact have that first-order belief. She only mistakenly believes that she has that belief. It is the presence or absence of the first-order belief that determines her behavioural and affective dispositions.

Although we admire Currie's basic hierarchical approach to delusions, we have doubts about his details. Currie acknowledges that his theory has problems explaining why some deluded patients do act or feel in ways appropriate to someone who has the relevant first-order belief, i.e. why some patients who have the delusion that the sky is falling seek cover and exhibit distress. His only suggestion here is that, perhaps the second-order belief that one believes that the sky is falling can, under certain conditions, cause one to come to first-order believe that the sky is falling.

However, there is another way to look at the situation, one that includes the insight that delusions are second-order attitudes, but that proposes two changes in Currie's account of delusions. First, we do not see why the patient's second-order belief has to be false. That is, we think that even a deluded patient might have an accurate appreciation of the character of her first-order attitudes. She might believe that she believes that the sky is falling, and this second-order belief might be true. She does believe that the sky is falling. Second, we do not think that the second-order attitude characteristic of delusions is best understood simply as a second-order *belief*. Indeed, we think that the second-order state involved in delusion is complex. So, we prefer to see the higher order state as a 'stance', i.e. a multifaceted disposition (which may include affective and mood dependent components on occasion) to respond in various ways to one's first-order state. We call this stance, as noted earlier, the 'delusional stance'.

Putting our proposal a bit more precisely, if still in a rather abstract form, we hold that a person has the delusion that *p*, if she adopts the delusional stance towards one (or more) of her first-order states that have the content that p. Or still more precisely and as expressed in DST-1:

> Delusions are second-order attitudes that constitute a kind of stance taken towards first-order mental contents or intentional states, which may be of a variety of different sorts (including, but not restricted to, beliefs).

Following Currie, we allow—DST-1 allows—that the relevant first-order state might not qualify as the first-order belief that p. In our view, the subject may adopt the delusional stance towards any of a variety of different first-order states. The deluded subject may be first-order believing that the sky is falling, or merely first-order considering the proposition that the sky is falling, or vividly first-order imagining (without believing) that the sky is falling. Indeed, we do not even require that the first-order state about which the patient takes the delusional stance has any coherent propositional content, i.e. any intelligible semantic interpretation. Perhaps the patient is fixated (as Berrios suggests) on some verbal formula (the sky is falling), though neither she nor anyone else can say anything helpful about what the formula might mean. In our account, one can adopt the delusional stance promiscuously towards many different sorts of first-order states.[7]

Again following Currie's lead, we allow that the nature of the relevant first-order state plays a central role in determining how a patient with the delusion that p will reason, act, and feel. A patient who has adopted the delusional stance towards a first-order belief that p, will be convinced of the truth of p and will act, reason, and emote as we would expect of someone who believes that p. By contrast, a patient in the delusional stance towards a first-order state in which she is merely entertaining the idea that p or, perhaps, imagining what it would be like if p were the case, may exhibit (in the manner of Sass's description) distant, 'ironic' attitudes towards p. She may signal in various ways that she's not really committed herself to believing that p. She will reason and act, not as one who believes that p, but as one who is considering or playing with the idea that p. If she is in the delusional stance towards a first order state that has for its content an empty verbal formula, she may repeat the formula 'significantly' for herself or to others. She feels that somehow it expresses something terribly important, but her attempts to say what it expresses will result in frustrated incomprehension on the part of her audience, and perhaps even in her own case, thus inviting the interpretation as empty speech act.

Thus, our account accommodates the clinical observation that patients to whom it seems appropriate to attribute the delusion that p in some instances exhibit and in other instances fail to exhibit the behaviour characteristic of someone who believes that p. One has the delusion that p if one adopts the delusional stance towards one's first order attitude that p, regardless of the character or attitude type of the first order attitude.

As we see it, then, to return momentarily to the case study that began the paper, Laura was not deluded because she believed that thoughts were being inserted into her mind or that she was being compelled to urinate on herself. Such beliefs are false and bizarre, to be sure, but they are not the proper basis of her diagnosis as delusional. Laura was delusional, and delusional in believing what she did, because of her delusional stance towards such lower order attitudes. It is higher not lower order attitudes that constitute delusion. We shall now offer a characterization of the delusional stance.

DST-2 and characteristics of the delusional stance

We turn now from the first part of DST to the second. What sort of (second or higher order) attitude towards a (lower) first-order attitude that p constitutes having the delusion that p? As we have said, we take the delusional stance to be a complex disposition to respond to or deal with a first-order state in various ways. The major components of this multi-track disposition are the following.

Self-identification

A person having the delusion that *p* identifies herself with the first order attitude that p. The term 'thought', as Crane (2001, p. 102) points out, 'can be used to apply to particular acts of thinking, or to the intentional content of such acts'. A person having the delusion that p not only experiences this intentional content, but she experiences it as her act of thinking. She regards thinking or entertaining, in some way, the thought that p as an expression of her agency or person. The thought is experienced or represented as the product of her psychological makeup or situation.

Of course this feature of self-identification or self-represented personal possession does not distinguish delusions from normal or non-pathological second-order attitudes. If we think about first-order attitudes at all, we prototypically second-order regard our thoughts as expressions of ourselves: as things that we ourselves think—actively. This feature, however, does distinguish delusions from various other pathological (or, at least, abnormal) ways of viewing one's first-order thoughts. For example, subjects who suffer from verbal hallucinations (voices) or experiences of thought insertion (in the manner of Laura) regard what are in fact their own thoughts or intentional contents as expressions of someone else's agency. Though they recognize that first-order thoughts or contents occur in their mind or stream of consciousness, they regard their 'voices' or inserted thoughts as alien to themselves: as something imposed on them as subjects by another. They admit that these 'alien' thoughts occur in them, but they deny that they *think* these thoughts (see Frith 1992; Cahill and Frith 1996; Campbell 1999; Gallagher 2000; Graham 2004; Stephens and Graham 2000).

In certain similar cases, the subject may feel that she does think (is the agent of) a given act of thinking, but still maintains that another is controlling or influencing her thinking. Here the other's control is (experienced as) less direct or intrusive than for inserted thoughts. Instead of the other (experienced as) thinking his thoughts in her mind, the other is (experienced as) influencing her to think these thoughts. In such cases of 'thought control' or 'thought influence', the subject also has the sense of being imposed on by another and does not regard the 'controlled' thoughts as fully her own: as expressions of her true self (Fulford 1994).

A more common, if still non-prototypical, attitude towards one's own thoughts is that, although they do not express someone else's agency, they also do not express my own agency. They occur in me willy-nilly, 'automatically', or otherwise out of my control. Here I regard these thoughts, not as my actions—as things that I *think*—but merely as things that happen to me. In extreme cases, such an uninvolved attitude towards one's own thoughts might be called 'depersonalization'.[8]

However, at least in unobtrusive doses, e.g. the idiotic jingle that 'runs through one's head', these occurrences are a periodic feature of our introspective experience.

The delusional subject, however, does not distance herself from the first-order thought that is the object of her delusion. She acknowledges or identifies with it, if not with enthusiasm, then at least with the firm conviction that it is a normal expression of her mental agency. She regards it as an integral feature of her personal self.

Of course, one may acknowledge that a thought is one's own—in the sense of being something one *thinks*—while also wishing devoutly that one did not think it. This seems to be the standard position or stance with regard to obsessive thoughts. The subject acknowledges her agentic involvement in and responsibility for thinking, for example, that the door is unlocked or that her mother is a monster. Nevertheless, obsessive patients generally recognize the inappropriate, irrational, or dysfunctional character of their obsessive thoughts and may feel that they are blameworthy for thinking them. Unfortunately, such insight does not enable them to avoid thinking the obsessive thoughts. The subject feels compelled to think the thought 'against her will', i.e. despite her recognition that it would be better for her not to think it. She may also find herself compelled to act in response to the thought. Sometimes such actions are rationally related to the thought, e.g. checking the lock on the door in response to the thought that the door is unlocked, but they also may be purely ritualistic, e.g. counting by twos to one hundred. Therein they serve only to reduce the anxiety produced in her by thinking the thought. Victims of obsessive thoughts generally claim that they do not really believe, for example, that the door is unlocked, but they cannot dismiss the thought or the anxiety that it produces.

In delusions there is no such resistance or feeling of helplessness regarding the first-order thought. It is no doubt often distressing to have the delusion that one is being commanded to pass urine while standing, but the source of the subject's distress is the prospect of external control, not that, under the circumstances, she is thinking about being externally controlled. Laura, for example, regards her first-order thought, 'I am being asked to pass urine', as a normal, understandable thought for her to entertain in the circumstances in which she finds herself. Laura does not regard the occurrence of her first-order thought as an indication that something is wrong with her, but as an indication that something is wrong with the situation in which she finds herself (Fulford 1994). Witness the following segments of a transcribed hospital interview of Laura (L) ('IN' is the interviewer) (Young and Leafhood 1996, pp. 102–103:

IN: I would like to thank you for agreeing to so this today after all the false alarms we've had so far. It is very good of you to agree to do it.

L: (Smiles) Shit happens.

IN: I'll start by . . .

L: . . . and then you die.

IN: Do you think you suffer from (schizophrenia)?

L: I think I just suffer from things that bother me—like trying to figure out who my mother is. I just think I am in here because doctors need money.

IN: Where do the voices come from?

L: Other people—other people around here are talking. I don't know how to explain it. Some people don't make a lot of sense when they are sick.

IN: Are your voices . . . an illness?

L: Myself, I don't think so.

Resistance

The subject who has the delusion that p, resists changing her first-order thought that p, clinging to it in the face of good reason for dismissing it.

The feature of the delusional stance to which we here refer is what Jaspers called the 'incorrigibility' of delusions.[9]

It is one of the most frequently noted characteristics of delusional thinking. Berrios's (1994) collection of nineteenth- and early twentieth-century writings on psychopathology includes citations to this effect.

Delasiaure says of delusions that 'their action is tyrannical, they are impervious to objection and surround themselves with childish defenses' (p. 99). Griesinger notes that 'the patient cannot get rid of them, they resist correction by the testimony of the senses and the understanding' (p. 102). Hart defines 'delusion' as 'a false belief which is impervious to the most complete logical demonstration of its impossibility and unshaken by the presence of incompatible or obviously contradictory facts' (p. 111).

Berrios's quotation from Hart illustrates the traditional understanding of delusional incorrigibility in epistemological or belief-based terms. It is a matter of continuing to believe that p in the face of overwhelming evidence that p is false. However this understanding of incorrigibility applies only to beliefs. In line with our contention that delusions may involve first-order thoughts that are not beliefs, we need a broader or more generic notion of incorrigibility, which includes but is not restricted to the epistemological notion. In the general sense, incorrigibility is a matter of persisting in an activity even when it is better, on the whole, not to do so. Certainly one sort of reason why it is better for me not to persist in believing that p, is that there is decisive evidence that p is false. However, not every strong reason for dismissing a thought is epistemological or evidential.

If I am merely entertaining the proposition that p, or imagining what it would be like were it the case that p, the fact that I have decisive evidence that p is false may not be a good reason for me to abandon the thought that p. For many reasons, it is quite legitimate to entertain a thought even though the thought is false. I may find joy, relaxation, or insight in imagining that, for example, an object can fall through the earth's atmosphere without encountering any resistance or that in the mountains of Tibet there hides a monastery filled with contented scholars who live to be 350 years old.

On the other hand, I may have good reasons not to entertain a first-order thought that has nothing whatsoever to do with whether the thought expresses a true proposition. For example, if I persistently imagine being a victim of a brain tumour, entertaining this thought may make me anxious or depressed or it may distract me from more profitable or necessary activities. It may be better for me, on the whole, not to think (or at least to dwell on) certain thoughts, even if I have good evidence that the propositions expressed in these thoughts are true.

Thus, the sort of incorrigibility characteristic of the delusional stance is, we contend, a matter of the subject's persisting in thinking certain thoughts when it would be better for the subject not to think them. Just whether some consideration constitutes a good reason for not thinking a first-order thought will depend, at least in part, on the type of first-order thought (belief, imaginative rehearsal, etc.) that is the object of the delusional stance. This good reason—depending on the corresponding type of first order thought—may be an epistemic or evidential matter or it may not.

We have the impression in reading the clinical literature, that even where a delusion involves a 'pretty convincing' example of being a false belief, the incorrigible subject may keep the belief isolated or encapsulated, as it were, from her other beliefs or attitudes, so as to help to maintain it. This may result from a desire not to test the belief by reflecting on its logical consequences or practical implications. Though we do not endorse any general psychodynamic explanation of delusions or of the possible motivational sources of incorrigibility, we suppose that some subjects may adopt the delusional stance towards a first-order thought because they are motivated to protect and preserve it. This could give rise to a tendency to wall off the first order thought from collision with her other attitudes and to allow it to manifest itself only under carefully controlled or circumscribed conditions.

Here it might be observed that it is a commonplace of epistemology and cognitive psychology that people tend to take a conservative attitude towards their beliefs and established patterns of thought. We do not like to have our mental lives disturbed and try to minimize any changes forced on us by circumstances. One might then wonder whether the sort of incorrigibility associated with the delusional stance really identifies a distinct feature of delusions (rather than of normal cognitive activity) and whether it can explain what's pathological about delusions.

We would respond that, as with distinguishing clinical depression from normal sadness, for example, delusion involves an intensification or excess of a normal tendency. The deluded are more attracted to the relevant first-order attitudes than is normal. There are different ways of exhibiting this more intense or excessive attachment to a first-order thought. As a victim of delusion, I might vigorously avoid (perhaps at some personal risk to myself) putting myself in situations that might lead to my re-evaluating or reflecting upon my reason for entertaining the thought. I might strenuously refuse to become involved in or seek to avoid circumstances where I must justify my thinking to others, though the circumstances are common and ordinarily quite harmless. Or I might retreat from even introspective examination of the question whether it is rational for me to persist in thinking along certain lines.

Delusional incorrigibility is not neatly walled off from normal commitment to first-order thoughts. But quantitative differences can amount to a qualitative difference. Pathology of delusion can turn out to be a matter of excess or degree.

Finally, we should note that just as not every delusion is a false belief, so, in our view, not every false belief is a delusion, not even if the belief in question is held by a person who is schizophrenic. Maher (1974, 1988) argues that at least some of the beliefs routinely described as delusions in the context of schizophrenia represent reasonable attempts to make sense of anomalous perceptual experiences. A patient suffering from auditory hallucinations, for example, may have some phenomenological or subjective basis for hypothesizing that unseen agents are communicating with her (Stephens and Graham 2000). Again: what determines whether a belief is delusional is not the content of the belief, but the stance or higher order attitude that the subject takes towards that belief. On occasion, a victim of schizophrenia may not be unreasonable or delusional in coming to believe that unseen agents are communicating with her, even though persisting in this belief in the teeth of strong contrary considerations is delusional.

Suppose that Laura believes that unseen speakers are commanding that she pace up and down the ward. Whether she is deluded in so believing does not depend on whether outside observers regard her convictions as bizarre or radically unsupported by the available evidence. Rather, it depends on how she relates to the belief—to the picture of reality that it presents to her. Does she test it: seeking evidence for or against its truth? Would she abandon it if she were presented with powerful counter-evidence or a more plausible alternative hypothesis? Does she consider it in the context of her other beliefs and is she prepared to accept its logical consequences? Or, does she compartmentalize it, avoiding situations where she might be forced to reconsider it? Does she appreciate the effects that this belief might have on the rest of her life? Does she persist in the belief in the face of strong reasons for abandoning it, or does she refuse to face such reasons? As we noted that Sass observes, and as remarked earlier in the chapter, it is the *way* one believes something and not *what* one believes that defines delusion.

Lack of insight

The delusional stance is characterized by a lack of insight concerning the first-order thought that is the object of the delusion. This feature of delusions, which is a pronounced or disturbing absence of first-person insight, is emphasized by Fulford (1989, 1994) and Currie (2000). For Fulford the insight lacking is a diagnostic insight. Just such an insight was lacking in Laura. When asked if she was sick, Laura said that she was suffering from things that bothered her. When asked, 'If you are not ill, why are you in the hospital?', she replied, 'I do not know'. However a year later—in a marked sign of her recovery—when asked about her delusions, she replied, 'I think I was getting sick at this point' (Young and Leafblood 1996, p. 107).

The deluded subject fails to recognize that the occurrence or persistence of the relevant first-order thought indicates that something is wrong with her (that she is sick) rather than with the world (that it is making her suffer). Again: my having the belief that my nurses are poisoning me should indicate to me that I am irrational or ill, not that my nurses are poisoning me.

My disinclination to abandon this belief should show me that I am not thinking straight, not that certain events are overwhelmingly confirming it.

Jones (1999) provides an interesting example of delusional lack of insight. It is part of the standard diagnostic criterion for delusion that delusions are beliefs at variance with the subject's cultural milieu and not generally accepted by the subject's peers (Gelder *et al.* 1996, p. 9). The usefulness and accuracy of this criterion has been questioned, but many delusions clearly are atypical and idiosyncratic. However, Jones (1999) notes that deluded subjects generally fail to recognize that their beliefs are regarded by others as aberrant or bizarre.

Currie (2000) supposes that deluded subjects are often, even typically, mistaken concerning the nature of their first-order states. They take themselves to believe that *p* when, in fact, they have no such first-order belief. They suffer, he argues, from 'cognitive hallucinations'. They mistake imagining something for believing it. Hence, they operate with a misleading conception of their cognitive economy and in consequence they are frequently unable to understand and predict their own behaviour.

Jones's (1999) study also provides evidence that deluded subjects may lack insight into the aetiology or origin of first-order thoughts (see also Vinogradov *et al.* 1998, p. 194). They tend to regard the first-order thoughts involved in their delusions as springing directly from perception or intuition. They do not see them as products of ratiocination, as deriving from other beliefs or influenced by motives or affective conditions. Such a lack of aetiological insight has been called a failure of 'source of information' monitoring.[10]

When Laura was asked, for example, why she believed that the voices that were emanating from the TV, sometimes appeared, to her, to be taking her (non-existent) boyfriends away from her, she said that this was because she saw them flirt, 'They do that even in shampoo commercials,' she replied (see Young and Leafhood 1996, p. 101).

Regardless of one's evaluation of these specific proposals regarding the exact sort of insight lacking in deluded subjects, we take the above proposals as general evidence of the following. There is clinical consensus that failure to appreciate the nature of one's condition is an essential feature of delusions. In general terms, we suppose that deluded subjects do not understand the costs of maintaining certain first-order thoughts, the place of these thoughts in their psychological economies, or the pathological character of their condition. When such insight is achieved—as it eventually was in the case of Laura— this constitutes a sign of recovery. 'I'd like to know where I get these ideas from,' Laura remarked as her general status improved and she began to describe her illness as an illness (see Young and Leafhood 1996, p. 108).

It is worth noting, for clinical comparison, that insight tends to be present in victims of obsessive thinking. Victims often lucidly appreciate the obsessive character of their thinking, and therein this helps to distinguish victims of obsessive thinking from deluded persons. Goodwin and Guze (1996, p. 4) note that if someone with obsessive thoughts clearly does not have insight into the abnormal nature of those thoughts, it may not be possible to confidently distinguish his or her obsessional disorder from schizophrenia.

So, to sum up, we propose that the delusional stance should be understood as follows (as stated in DST-2). The higher order or delusional stance involves the deluded person's identifying himself or herself with the relevant first-order contents, so much so that he or she persistently maintains those contents, incorrigibly, in the face of strong counter-considerations and with a disturbing lack of diagnostic or first-person insight.

Schizophrenia and delusion

What do delusions suggest about the cognitive pathology of schizophrenia? In this final section of the chapter we will sketch in fairly broad strokes some implications of DST for understanding schizophrenia. We shall attempt to bring out these implications by comparing delusions, as understood in DST, with verbal hallucinations, another prominent symptom of schizophrenia, and with obsessions, another disorder of thinking.

In addition to attacks on the traditional conception of delusions, the current literature on psychopathology also features an extensive critique of the traditional understanding of 'voices' or verbal hallucinations. According to the traditional picture, verbal hallucinations are pathological sensory experiences. Subject's who 'hear voices' are supposed to mistake their awareness of their own thoughts or inner speech for auditory perception of another's overt speech. Such mistakes are seen as failures of 'reality testing', that is, an inability to discriminate, at the perceptual or introspective level, what one imagines from what one actually perceives, and they are supposed to be explained by reference to an abnormal phenomenology in the hallucinator's experience of his inner speech (see Slade and Bentall 1988). In this view, the primary question about schizophrenia raised by verbal hallucination concerns the nature of the underlying perceptual processes that produce such bizarre experiences.

In rejecting the above model, Junginger (1985; also Junginger and Frame 1986) and Hoffman (1986) argue that hallucinators do distinguish their 'voices' from normal perceptual experiences. Hoffman maintains that reference to the phenomenology of the hallucinatory experience does not explain the subject's conviction that the voice comes from the outside: rather the reverse—that the subject's initial impression that the voice is of non-self origin explains or induces the distinctive features of the phenomenology. Hoffman as well as Frith (1992) insists that a voice appears alien to the subject because he fails to detect the role of his personal agency or intentions in its production. The pathological condition responsible for verbal hallucinations is a breakdown, not at the level of sensory experience, but in the processes involved in the subject's awareness of or monitoring of his own cognitive activities.[11]

DST offers a similar construal of the pathological character of delusions. There may be nothing bizarre or pathological about the beliefs or other first-order states or attitudes that serve as objects of the delusional stance. Consequently DST does not expect to find the cognitive dysfunctions that operate in delusions in the processes by which the subject acquires those first order states. Rather, DST looks for the pathology temporally downstream in the processes that give rise to the attitudes and habits that constitute the delusional stance. According to DST, the questions we need to answer in order to explain the pathological significance of the delusion that the sky is falling are not likely to be questions about how the patient came by the first-order thought that the sky is falling.[12]

Rather, they will be questions about how and why the patient came to identify with the thought, to be incorrigibly committed to maintaining it, and why he fails to grasp or to have insight into its role in his psychological economy.

Earlier we contrasted delusions with obsessional thoughts. The subject who suffers from obsessional thoughts does not embrace or identify with them even if he acknowledges them as his own. He recognizes their 'unhealthy' character and struggles against them. The deluded patient, on the other hand, identifies with the relevant first-order thoughts, does not see their occurrence as a problem for him, and lacks insight into the costs of maintaining them.

Despite these differences, however, we believe that the sorts of problems delusions impose on those who hold them are quite similar to the problems imposed by obsessions. Subjects are said to suffer from obsessions primarily because dealing with obsessions draws energy and attention away from more useful projects. They distract the subject from, and hinder his pursuit of, the tasks required for living a satisfactory life. Delusions likewise represent harmful preoccupations. They channel the subject's cognitive activities into unproductive patterns. They prevent him from fully engaging with the problems of day-to-day living. Indeed, delusions typically are more insidious than obsessions, since the patient fails to recognize their costs and is not motivated to escape them.

Even where delusions involve false first-order beliefs, the problems presented by delusions are distinct from, and may operate independently of, problems normally associated with false beliefs. The latter problems centre on the subject's failure to achieve the ends of particular actions (those actions which require true beliefs) and conflicts with persons who do not share the subject's beliefs. The former problems involve a much more general failure to organize one's cognitive activities in an efficient and productive manner. Various forms of schizophrenia, in which delusions of imprudent sorts predominate, are especially vivid illustrations of this failure of efficiency and productivity. Victims of paranoid schizophrenia, for example, may suffer from dramatic inability to efficiently negotiate the social world and to effectively maintain social relationships and responsibilities.

Not that a paranoid's failure is self-appreciated. The delusional stance ensures that the inefficiency of one's actions may be hidden from the subject's recognition or acknowledgement. As one desultory post-delusional patient put it, after recovery from a religious delusion, 'I always felt that everything I said was worthless, but as Jesus everything I said was important—it came from God' (Bolton and Hill 1996, p. 341).

To summarize, DST says that the victim of delusion suffers less from a failure to accurately represent the state of the world than from a failure to understand the nature and consequences of her own mental activities. DST locates the pathological character of delusions in the subject's attitudes toward and ability to manage her first or lower order cognitive activities. DST takes the association between schizophrenia and delusions as an indication that, whatever other dysfunctions may be present, schizophrenia involves a failure of self-knowledge and self-control regarding one's first order thinking. One of the misfortunes of schizophrenia is having one's lower order thoughts caught in the grip of the delusional stance.

Endnotes

1. This is a thoroughly co-authored paper. The order of authorship has been determined randomly. Occasionally the first-person pronoun is used as a stylistic device. See also Stephens and Graham (2004). We owe thanks to a number of people who shared reactions to various ideas in this or the 2004 paper. These include Tim Bayne, Stephen Braude, and Jennifer Radden.
2. In the statements to follow, the names of Laura's delusion types are indicated in parentheses.
3. By 'voices' we mean what are usually designated as verbal hallucinations. We interpret voices to be quite similar to delusions of thought insertion and hence refer to them here as delusions rather than hallucinations. See Stephens and Graham (2000).
4. See Berrios (1996, chap. 5) for a chronologically organized discussion of attempts to characterize delusions.
5. For reasons of expository convenience, hereafter we speak of the higher order as 'second order' and of the lower order as 'first order'. Two qualifications must be noted in doing this, however. The first is that some delusions involve third-order attitudes towards second-order content. The second is that we do not mean to suggest that first- or lower order thoughts are singular in number or of one and the same psychological type. Multiple lower order contents and sometimes of quite different types, including not just beliefs but also emotions, acts of imagination, and so on, may be involved in the lower order manner in delusions.
6. Sedler quote and citation taken from Vinogradov et al. (1998), p. 190.

7. Also, as suggested in footnote 5, some delusions invite construal as attitudes not to first-order but to higher order states. Thought insertion, suffered by Laura, is a third-order delusion. That is, speaking from the point of view of the victim, the thought that is the object of the delusion that another is inserting thoughts into my mind, is the second-order thought that 'Another is inserting thoughts into my mind'. The subject adopts the delusional stance towards this thought and, as we explain later in the body of the paper, identifies herself with it. So, although we here state DST as a thesis about first and second order, this is for ease of exposition only. The main DSM-1 point is that a delusion is a kind of stance taken towards what one believes or thinks is going on in one's lower order psychological economy.

8. Gerrans (2000, pp.116-117) claims that such experiences of depersonalization may be central to the aetiology of the Cotard delusion.

9. As quoted in Sass (1994), p. 5.

10. Failure of source of information monitoring has been associated in the neuroscience literature with the neuromodulatory effects of dopamine in the prefrontal cortex. Various kinds of dopaminergic activity may perhaps contribute to diminishing the deluded person's attention to or memory of the overall evidential context in which thought content originates or first occurs (Vinogradov *et al.* 1998).

11. See Stephens and Graham (2000) for a detailed exposition and defence of this 'non-traditional' account of verbal hallucinations. One of the consequences of the account is that it forges a close association, conceptually, between verbal hallucinations and the delusion or phenomenon of thought insertion.

12. Perhaps the patient had a bizarre perceptual experience and thinks that the sky is falling because of that experience.

References

American Psychiatric Association (APA). (1994). *Diagnostic and statistical manual of mental disorders* (4th edn). Washington DC: APA.

Bayne, T. and Pacherie, E. (2005). In defense of the doxastic conception of delusions. *Mind and Language*, **20**: 163–188.

Berrios, G. (1991). Delusions as 'wrong beliefs': a conceptual history. *British Journal of Psychiatry*, **159**: 6–13.

Berrios, G. (1996). *A history of mental symptoms: descriptive phenomenology since the nineteenth century*. Cambridge: Cambridge University Press.

Bolton, D. and Hill, J. (1996). *Mind, meaning, and mental disorder: the nature of causal explanation in psychology and psychiatry*. Oxford: Oxford University Press.

Cahill, C. and Frith, C. (1996). False perceptions or false beliefs: hallucinations and delusions in schizophrenia. In: *Method in madness: case studies in cognitive neuropsychiatry* (ed. P. Halligan and J. Marshall), pp.267–291. East Sussex, UK: Psychology Press.

Campbell, J. (1999). Schizophrenia, the space of reasons, and thinking as a motor process. *The Monist*, **82**: 609–625.

Chen, E. and Berrios, G. (1998). The nature of delusions: a hierarchical neural network approach. In: *Neural networks and psychopathology: connectionist models in practice and research.* (ed. D. Stein and J. Ludik), pp.167–188. Cambridge: Cambridge University Press.

Crane, T. (2001). *Elements of mind: an introduction to the philosophy of mind.* Oxford: Oxford University Press.

Currie, G. (2000). Imagination, delusion, and hallucinations. In: *Pathologies of belief* (ed. M. Coltheart and M. Davies), pp.167–182. Oxford: Basil Blackwell.

Frith, C. (1992). *The cognitive neuropsychology of schizophrenia.* Hillsdale, N.J.: Erlbaum.

Fulford, K.W.M. (1989). *Moral theory and medical practice.* Cambridge: Cambridge University Press.

Fulford, K.W.M. (1993). Thought insertion and insight: disease and illness paradigms of psychotic disorder. In: *Phenomenology, language, and schizophrenia* (ed. M. Spitzer, F. Uehlin, M. Schwartz, and C. Mundt), pp.1–17. New York: Springer-Verlag.

Fulford, K.W.M. (1994). Value, illness, and failure of action: framework for a philosophical psychopathology of delusions. In: *Philosophical psychopathology* (ed. G. Graham and G.L. Stephens), pp.205–233. Cambridge, USA: MIT.

Gallagher, S. (2000). Self-reference and schizophrenia: a cognitive model of immunity to error through misidentification. In: *Exploring the self: philosophical and psychopathological perspectives on self-experience* (ed. D. Zahavi), pp.203–239. Amsterdam: John Benjamins.

Garety, p. A. and Hemsley, D.R. (1995). *Delusions: investigations into the psychology of delusional reasoning.* Oxford: Oxford University Press.

Gelder, M., Gath, D., Mayou, R. and Cowen, P. (ed.) (1996). *Oxford textbook of psychiatry* (3rd edn). Oxford: Oxford University Press.

Gerrans, p. (2000). Refining the explanation of Cotard's delusion. In: *Pathologies of belief* (ed. M. Coltheart and M. Davies), pp.111–122. Oxford: Basil Blackwell.

Goodwin, D. and Guze, S. (1996). *Psychiatric diagnosis* (5th edn). New York: Oxford University Press.

Graham, G. (2004). Thinking inserted thoughts. In: *Oxford companion to the philosophy of psychiatry* (ed. J. Radden), pp. 89–105. New York: Oxford University Press.

Graham, G. and Stephens, G.L. (1994). Mind and mine. In: *Philosophical psychopathology* (ed. G. Graham and G.L. Stephens), pp.91–109. Cambridge, USA: MIT.

Halligan, P. and Marshall, J. (ed.) (1996). *Method in madness: case studies in cognitive neuropsychiatry.* East Sussex, UK: Psychology Press.

Hoffman, R. (1986). Verbal hallucinations and language production processes in schizophrenia. *Behavioral and Brain Sciences,* **9**: 503–517.

Jones, E (1999). The phenomenology of abnormal belief: a philosophic and psychiatric inquiry. *Philosophy, Psychiatry, and Psychology,* **6**: 1–16.

Jones, E. and Watson, J. (1997). Delusion, the overvalued idea, and religious beliefs: a comparative analysis of their characteristics. *British Journal of Psychiatry,* **170**: 381–386.

Junginger, J. (1985). Distinctiveness, unintendedness, location, and non-self attribution of verbal hallucinations. *Behavioral and Brain Sciences,* **9**: 527–528.

Junginger, J. and Frame, C. (1986). Self-report of frequency and phenomenology of verbal hallucinations. *Journal of Nervous and Mental Disease,* **173**: 149–155.

Maher, B. (1974). Delusional thinking and perceptual disorder. *Journal of Individual Psychology,* **30**: 98–113.

Maher, B. (1988). Anomalous experience and delusional thinking. In: *Delusional beliefs* (ed. T. Oltmanns and B. Maher), pp. 260–268. New York: Wiley.

Marshall, J. and Halligan, P. (1996). Towards a cognitive neuropsychiatry. In: *Method in madness: case studies in cognitive neuropsychiatry* (ed. P. Halligan and J. Marshall), pp. 3–11. East Sussex, UK: Psychology Press.

McKay, A., McKenna, p. , and Laws, K. (1996). Severe schizophrenia: what is it like? In: *Method in madness: case studies in cognitive neuropsychiatry* (ed. P. Halligan and J. Marshall), pp. 95–122. East Sussex, UK: Psychology Press.

Mellor, C. (1970). First rank symptoms of schizophrenia. *British Journal of Psychiatry*, **117**: 15–23.

Sartorious, N., Jablensky, A., Korten, G., Ernberg, G., Anker, M., and Cooper, J.E. (1986). Early manifestations and first-contact incidence of schizophrenia in different cultures. *Psychological Medicine*, **16**: 909–928.

Sass, L. (1994). *The paradoxes of delusion: Wittgenstein, Schreiber, and the schizophrenic mind.* New York: Cornell University Press.

Sedler, M.J. (1995). Understanding delusions. *Psychiatric Clinics of North America*, **18**: 251–62.

Slade, P. and Bentall, R. (1988). *Sensory deception: a scientific analysis of hallucinations.* Baltimore: Johns Hopkins University Press.

Stephens, G.L. and Graham, G. (2000). *When self-consciousness breaks: alien voices and inserted thoughts.* Cambridge, USA: MIT Press.

Stephens, G. L. and Graham, G. (2004). Reconceiving delusion. *International Review of Psychiatry*, **16**: 236–241.

Vinogradov, S., Poole, J. and Willis-Shore, J. (1998). 'Produced by either God or Satan': neural network approaches to delusional thinking,' In: *Neural networks and psychopathology: connectionist models in practice and research* (ed. D. Stein and J. Ludik), pp. 189–230. Cambridge: Cambridge University Press.

Young, A. (1999). Delusions. *The Monist*, **82**: 571–589.

Young, A. and Leafhood, K. (1996). Betwixt life and death: case studies of the Cotard delusion. In: *Method in madness: case studies in cognitive neuropsychiatry* (ed. P. Halligan and J. Marshall), pp. 147–171. East Sussex, UK: Psychology Press.

11   Against the belief model of delusion

Andy Hamilton

Psychotic and non-psychotic delusions

The central aim this article is to criticise the received opinion that delusions are beliefs. I will argue that in many psychotic and non-psychotic cases, the basic level of description of delusion falls short of the ascription of belief. In monothematic, behaviourally inert cases at least, I maintain that although the delusion shares some features of belief, the disanalogies are sufficient to justify withholding a clear belief-attribution. My thesis is not quite that in many cases delusions are not beliefs; rather, it is that there is no fact of the matter concerning whether S believes that p.

In this opening section, however, I will also question the usual concentration—by philosophers as well as psychiatrists and psychologists—on psychotic delusion. Psychotic cases are the most fascinating, but in ignoring non-psychotic delusion, one loses a wider perspective which, I believe, tends to support the central thesis of this article, that many delusions are not beliefs. In a range of non-clinical cases we speak of people being deluded. These include conditions such as self-deception and wishful thinking, where in contrast to many psychotic delusions, there is nothing bizarre about the proposition that is allegedly believed. The self-deceiver is deluded when, against the evidence, she apparently gets herself to believe that her partner is not being unfaithful. The thirsty, exhausted desert traveller is deluded when wishful thinking makes him disregard the likelihood that the oasis is just an optical illusion; even someone unfamiliar with this kind of optical illusion, and therefore epistemically relatively blameless, could be described as deluded. When Lord Archer, whose confabulations have so enlivened British public life in recent decades, says that he gained a degree from an American university, or denies that he was ever arrested for shop-lifting, there is the feeling that he is not just lying for reasons of self-advantage, but is deluded—he is a fantasist.

Non-psychotic delusions mostly fall under the heading of motivated irrationality. But in colloquial usage the scope of non-psychotic delusion may appear broader still. People are ready to describe as delusory many religious or political beliefs which they reject—for instance the Roman Catholic belief that the bread and wine in the Eucharist are converted into the body and blood of Christ—but this is a metaphorical use. For the description to be more than metaphorical, an ideological critique along the lines suggested by Freud or Marx would have to be endorsed. A delusion is not simply a groundless framework principle that one does not accept; to call something a delusion is to imply that it is more than a simple error. It is essential to distinguish delusions, especially psychotic cases, from mere mistaken belief. J.L. Austin remarked that the presence of delusion indicates that something is wrong with the subject, whereas the explanation for illusion lies in the world (Austin 1962, pp. 20–25). However, non-perceptual illusions are often assimilated with delusion; an illusion, except when perceptual, is always a positive belief, something that one wishes to believe, while delusion is neutral. Hence Freud in 'The future of an illusion' refers to religious beliefs as illusions rather than delusions: 'not precipitates or end-results of thinking: they are illusions, fulfilments of the oldest, strongest and most urgent wishes of mankind' (Freud 1953, p. 30). Ian Kershaw describes Hitler in 1944 as believing unshakeably that 'the strength to hold out would eventually lead to a turning of the tide, and to Germany's final victory...he expressed his unfounded optimism through references to the grace of Providence...the self-deception involved was colossal. Hitler lived increasingly in a world of illusion, clutching as the year wore on ever more desperately at whatever straws he could find' (Kershaw 2000, pp. 609–610). Both of the latter cases could be described as delusion.

In contrast, psychotic delusions are never described as illusions. They include Cothard's and Capgras' delusions, and schizophrenic delusions; under this heading would be included Descartes's examples of subjects who believe that they are made of glass, that they are a pumpkin, and so on. Some psychotic delusions are caused by brain injury, or are otherwise organic, others are not.[1] Capgras' delusion seems to fit into the former category, since it occurs after right-hemisphere brain damage; while many drugs cause psychotic episodes involving delusions. The hallucinating subject is deluded if they believe that there really are pink rats, that is, where the hallucination is not 'lucid' in the manner of lucid dreaming. (Most cases of hallucination involve either psychosis, or drug-induced psychotic episodes; but hearing voices may, in some cases, be a non-psychotic hallucination.)

The account presented here allows for a vague boundary between psychotic and non-psychotic cases. But the very distinction between psychotic and non-psychotic may be tendentious, since it implies a medical model of mental illness. Although the anti-psychiatry debate is not addressed directly here, the arguments presented will have implications for it. In particular, in criticizing the assumption that all delusions are beliefs, and offering a deflationary analysis of the phenomenon of delusion, the present account may undermine the standard medical model of psychosis as involving 'poor reality-testing'. It should also be noted that the analysis offered here treats work in scientific psychology and psychiatry as useful data rather than theoretical support for philosophical conclusions.

It might be argued that psychotic delusions, as the results of mental illness or brain damage, are the only genuine, objective cases of delusion. This is a tempting position, especially for those who regard delusion as loss of reality-testing and thus as defining madness or psychosis, since those who are deluded in the non-psychotic sense have lost this contact with reality only in a relatively mild way. The position seems to have wide support. For Lacan, 'the clinical characteristic of the psychotic is distinguished by this profoundly perverted relation to reality known as delusion' (Lacan 1993, p. 44); G. Lynn Stephens writes that 'delusion does more than serve as a sign of madness: it is constitutive of madness, or at least of some forms of madness' (Stephens 1999, p. 25).[2]

Proponents of this view regard non-psychotic delusion as secondary. Psychiatrist Anthony David evidently assumes that all delusions are psychotic. He provides an interesting list of false beliefs found in anorexics, sufferers from Chronic Fatigue Syndrome, anosognosia, and other conditions, which he claims illustrate our inconsistency in applying the concept of delusion; claiming to be overweight and denying the fact that one is dangerously thin is regarded merely as an 'overvalued idea', and claiming that Elvis is still alive is regarded as daft, and not a delusion (David 1999, p. 18). But if one allows that there are non-psychotic delusions, then most of the cases that David cites will count as delusions in this broader sense. (The anosognosic patient who denies that they are paralysed on their left side is an interesting case, perhaps closer to Ignorance than delusion.) It is hard to judge which position is correct, and here I leave the question open. The most important criterion of delusion is that in neither the psychotic nor the non-psychotic sense does it involve a simple error; the attribution of delusion implies that there is something fairly serious wrong with the subject.

The status of non-psychotic delusion bears on the question of whether delusion is something that is not accepted by others in one's culture or sub-culture, and the related question of the contrast between bizarre and more mundane delusions. DSM-IV contrasts mundane delusions—the delusion that one is being followed or that one's spouse is having an affair—with bizarre delusions such as that one's internal organs have been removed or that one's partner has been replaced by a double. According to DSM-IV, bizarre delusions are generally impossible, non-bizarre delusions are merely improbable. (Presumably the impossibility could be either physical or conceptual.) Clearly there is a vague boundary between these categories. However, DSM-IV also claims that a delusion is a belief not 'ordinarily accepted by other members of the person's culture or subculture (e.g. it is not an article of religious faith)' (APA 2000, p. 765).

The apparent conflict between these criteria—if something is merely improbable why could it not be accepted by others who are sane?—is resolved when one recognizes that it is the perplexing relation to a ground as well as any bizarre propositional content which makes something a delusion. Thus the propositional content of a mundane delusion may very well be accepted by others in one's culture or sub-culture, but on a rational basis. What DSM-IV should say, therefore, is that in psychotic cases, if the delusion is bizarre, it is not accepted by (normal) others at all; if mundane, it is not accepted in the way that the psychotic subject appears to accept it, that is without grounds. It may be felt that the bizarreness of a bizarre delusion has to be culture-relative; but the essential claim is that the delusion is bizarre relative to the prevalent beliefs of the subject's own culture. It might be argued that Capgras' delusion, where the patient says that their partner has been replaced by a double, is not intrinsically bizarre; recall the films *The Return of Martin Guerre* and *Sommersby*, where the long-lost husband turns out to be an imposter. The question is whether the subject says that their partner is an imposter or a double (a replica).[3] Bizarre delusions such as 'I am the Virgin Mary' may be characterized as those which cannot properly be acted on, while mundane delusions, which might be acted on, are often curiously inert—or so I will argue.

The DSM-IV claim that the delusory belief is not accepted in one's own culture remains problematic, however. It is not just that the belief, if it is a belief, is not accepted by others—it is not even understood by them. More-over, it is not clear that culture-wide delusion is impossible. Collective hallucinations have resulted in collective delusion, for instance when troops in battle report that angels appeared from the clouds and fought on their side. The idea of a collective delusion seems more plausible when a physical cause is implicated, for instance ergotamine poisoning from eating bread made from rye flour infected with ergot, which on one analysis contributed to causing the First Crusade; mass hysteria and other infectious delusions are also exogen-ous, if not within the sphere of reasons. Culture-wide delusions such as 'The end of the world is nigh' will not be bizarre in the sense of 'I am the Virgin Mary'; and a culture cannot be collectively interpreted as 'insane'.

The diverse range of delusions implies differences in philosophical treat-ment. Non-psychotic delusions, I will argue, fall within the sphere of reasons, broadly construed, and only in these cases can one speak of a bias in reason-ing—the subject's beliefs are motivated by their desires or wishes. Psychotic delusions, in contrast, do not fall within the sphere of reasons, and so a reasoning bias explanation is not appropriate. However, this claim does not imply that the deluded subject does not really understand what they are saying. That would be one possible thesis, and I will discuss it shortly. The alternative thesis to be defended here is, to reiterate, that in many psychotic and non-psychotic cases, the basic level of description of delusion falls short of the ascription of belief. Such cases include self-deception and monothematic delusion, where apparently only a single belief is affected, and the delusion tends to be behaviourally inert; in contrast, wishful thinking and polythematic delusion, where patients tend to be delusional about anything that attracts their attention, are closer to belief-status. I argue that at least in monothematic, behaviourally inert cases, although the delusion shares some features of belief, the disanalogies are sufficient to justify withholding a clear attribution.

I have argued elsewhere, in an analysis of self-deception, that it is not clear-cut that the self-deceiver believes both that p and that not-p, where p is for instance 'My partner is being unfaithful'; rather, there is evidence that they believe that p, and evidence that they believe that not-p. In such cases one should take as basic the conflict of evidence concerning whether X believes that p or not-p, and not assume a further, possibly evidence-transcending fact of the matter concerning their belief (Hamilton 2000). Here I argue that in the case of monothematic psychotic delusion also, there can be no clear ascription of belief. Rather, what one should take as basic is that there is evidence that X believes that p and evidence that X does not believe that p, in contrast to self-deception where there is evidence that X believes that p and evidence that X believes that not-p. The evidence for the ascription of a (delusory) belief is that the subject, apparently without intending to deceive, repeatedly asserts p; the evidence against such an ascription is that they act on the putative belief in rather circumscribed ways at best, and seem not to hold it on the basis of reasons. In self-deception, in contrast, there is a question in a different way about whether the subject believes that p, since here, the opposed evidence indicates not that they have no belief on the matter, but that they have the contrary belief. The situation is quite different in the case of wishful thinking, where the subject does indeed believe that p; likewise, arguably, in the case of polythematic delusion.

Thus, to reiterate, my thesis is not quite that in many cases delusions are not beliefs; rather, it is that there is no fact of the matter concerning whether S believes that p. This position is subtly different from that of a number of recent writers who have argued that delusions should not be regarded as beliefs.[4] It also offers a less radical alternative to the thesis that the deluded subject has lost understanding of the terms they are using. This thesis, defended recently by John Campbell, is one that I will be concerned to undermine; but first some scene-setting of the contemporary terms of debate is required.

Delusions, reasons, and causes

Henceforth, while noting the existence of non-psychotic cases, I will focus on psychotic delusion; 'delusion' will generally function as a contraction of 'psychotic delusion'. Accounts of psychotic delusion have tended to follow two opposed tendencies—rationalist and irrationalist. The irrationalist tendency is exemplified by Jaspers' pioneering treatment in *General psychopathology* (1963, first published 1923), which argued that schizophrenic delusions are not comprehensible—that is, they do not have a rational explanation in terms of common-sense psychology, only a causal explanation in terms of brain disease. In the rationalist camp, in contrast, belongs the extensive recent psychological research that regards deluded subjects as having a general tendency to faulty inference and biased reasoning. An example is the work of Davies and Coltheart, although their commitment to a reasoning bias explanation is tempered by adducing a tendency towards self-serving bias of the kind often regarded as a mechanism for maintaining self-esteem. They allow that such biases will not by themselves explain delusional beliefs, and claim that some delusional beliefs may be arrived at by taking an illusory experience to be veridical (Davies and Coltheart 2000, p. 13). But the general tendency of rationalist views is to assimilate delusions to mistaken beliefs based on faulty reasoning; and conversely, perhaps, to exaggerate the extent of irrationality in everyday thinking.

Both rationalist and irrationalist accounts should be rejected, I believe. Psychotic delusions are not beliefs explained by reasoning biases within the scope of common-sense psychology, or by rational reactions to bizarre experience; but nor should one concede that they involve mental attitudes subject only to causal explanation. My main target is the rationalist account, however, and here I simply emphasize that in rejecting it, one is not committed to the position of Jaspers and the irrationalists. (Here I make no particular comments about schizophrenic delusion, thought-insertion and control.) The latter are mistaken in dismissing the possibility that delusions express the individual's psychology or personality—though it should be conceded that the more the delusion does express this, the less it will be regarded as psychotic. There is an important distinction between explaining why the subject comes to have delusions, and why they come to have the kind of delusions that they do. The latter explanation might be individual, in terms of depth psychology, but it will have a social and cultural dimension also—for instance only in industrialized societies, which have television and the internet, could subjects believe that their thoughts are controlled through these media. A depth-psychological explanation would however be incompatible with causal explanation in terms of brain disease.

The problem with rationalism is that it makes psychotic delusions appear too comprehensible. Some cases cited by rationalists seem too 'rational' to be psychotic delusions at all, while genuine psychotic delusions are interpreted as a kind of error in thought. In the former category is Sedler's example of a woman who 'in the wake of an automobile accident in which [her] husband and child are killed...develops the conviction that she caused their deaths; later, she comes to believe that she is evil and must be destroyed, and, therefore, attempts suicide; finally, she is improved after a course of electro-convulsive therapy'. Sedler comments that at the level of manifest content the delusion seems neither random nor empty of significance. There may be a pre-existing dynamic—unconscious guilt, a forgotten wish to kill her father, or a more proximate wish to divorce her husband—or the psychosis may create a delusion that incorporates in distorted form the affects naturally arising out of the trauma; individual cases may differ, Sedler concludes (Sedler 1995, p. 258).

I would comment that as the case is presented, the woman's belief that she is evil is a comprehensible result of a sequence of events, and seems to lie close to the sphere of reasons. More detail is required—clearly it makes a difference whether the woman was driving the car and was therefore causally responsible for her husband's and child's deaths. If the woman believes that she is responsible morally and not just causally, this seems like a non-psychotic delusion; while even the delusion that she was evil might not count as psychotic. There are parallels with a real-life case reported some years ago in the British press, in which a woman ran over and killed a child who had suddenly run into the road. The woman had a strong Christian belief, and developed overwhelming feelings of guilt, including guilt that her own child, who was not involved in the accident, was still alive—that another parent and not herself had been bereaved. She came to believe that she must be evil and was suffering divine punishment. Such feelings and beliefs would not be incomprehensible even within the religiously moderate Anglican subculture. The women in both examples might benefit from psychotherapy, and it is Sedler's tendentious introduction of ECT treatment that helps to skew his example towards the psychotic.

The preceding cases are, I have argued, too comprehensible to count as psychotic delusions. The converse error made by rationalists is to attempt to explain genuinely psychotic delusions in a way that renders them too readily comprehensible. Proponents of reasoning bias fail to recognize that the 'conclusions' characteristic of bizarre psychotic delusion are so wayward that one cannot speak of a process of reasoning at all. As Wittgenstein would have put it, the alleged error of the psychotically deluded is 'too big for a mistake'. In *On certainty*, he comments on the distinction between mistakes and mental disturbances (Wittgenstein 1969, paras 71, 74):

> If my friend were to imagine one day that he had been living for a long time past in such and such a place, etc., etc., I would not call this a *mistake*, but rather a mental disturbance, perhaps a transient one. ...Can't we say: a *mistake* doesn't only have a cause, it also has a ground? I.e. roughly: when someone makes a mistake, this can be fitted into what he knows aright.

I take it that Wittgenstein means that where the subject is mistaken, one can for instance describe their faulty steps of reasoning, or their inattentive observation, which takes them from 'what they know aright' to an erroneous conclusion; the mistakes are, at least to some extent, understandable ones to make, if they are pointed out with enough patience and clarity, the subject will acknowledge them, and so on. This would not be possible in the case of psychotically deluded subjects. Delusion may be described as a failure of reason, but to say that someone has lost their reason is not to say that they reason badly; indeed, psychotic patients seem to fare no different to others in standard tests of reasoning.

Wittgenstein's remarks are cited in the recent discussion by John Campbell (2001a) and Naomi Eilan (2001). Campbell classifies recent psychological accounts of delusion under the headings of 'empiricist' and 'rationalist', although in the terms that I have been using, both accounts are rationalist in assimilating delusions with ordinary error. Empiricists, for Campbell, are those who regard the patient as making a broadly rational response to some very unusual (presumably hallucinatory) experiences.[5] According to empiricist accounts of Cothard's or Capgras's delusion, then, it is an abnormal lack of perceptual affect that causes the patient to think that they are dead or that their partner has been replaced by a double. On rationalist accounts, in contrast, there is a 'top-down disturbance in the subject's beliefs', which explains the change in affect. On this view, the Capgras' delusion 'My partner has been replaced by a double' becomes a local 'framework proposition' in the sense of Wittgenstein's *On certainty*—a proposition that is groundless and foundational to a practice.

Most important for present purposes is Campbell's characterization of the basic philosophical problem raised by delusion: In general we have to ascribe meaning to utterances in a way that makes the subject rational, yet in the case of the psychotic patient, we seem unable to formulate the content of their delusion; it seems that they do not retain a stable grasp of meaning through the mental disturbance (Campbell 2002, p. 91). I will call this 'Campbell's Problem', and clearly it does not apply to non-psychotic delusions. Eilan believes that Campbell's Problem yields a criterion for distinguishing (psychotic) delusions from mere mistakes, viz., 'We are in the realm of delusion rather than mistake when the failure of reason is such as to put into doubt the subject's understanding of the terms used to express his purported beliefs' (Eilan 2001, p. 123). (One should note that this criterion would make non-psychotic delusions into mere mistakes, and so for that reason alone would require qualification.)

Campbell's analysis is that the Capgras' patient no longer grasps what he terms the memory demonstrative 'that [remembered] woman'.[6] Thus when the patient says 'That [currently perceived] woman is not my wife', the underlying delusion is 'That [currently perceived] woman is not that [remembered] woman', while the patient also has the presumably correct belief that 'That [remembered] woman is my wife'. And yet, Campbell continues, the patient does not in any way try to verify the negated identity statement—notably by checking whether the woman he currently perceives shares memories of events in which he and his wife took part. Campbell asks how the patient can be said to retain a grasp of the meaning of their remarks, in particular the memory-demonstrative, when they use words in such a deviant way? He has a similar view of the schizophrenic patient who looks at a row of empty marble tables in a cafe and apparently becomes convinced that the world is coming to an end, commenting that it is problematic how any experience at all, let'alone one of marble tables, could be relevant to verifying the proposition 'The world is ending'. Campbell concludes that there must be 'top-down loading' of the experience by the patient; the consequence is that in expressing their delusion, the patient has lost an understanding of the words they use.

My position, in contrast, is that the claim of loss of understanding is too radical, and I will argue instead that there should be no clear attribution of belief to the subject. However, features that may be cited in support of Campbell's thesis—principally that the belief is groundless and behaviourally inert—also support the view that delusions are not genuine beliefs. (Indeed behavioural inertia is cited by Campbell.) I will present these features and then show why one should not conclude the loss of understanding thesis from them; finally I will try to defuse some objections to a non-belief model of delusion.

Non-belief-like features of delusion

(a) Groundlessness

It is a notable feature of psychotic delusion that either the patient offers no grounds for their delusion, or that if they do, they seem not to take them seriously. More mundane delusions, which share their propositional content with ordinary empirical beliefs based on grounds, are distinguished by being ungrounded. The psychotic patient seems convinced that they are the Virgin Mary or whatever, but the justifications that they offer carry the flavour of confabulation; they seem to be thought up after the question, and appear arbitrary, and psychiatrists comment that 'They don't mean anything to the patient'.[7] The reasons that the subject gives when questioned seem not to be operative. The self-deceiver recognizes that evidence is applicable, but has a curiously selective way of interpreting it; the psychotic patient, in contrast, seems not to recognize that evidence is applicable at all. This appearance contributes to what Jaspers called the 'axiom of the abyss', a therapist's feeling of encountering in the patient an absolutely enigmatic way of life; for him this was the central criterion for diagnosing schizophrenia.

It might be said against these arguments that at least in making past-tense claims about events apparently witnessed or experienced, the psychotic patient does not have to offer justifications, but simply has to report them in the way that people normally do. Memory is direct knowledge of the past, and so the subject need offer no justification beyond the claim 'I remember . . . '. Thus, the objection continues, the schizophrenic patient who recalls having an abortion in Buckingham Palace, says what anyone would say if they remembered such an event clearly. But though I would concur that memory is direct knowledge, and that memory reports do not require the justifications postulated by inferential accounts of personal memory, it is not obvious that the psychotic patient does say what others do when making personal memory-reports. Memory-judgements have a distinctive expression involving the continuous-verb form, which implies the possibility of a spontaneous manifestation or willed rehearsal of the remembered events in the form of memory images or memory-experience.[8] For the objection to be convincing, therefore, the schizophrenic patient would have to say, for instance, 'I distinctly remember being shown into the reception area, and taken by medical staff to the West Wing . . . '. It is doubtful that such patients would present their putative memory-delusions using the continuous verb form in this way. More generally, it is sometimes argued by proponents of reasoning bias explanation that many people believe things on little or no evidence. Clearly this is an issue that requires lengthy consideration, but I would suggest that such people are at least prepared to accept the appropriateness of reasons; the behaviour of psychotic patients implies a more radical estrangement.

(b) Behavioural inertia

Many delusions exhibit relative behavioural inertia, and are not fully acted on. As Bleuler commented (1950, p. 129), although many schizophrenic subjects have delusions that they are great leaders, 'None of our generals has ever attempted to act in accordance with his imaginary rank and station'. Similarly, sufferers from Capgras' delusion, which is relatively monothematic, often fail to express curiosity or form beliefs about where their spouse has gone, whether they are alive or dead, and so on. The delusion is avowed, and anger or irritation may be expressed towards the double; but often no attempt is made to get rid of them, or to search for the genuine spouse, and the subject may even be actively friendly. It is true that in some cases the delusion is acted on with tragic consequences, and here it is closer to a belief. But as Young notes (2000, p. 53), even when acted on 'there are often inconsistencies in accompanying affect and a curiously circumscribed quality to the delusion itself'. Sass comments on schizophrenic patients' tendency to 'double book-keeping'; their delusory utterances contrast with other statements, which suggest an accurate grasp of their situation. For instance, the patient who denies that she has children will give their names when asked (Sass 1994, p. 21). Jaspers contrasts the 'specific schizophrenic incorrigibility' with the normal dogmatism of fanatics or of manic-depressives. The schizophrenic's delusion is quite unshakeable, he explains; yet in contrast to dogmatics, their attitude to the delusion is 'peculiarly inconsequent at times', and such delusions often do not lead to action (Jaspers 1963, p. 4). It is definitive of schizophrenia that the delusions are often not accompanied by an emotional state appropriate to their content; for instance, a schizophrenic patient may report that others are trying to kill them, while apparently remaining completely indifferent to this prospect.

The distinction between mundane and bizarre delusions is relevant to the question of behavioural manifestation. There are limits to acting on bizarre delusions, which arise from their very unfeasibility; indeed 'The belief is not feasible' may just amount to 'It cannot be acted on'. It may be that nothing could count as acting from a bizarre delusion, since the attempt to do so would conflict with other everyday beliefs and behaviour. How could the belief that I am a tree or a pumpkin be consistent with walking downstairs, for instance? The English patient who claimed to be working for President Bush sen.—a relatively mundane delusion in the present context—did to some extent act on his belief; his flat contained material on US government and politics, and so on. A patient with the bizarre delusion that he was the Virgin Mary acted in accordance with it perhaps as far as one could—he dressed with a veil, spoke softly, and so on. But how could he express concern about Joseph, for instance, unless the delusion was broadened so that other individuals assumed Biblical identities? (This is to assume that the patient has the delusion that he really is the Virgin; perhaps if pressed he may admit that he is merely acting like her.)[9]

(c) The 'web of belief'

The final reason for questioning the comprehension or belief-status of delusions is that attribution of belief is governed by a constraint of rationality or reasonableness. Davies and Coltheart concede that if one cannot make any sense of how someone could reasonably have arrived at a particular belief on the basis of experience and inference, then this counts at least provisionally against the attribution of that belief to them (Davies and Coltheart 2000, p. 2). They comment that we expect to find an intelligible link between belief and experience, and that the subject's beliefs fit together tolerably well. Yet as Young (2000) notes, monothematic delusions are not readily compatible with holistic theories, which emphasize the importance of an integrated 'web of belief'. This fact is, I would argue, a further reason for denying belief-status to such delusions.

Against the "loss of understanding" thesis

To reiterate, these data—groundlessness, behavioural inertia, and failure to fit the web of belief—yield support both for a loss of understanding thesis and for a non-belief account. So it is necessary to show why the latter approach should be preferred. As noted earlier, Eilan claims that error becomes delusion 'when the failure of reason is such as to put into doubt the subject's understanding of the terms used to express his purported beliefs'. Her reference to a 'failure of reason' shows that she recognizes that it is not just any doubt about someone's understanding that implies the presence of delusion; they may attempt to express a belief using words which it is clear they do not understand, without this counting as a delusion. Eilan develops her position by suggesting that we are in the realm of delusion when we encounter doubt or denial of a framework proposition; she argues that this can never count as a mere mistake because such propositions are not accepted on the basis of reasons or evidence in the first place. Eilan glosses what Campbell terms 'top-down loading' of the experience as a change of framework belief rather than loss of understanding.[10]

It is evident that Eilan and Campbell at different times propose two distinct analyses:

(1) that the subject has no understanding of the words they use; and
(2) that they have a deviant understanding ('deviant' in the sociologist's non-evaluative, statistical use of the term).

Neither the loss of understanding nor the deviant understanding thesis is plausible, I believe, and each will be criticized in turn. The claim of loss of understanding is not tenable because the loss is not a general one; a local loss of understanding is implausible, and indeed may make no sense. The Capgras' patient has not lost a general understanding of the memory demonstrative or any other term, since in other contexts they grasp what 'my wife' and 'that woman' refer to, and what 'replaced by a double' means. Similarly, a schizo-phrenic patient has been using the words 'the world' and 'ends' correctly most of their life. In the latter case a loss of understanding is even less plausible since it would have to be intermittent, occurring only during florid phases of the illness. Conceptual role semantics, which argues that an understanding of a sentence consists principally in a grasp of its role in inference, provides no support for Campbell's position. The schizophrenic patient may well be able to infer from, for instance, 'The marble tables tell me that the end of the world is coming' to 'Something tells me that the end of the world is coming'. Many bizarre delusions—perhaps by definition all—seem to exemplify what Ryle (1949) termed a category-mistake. 'My internal organs have been removed', 'I am made of glass', and 'I am a pumpkin' look like category-mistakes; 'My wife has been replaced by an imposter' or 'I am working for President Bush', in contrast, do not. Now the person who regards the University as a mysterious entity separate from its component faculties, or the mind as a mysterious entity separate from the body—to take Ryle's own examples—is meant to have a pervasive misunderstanding of 'university' or 'mind' (Ryle 1949, pp. 17–25 and passim). On Campbell's thesis, in contrast, the psychotic subject's mis-understanding is purely local; they understand 'that woman' in most contexts except those featuring in the delusion itself.

The idea of a local category-mistake, and—it would follow—Campbell's thesis itself, may in fact be encouraged by a too-literal interpretation of Wittgenstein's remarks in *On certainty* concerning G.E. Moore's attempt to refute the sceptic. Eilan treats these remarks as supporting Campbell's thesis.

Moore based his refutation on apparently commonsensical claims such as 'I know that I have a hand', but Wittgenstein wishes to undercut the debate between the 'common sense' philosopher and the sceptic: ' "I don't know if this is a hand". But do you know what the word "hand" means?' (Wittgenstein 1969, para 306). That is, he suggests, if someone attempts to debate whether this is a hand, whether they are a sceptic or an opponent who believes that they are defending common sense, they put into question whether they really understand the word 'hand'. Note that this is a sceptical doubt concerning a framework proposition, a category into which many bizarre psychotic delusions fall, for instance the delusion that the inside of my skull is empty. G.E. Moore assumes that in entertaining the sceptical doubt he is saying something intelligible; Wittgenstein's response, 'But do you know what the word "hand" means?', questions this assumption.

However—and this is where Eilan goes wrong, I think—Wittgenstein is not claiming that it really is likely that a reasonably sane person such as Moore, in the course of philosophical discussion, has suffered a local loss of understanding of the word 'hand'. 'You have not given your words a clear meaning' does not imply 'You do not know what the word "hand" means in this context'; the most that one could say is that it is *as if* the philosopher does not understand what 'hand' means. Hence, although a temporary loss of understanding may perhaps be possible, there is no such thing as a 'local' loss of understanding. One cannot make a local category-mistake. Indeed Wittgenstein would be more likely to favour the Humean view that the sceptic does not really doubt that the best way to leave the room is by the door, rather than claiming that they do not understand what they are saying. This Humean view has obvious affinities with the position which I am defending, that there should be no clear ascription of belief in the case of many delusions.

The alternative thesis of a deviant understanding is even less plausible than that of a loss of understanding. It implies what may be termed the *lost tribe Romantic* or anthropological view concerning mental illness and psychotic delusion.[11] This position is exemplified by writers such as Foucault and R.D. Laing, and constitutes a branch of the anti-psychiatry movement that contrasts with Thomas Szasz's libertarian wing. Laing and Foucault think of psychotic delusion as expressing a genuine, deviant vision; the deviant subject does not speak gibberish, but uses a linguistic code which non-deviants have not grasped, and has an alternative rationality. For proponents of the anthropological view, there is a continuity between psychotic and non-psychotic delusion; the only real difference between allegedly psychotic delusions concerning the end of the world and the widespread belief in some parts of the United States that 9/11 was a portent of Armageddon is that the latter is more prevalent. Indeed Romantics must say that there is no such thing as psychotic delusion, for by his or her own lights the psychotic subject is rational; so it looks as if the deviant understanding thesis could not be a response to Campbell's original problem. Certainly Romantics are as mistaken as rational psychologists in assimilating psychotic delusion with the propositional attitudes of common-sense psychology. But a proper assessment of the anti-psychiatric position is beyond the remit of this article.

In fact, Eilan's suggestion of a deviant understanding seems to conflate two claims:

(1) the Capgras patient has deviant beliefs, so that 'This woman is a double of my wife' becomes a framework principle; and

(2) they have a deviant understanding, such that 'This woman is a double' means in non-deviant terms, say, 'God is evil'.

The second claim does not imply that the patient speaks Capgras-ese rather than English, but that they have a different understanding of certain concepts, just as individuals may have different understandings of '*hoi polloi*' or 'the moral sciences'. However, this deviance in understanding would have to be local, and locally deviant understanding is no more plausible than local loss of understanding. (In fact the well-defined brain pathology of Capgras' syndrome means that such patients are not ideal material for the anti-psychiatry case.) There is the further objection that delusions cannot be regarded as expressing alternative framework principles in Wittgenstein's sense, as Eilan proposes, since not all of them are candidates for framework status. Even those that are candidates exhibit groundlessness in a different way to ordinary framework principles. Such principles—which are better described as framework assumptions—constitute a basis for a wide range of the subject's beliefs; they are not behaviourally inert, though their behavioural manifestation requires careful presentation. Many delusions, in contrast, seem to ground a very restricted range of attitudes, if indeed they ground these at all. Campbell's thesis of loss or change of understanding is therefore implausible.

Delusions distinguished from beliefs

In an earlier defence of the authority of avowals of belief, I questioned the alleged holism of belief and desire in the explanation of action (Hamilton 2000). It is a by-product of the present article that another Davidsonian holism, that of belief and understanding, is also questioned. In this case, however, the authority of avowals—often called first-person authority—is not implicated; self-ascriptions of understanding are not authoritative, for clearly the subject may be mistaken in thinking that they understand a word correctly. Campbell's position, in contrast, may be consistent with the holism of belief and understanding—since if the subject does not understand what they are saying, presumably there is no belief which can be ascribed to them either.[12]

In support of the holistic claim is the fact that it may be difficult in some cases to decide whether the subject has lost understanding of the words they use, or whether no belief should be attributed. The general problem of interpretation involves an unclarity about what consequences to draw concerning how the subject will behave, what claims they will infer, and so on. But if my position is correct—that in bizarre cases a subject may be said to understand what they are saying without it being clear that they believe it—belief and understanding may be attributed separately, and so there is no holism.

The position I wish to defend, which questions whether the psychotic patient really believes what they say, is less radical than Campbell's. Furthermore, to reiterate, my argument is not that psychotic delusions are never beliefs. Monothematic, behaviourally inert delusions should be denied belief-status, while polythematic, behaviourally active delusions are more belief-like. Where nothing could count as acting from a bizarre delusion, it is correspondingly less plausible to classify such delusions as beliefs. (Insofar as the grounds for a loss of understanding thesis coincide with those for rejecting the belief-status of delusions, perhaps Campbell would allow that polythematic, behaviourally active delusions involve no loss of understanding.) As noted earlier, the distinction between belief-like and non-belief-like delusions is present in non-psychotic cases also; in the case of self-deception, for instance, there is no clear belief. A further, essential feature of the position which I am defending may also be overlooked. It is the following. My conclusion is not quite that the patient does not believe that their partner has been replaced by a double. Rather, it is that there is evidence that the subject believes that p, and evidence that they do not believe that p, and no way of resolving the conflict. In everyday cases, it is possible that even if X believes something firmly without it being any kind of delusion, there still could be evidence against the fact that they believe it. But we usually think that the question concerning what X believes can be settled, and that any undecidability reflects X's own indecision. In the case of many delusions, in contrast, the question cannot be resolved. 'What do they believe, then?' is the wrong question. There is a proposition concerning which there is evidence that the subject believes it, and evidence that they do not, and that is the best that can be said—a puzzling phenomenon.

Thus if one asks 'What is the problem with this person?', three kinds of answer may be given:

1. He believes that his wife has been replaced by a double.

2. He claims, without intending to deceive, that his wife has been replaced by a double, but he does not believe it because he does not act in ways consistent with the belief, does not base it on grounds, and so on.

3. He claims, without intending to deceive, that his wife has been replaced by a double, but we cannot say that he believes it because he does not act in ways consistent with the belief, does not base it on grounds, and so on. There is no fact of the matter about whether he believes it or not.

I am proposing the third answer.

It may be felt that the basic level of description in such cases cannot be evidential, since the very use of the term 'evidence' points to a more basic level—that which the evidence is evidence for. Clearly this is normally so. But in the case of the puzzling phenomena of self-deception and psychotic delusion, the two sets of criteria for the ascription of belief, involving verbal and non-verbal behaviour respectively, do not cohere. These criteria also diverge when philosophers profess Pyrrhonian scepticism, or claim that they are essentially disembodied, yet continue to act purposefully. In such cases I do not argue that the question is indeterminate, but instead follow Hume in claiming that the subject does not really believe what they say; however, in these cases there is the possibility of some kind of insincerity or bad faith.

In discussing the behavioural inertia of many delusions, I cited Louis Sass, who offers one of the most developed accounts to distinguish delusions from genuine beliefs. Sass is concerned to reject 'poor reality-testing' as the fundamental sign of madness and the basic principle of psychiatry, and in this he agrees with lost tribe Romantics such as R.D. Laing. He argues, for instance, that many schizophrenic patients experience their delusions or hallucinations as having a special quality, which sets these apart from their 'real' beliefs, or from reality as experienced by a 'normal' person (Sass 1994, p. 3). Although the account that I am defending does not imply lost-tribe Romanticism, I agree with Sass in questioning the medical model of 'poor reality-testing'; as a result the phenomenon of delusion is deflated. Some delusions may retain belief-status, but nonetheless the DSM-IV definition of delusion—'A false belief based on incorrect inference about external reality that is firmly sustained despite what almost everyone else believes and despite what constitutes incontrovertible and obvious proof or evidence to the contrary . . . ' —is mistaken in most aspects, not least in accepting without question the belief-status of delusion (APA 2000. p. 765).[13] That assumption should certainly be questioned.

Endnotes

1. Young (2000, pp. 50–51) presents some examples of delusion arising from brain injury.
2. Anthony David comments that 'delusion is the hallmark of psychosis' (David 1999, p.17).
3. 'Imposter' is often used in the literature on Capgras, but it implies hostility by the subject, which fits only a range of cases; hence the more neutral 'double' is preferable as a general description.
4. For instance Currie (2000), Graham and Stephens in this volume.
5. For instance Ellis and Young (1990); a similar approach is endorsed by Radden (1985), who writes that the delusion of the psychotic patient may be 'based upon

idiosyncratic ... ''evidence'' provided by hallucinations' or 'a private hallucinated world' (pp. 68–69).
6. The 'memory demonstrative' is discussed more fully in Campbell (2001b).
7. Comment to the author by Anthony David.
8. A claim defended in Hamilton (2003) and Hamilton (forthcoming).
9. These cases are discussed in Chung (1992), pp. 395–429, 362–392.
10. Campbell (2002), p. 95.
11. I take the term from Squires (unpublished).
12. He refers to 'perfectly sincere assertions made by people who seem to understand what they are saying, who may indeed act on the basis of what they are saying' (p. 91).
13. In writing this article I am indebted to comments from Matthew Broome, Man Chung, Tony David, George Graham, Lucy O'Brien and Roger Squires, and from an audience at the Australasian Association of Philosophy Conference in Adelaide, 2003. I am grateful for support from the British Academy which enabled me to attend this conference.

References

American Psychiatric Association (APA) (2000) *Diagnostic and statistical manual of mental disorders* (DSM-IV-TR), (4th edn, revised). American Psychiatric Publishing Inc.

Austin, J.L. (1962). *Sense and sensibilia*. Oxford: Oxford University Press.

Bleuler, E. (1950). *Dementia praecox or the group of schizophrenias* (trans. J.Zinkin). New York: International Universities Press.

Campbell, J. (2001a). Rationality, meaning and the analysis of delusion. *Philosophy, Psychiatry, and Psychology,* 8(2/3): 89–100.

Campbell, J. (2001b). Memory demonstratives. In: *Time and memory: issues in philosophy and psychology* (cd. C. Hocrl). Oxford: Oxford University Press.

Chung, M. (1992). Social non-complicity of schizophrenia. Unpublished PhD thesis. University of Sheffield.

Currie, G. (2000). Imagination, delusion and hallucination. *Mind and Language.* 15(1): 168–183.

David, A. (1999). On the impossibility of defining delusions. *Philosophy, Psychiatry and Psychology.* 6(1): 17–20.

Davies, M. and Coltheart, M. (2000). Pathologies of belief: introduction. *Mind and Language.* 15(1): 1–46.

Eilan, N. (2001). Meaning, truth and the self: a commentary on Campbell and Parnas and Sass. *Philosophy, Psychiatry, & Psychology,* 8(2/3): 121–132.

Ellis, A.W. and Young, A.W. (1990). Accounting for delusional misidentifications. *British Journal of Psychiatry,* 157: 239–248.

Freud, S. (1953). *The standard edition of the complete psychological works of Sigmund Freud,* vol.21. London: Hogarth Press.

Graham, G. and Stephens, L. (ed.) (1994). *Philosophical psychopathology.* Cambridge MA: MIT Press.

Hamilton, A. (2000). The authority of avowals and the concept of belief. *European Journal of Philosophy,* **7**(2): 20–39.

Hamilton, A. (2003). 'Scottish commonsense' about memory: a defence of Thomas Reid's direct knowledge account. *Australasian Journal of Philosophy,* (In press).

Hamilton, A. (forthcoming). *Memory and the body: a study of self-consciousness.*

Jaspers, K. (1963). *General psychopathology* (trans. J.Hoenig *etal.*). Manchester: Manchester University Press.

Kershaw, I. (2000). *Hitler 1936–45: nemesis.* London: Penguin.

Lacan, J. (1993). *The psychoses: the seminar of Jacques Lacan, Book III 1955–1956* (trans. R. Grigg). London: Routledge.

Radden, J. (1985). *Madness and reason.* London: George Allen & Unwin.

Ryle, G. (1949). *The Concept of mind.* London: Hutchinson.

Sass, L. (1994). *The paradoxes of delusion.* Ithaca: Cornell University Press.

Sass, L. and Parnas J. (2001). Self, solipsism and schizophrenic delusions. *Philosophy, Psychiatry and Psychology,* **8**(2/3): 101–20.

Sedler, M. (1995). Understanding delusions. *The Psychiatric Clinics of North America,* **18**(2): 251–262.

Squires, R. (unpublished). Mental disorder.

Stephens, G. (1999). Defining delusion. *Philosophy, Psychiatry and Psychology,* **6**(1): 17–20.

Wittgenstein, L. (1969). *On certainty.* Oxford: Basil Blackwell.

Young, A. (2000). Wondrous strange: the neuropsychology of abnormal beliefs. *Mind and Language,* **15**(1): 47–73.

12   The clinician's illusion and benign psychosis

Mike Jackson

This chapter develops the concept of the 'clinician's illusion', and considers its implications for our view of schizophrenia and the psychoses. In particular, it is suggested that both our clinical and our theoretical perspectives on psychosis are restricted by a focus on disorder and dysfunction, rather than being informed by an 'empirical, agnostic approach to the study of delusions and hallucinations' (Delespaul and van Os 2003). By contrast, a 'fully dimensional' conceptualization of the psychosis continuum (Claridge 1997) encompasses benign psychotic states, and invites the consideration of theoretical models from beyond the clinical domain.

The clinician's illusion

The clinician's illusion in its general form can be defined as the tendency of those who work in mental health services and clinical research to form a view of mental illness that is biased by their restricted role and perspective. The best recognized examples of this effect are forms of sampling bias imposed by the demands and characteristics of mental health services. 'Treatment seeking bias' (Berkson 1946) is the tendency to consider only those who seek the help of services, and 'Neyman bias' is the tendency to focus on those with more chronic conditions (Cohen and Cohen 1984), rather than those who make partial or full recoveries. A further filtering factor in services for people with psychoses is towards those who tend to involuntarily 'come to the attention' of services, by getting into social or forensic crises.

These filters on the wider population of people experiencing psychotic symptoms produce the 'clinical sample' from which most of our experience of these disorders is drawn. From the clinician's perspective, people who have psychotic symptoms, but do not seek help, and manage not to get into critical situations that bring them to the attention of services, or recover enough ability to function to disengage with services and avoid further contact, are effectively invisible. Within the clinical sample, those who are available for research, consent to participate, and complete research protocols without dropping out, constitute the more restricted research sample, on which our empirical understanding of the psychoses is based. The illusion takes effect when those characteristics of our clinical or research sample, which are artefacts of these selecting factors, are incorporated into our understanding of psychotic disorder, or contribute to the outcome of research studies. 'The biased and selective focus on the extremes of the psychosis distribution, continues to portray schizophrenia as a chronic incurable condition, drawing away hope from patients and carers alike' (Delespaul and van Os 2003).

While the concept of a psychosis continuum is widely accepted, there are competing views on how it should be conceptualized (Claridge and Beech 1994). Quasi-dimensional models define the continuum in relation to psychotic disorders, and milder expressions of psychosis are seen as indicating latent or sub-clinical disorders. Fully dimensional models aim to define it in terms of individual differences within the normal population, and thus to separate the concept of psychosis from that of disorder. 'Psychotic characteristics are not the prerogative of the classically diagnosable psychotic patient but form, instead, part of the array of psychological and biological features that impart individual variation to the human species' (Claridge and Broks 1984).

While there is a substantial body of evidence supporting the fully dimensional approach, it represents a radical conceptual leap, which contemporary psychological models of psychosis have arguably failed to make. It is suggested here that the assumption that *psychosis implies disorder* is a further layer of the clinician's illusion, which still pervades our reconstructed dimensional, biopsychosocial understanding of psychosis. This 'pathologizing bias' restricts our perspective by excluding benign psychosis from clinical or theoretical consideration; reducing benign features of psychotic disorders to 'symptoms' of underlying disorder; and limiting the search for explanatory concepts to the domain of clinical theories of disorder.

The psychosis continuum

Schizotypy questionnaire studies have established that items describing mildly psychotic experiences are widely endorsed in the normal population (Bentall *et al.* 1989; Joseph and Peters 1995). Psychometric analyses of these questionnaires (Mason *et al.* 1995), have identified a reasonably consistent profile of underlying schizotypal traits, such as Unusual Experiences (hallucinations, magical thinking, etc.), Cognitive Disorganization (impaired attention and decision making, purposelessness), and Introvertive Anhedonia (dislike of intimacy, lack of enjoyment). These map onto factor analyses of symptoms in schizophrenia, which have produced factors such as Reality Distortion, Disorganization, and Psychomotor Poverty (Liddle 1987), and they show associations with cognitive and neuropsychological variables which are predictable from findings in schizophrenia research (Claridge 1997). While this body of research supports a fully dimensional model, it is not clear from fixed response questionnaire data how far the experiential variables measured by these questionnaires relate to psychotic disorder. A 'Yes' response to an item such as 'Are your thoughts sometimes so strong that you can almost hear them?' (OLIFE questionnaire, Mason *et al.* 1995) or 'Do you ever feel as if someone is deliberately trying to harm you?' (PDI questionnaire, Peters *et al.* 1999) could refer to a wide range of experiences, many of which may not be remotely psychotic.

More methodologically sophisticated studies have addressed this issue, using standardized psychiatric interviews in epidemiological samples (Kendler 1996; van Os *et al.* 2000; Verdoux and van Os 2002; Johns *et al.* 2004). In each, the estimated prevalence of formal psychotic symptoms in the normal population substantially exceeds the prevalence of recognized psychotic disorder, varying between 5.5% in the British National Survey of Psychiatric Morbidity, to 17.5% in the Dutch NEMESIS study. The NEMESIS study had broader inclusion criteria, employing a category of 'symptom present, but Not Clinically Relevant' (NCR: 'not bothered by it and not seeking help for it'). This type of 'symptom' was considerably more common than 'true' symptoms (3.3% of their large sample had a 'true' delusion, vs. 8.7% who had a NCR delusion; 1.7% had a true hallucination vs. 6.2% NCR). In both of these studies, undetected psychotic symptoms were associated with the same demographic and environmental risk factors as formal psychotic disorders. Furthermore psychotic symptoms were associated with relatively low quality of life scores and neurotic symptoms.

These studies establish the existence of a symptomatic continuum between the normal population and formal psychotic disorders. The continuum revealed, however, appears to be quasi-dimensional, in that it is restricted to a small, and apparently mildly disordered, proportion of the population. However, this effect could be seen as a function of the methodology: the use of psychiatric interviews to elicit participants' psychotic experiences, whilst appropriate for the purposes of the research, introduces a pathologizing perspective on this domain of experience, which may inhibit disclosure, particularly of more benign psychotic experiences. If we are to fully pursue an 'agnostic approach to the study of delusions and hallucinations', we need to look beyond the clinical frame, at individuals who have psychotic experiences that may not meet psychiatric definitions, and may be benign rather than disordered. This requires different ways of identifying and eliciting experiences, which avoid pathologizing implications.

Benign psychosis?

Auditory hallucinations, volitional passivity, referential experiences, delusional beliefs, and other 'symptoms' (or more neutrally 'characteristics') of psychosis, can be observed in various domains of experience, beyond the clinical context. Examples considered in the following include spiritual experience, survival in extreme situations, and creative inspiration. Of these, spiritual experience is the most extensively researched, in that a number of large scale surveys, and detailed interview studies have been conducted in this area (Starbuck 1901; Greeley and McCready 1974; Hay 1987). Rather than rating symptoms in the context of a psychiatric interview, however, these surveys have been conducted in the context of broader research on attitudes and experiences, and responses have been elicited by more neutrally or positively framed questions, such as:

'Have you ever been aware of, or influenced by, a presence or a power, whether you call it God or not, which is different from your everyday self?'

Surveys using this question have found that between 30 and 40% of the normal population answer affirmatively (Hay and Morisy 1978). Analysis of a self-selected sample of written accounts of spiritual experiences revealed a wide spectrum of experience, including relatively mundane and 'culturally sanctioned' religious feelings, religious conversion experiences, life-changing mystical experiences, paranormal experiences, and some frankly psychotic experiences (Hardy 1966; Maxwell and Tschudin 1990). Whilst many of these experiences appear to include considerable psychotic phenomenology, they are usually described as having been of profound personal significance, and as having had important positive benefits for the individual's well-being. One of the most frequently described examples is the experience, following bereavement, of a comforting external presence, usually identified either as the deceased, or a benign spiritual figure.

A number of respondents to this survey question were followed up in a qualitative study of spiritual experience and psychosis (Jackson 1991, 1997). In-depth interviews were conducted with undiagnosed individuals who were selected because their written accounts suggested psychotic phenomenology and, for comparison, with individuals who had received a diagnosis of psychotic disorder, but regarded their illness in spiritual terms. The interviews were explicitly part of a larger study of spiritual experience, and special care was taken to respect participants' spiritual values and beliefs. Two examples from the undiagnosed group are given here to illustrate benign psychosis:

'Sara' described the following experience, which occurred while she was waiting at a traffic light on her way to work. At the time, she was disillusioned with her career, and uncertain about what to do with her life.

> I heard a voice say 'Sara, this is Jesus. When are you coming to work for
> me?'. And my first reaction was, I honestly thought it was my brother hidden

in the back of the car.... I thought he was having me on. I turned round to look and there was nobody there. I turned back and thought 'He's put a tape in the car' because it was so real and there was nothing there. Then I heard it again.

This was the first of many intense spiritual experiences which led to her giving up her successful management career to work on a voluntary basis with her local church. She was encouraged in this by her priest, who advised her that the voice was authentic, and that she should follow its promptings. At the time of interview she was stable and happy, and she described herself as deeply fulfilled by her work.

'Sean' also described having reached a point of crisis in his life through redundancy and illness, when he had the following experience:

> I heard words not of my choice, but like another voice within me saying my name—'Sean, none of this matters. You will always have what you need.... This is the beginning of things. Have no worries because... you are living in a timed existence now. That will pass, and this is the beginning of eternity.... We are all part of one another. Our intelligence is all linked.'

The voices continued to speak for long periods 'almost daily', for about nine months. He described the experience as:

> ... like coming through a headset... it was not my voice, not my sound of voice... everything was so simply said and yet directly to the point. The meaning was there with few words and... not clever words but a phraseology that I wouldn't normally use... I am sent the knowledge and it turns into a voice within me.

He identified the voices as 'the cosmic CIA', and felt that they had profoundly benefited his quality of life:

> ... it turned me upside down in many ways. It altered my views completely... [I] live life now as far as I can by what I'm learning... I think I have support and guidance, so nothing in this world can worry me.

Sean had never discussed the voices with anyone, and he commented:

> I know me, I ain't no loony, I don't go and do crazy things... I am definitely sure that I am open to hear things that most people aren't....

While these experiences involve relatively strong psychotic phenomena, the general experience of a benign authoritative presence is a central feature of most accounts of spiritual experience in the normal population (Beardsworth 1977). It is also a striking feature in some accounts of survival in extreme circumstances, two of which are briefly presented here.

Survival in extreme circumstances

These extracts are taken from Steven Callahan's (1986) account of being adrift alone in a fragile life raft for 76 days. During the period described, he was chronically fatigued, malnourished, and most pressingly, dehydrated. He was also highly stressed by the almost insurmountable tasks involved in survival—his inflatable life-raft was punctured and required frequent repair, he was threatened by severe weather, and capsized many times, his water distillation system required constant attention, and he had to catch fish with inadequate equipment in order to survive. He was frequently frightened, and conflicted about why he was continuing to struggle on against such odds.

> Day 59
>
> I have the nagging feeling that I am accompanied by someone. As I doze off, my companion assures me that he will keep watch or work on a project. Sometimes I remember conversations that have been shared, confidences, advice. I know it could not have happened, but the feeling persists. Fatigue is growing dangerous. My companion assures me I can last till April 20th.
>
> (Callahan's 1986, p. 181.)
>
> Day 67
>
> Maintaining discipline becomes more difficult each day. My fearsome and fearful crew mutter mutinous misgivings in the fo'c's'le of my head. Their spokesman yells at me.
>
> 'Water, Captain! We need more water. Would you have us die here, so close to port?'
>
> 'Shut up!' I order, 'We don't know how close we are...'.
>
> They gather together, mumbling amongst themselves....
>
> (Callahan's 1986, p. 194.)

The psychotic features of this harrowing account, which are only briefly illustrated here, probably result from his bad physical condition, particularly dehydration, and as such, should probably be regarded as a form of organic psychosis. Reading his account, however, it is hard not to feel that a more 'sane' response would have been to have given up, far earlier in the sequence of apparently impossible problems and hardships that he encountered, and overcame. As he describes it, his psychotic experiences appeared to play a critical role in keeping him struggling on, by providing external encouragement and support, a sense of companionship, and at times, useful suggestions.

A further example of this kind of constructive hallucinatory experience in similar circumstances is given in Joe Simpson's account of his dramatic descent down a glacier, in extreme conditions of fatigue and dehydration, alone, with a badly broken leg, having been given up for dead by his companion (Simpson 2004). He describes how, trying to accept that he was alone and what he had to do:

> A voice in my head told me that this was true, cutting through the jumble in my mind with its coldly rational sound. It was as if there were two minds within me arguing the toss. The voice was clean and sharp and commanding. It was always right and I listened to it when it spoke, and acted on its decisions. The other mind rambled out a disconnected series of images and memories and hopes, which I attended to in a daydream state, as I set about obeying the orders of the voice.
>
> (Simpson 2004, p. 141.)

This experience would be classified as a pseudohallucination, in that he is clear that it was 'a voice in my head', and, like Steven Callahan's experience, it was probably caused by physical factors. Again, it has the characteristics of feeling separate from himself, authoritative, and benign. Following its instructions literally saved his life.

Benign features of psychotic disorders

In psychotic disorders, the sense of authority and significance attributed to an autonomous agent is also a central feature, although it tends to be described clinically in pathological terms. This 'sense of presence' is implicit in many of the positive symptoms of schizophrenia—hearing voices, feeling controlled from outside, being watched, and so on. When the spiritual experience survey question cited above was administered in a psychosis self help group, 89% responded affirmatively, compared with 28% in the control sample (Jackson 1991, 1997). The experience of a sense of presence then, appears to be both common in the normal population, and almost universal in psychosis, (although the survey result alone does not establish how far the same kind of experience is being described in these different samples).

Other features of benign spiritual experience find strong parallels in psychotic disorders:

> In delusional insanity, paranoia as they sometimes call it, we may have a kind of diabolical mysticism, a sort of religious mysticism turned upside down. The same sense of ineffable importance in the smallest events, the same texts and words coming with new meanings, the same voices and visions and leadings and missions, the same controlling by extraneous powers. . . .
>
> (James 1902, p. 401.)

There is a substantial body of research that broadly supports the claims James makes here, for the strength of the parallels between 'mysticism' and 'delusional insanity' (James 1902; Underhill 1930; Boisen 1952; Jung 1960; Laing 1967; Campbell 1972; Arieti 1976; Prince 1979; Buckley 1982; Watson 1982; Lenz 1983; Wootton and Allen 1983). His conclusion is that the same psychological processes are occurring in benign and pathological psychoses, but that they can be distinguished by their emotional tone and their consequences for the individual.

> ...only this time the emotion is pessimistic: instead of consolations we have desolations; the meanings are dreadful; and the powers are enemies to life. It is evident that from the point of view of their psychological mechanism, the classic mysticism and these lower mysticisms spring from the same mental level...that region contains every kind of matter: seraph and snake abide there side by side.
>
> (Ibid.)

In many cases, James's distinction concerning the positive or negative emotional quality of the experience may be accurate. Even in the context of diagnosed psychotic disorder, however, it is not hard to find examples of subjectively positive phenomena, which suggest strong parallels with the benign psychosis examples cited above.

Mania and hypomania are the most obvious examples of psychotic states involving strongly positive subjective experiences. While there are often the dreadful overtones suggested by James, some manic episodes involve profoundly positive states described in terms of ecstasy, bliss or joy:

> Without warning I was projected out of my own familiar space. I seemed to be beside myself. An expansion of mind; the skull felt as if it had been opened and all the contents were streaming out into this splendour of light. I felt a physical bliss, piercing pulsating, a rising crescendo of sensation, not erotic but somehow like that. If it was like anything it was like a climax of physical love, a magnificent orgasm. But it wasn't that. The feeling of body and mind soared, then a vibration of sound somewhere, a high bell-like infinite sound, very fine and clear, attenuated. It was as if I was a telescope, body and mind, and that I was being focused, turned towards a brilliant light which burst upon me in full flood for a moment. Some white sea-birds swung across the road, bright against the clouds, and soared high. I felt like them, with them. Light, airborne, higher soaring and higher. My mind burst like an exploding shell in a spasm of radiance, whiter than doves wings; a sound in my head, a note higher and sweeter and more distant than the pitch of words to tell, hovering, wind-like, a kite-bird. Bliss, blossoming in showers of white and gold...then we came to the turning in the road, and I was returned.
>
> ('Penny', quoted in Jackson 1991.)

The existence of ecstatic feelings is well-recognized in mania, and it can be a feature of other psychotic disorders. The experience of intense pleasure is a strange characteristic for an illness to have, even when it also involves a sense of distress, or adverse consequences. This is also true of the sense of profound meaning and significance which characterizes most psychotic disorders, described by Jaspers as 'a direct experience of meaning', or 'a seeing of meaning' (Jaspers 1963). This characteristic pervades psychotic disorders, from the sense of heightened significance ('delusional mood') of prodromal states (Boisen 1947; Freedman and Chapman 1973; Moller and Husby 2000), through the intensity of primary psychotic experiences in acute episodes, to the dogmatic certainty of a stable, systematized delusional belief (Watson 1982). These features are usually regarded as essentially pathological, although, as James observed, strong parallels are found in benign psychosis.

The sense of authority and conviction associated with spiritual experience can be seen as positive features, which help the individual to find meaning and purpose in their lives (Hay 1987). Interestingly, the altered sense of meaning in psychosis can have apparently similar effects, although often with much higher social costs to the individual. Roberts (1991) found that people with systematized paranoid delusions scored highly on a measure of meaning and purpose in life, and had low scores on a measure of depression. Their scores were similar to a group of Anglican ordinands, and contrasted strongly with a psychotic group whose delusions were 'in remission', and with psychiatric staff, both of which scored lower on purpose in life, and higher on depression.

> The only subject to return a maximal score on Purpose in Life Test, with a zero depression rating, was a well known vagrant, who dines out of dustbins and controls the world from a makeshift tent, but has no contact with psychiatric services.

The defensive function of paranoid delusions in masking underlying depression (Winters and Neale 1985) has been incorporated into some contemporary psychological theories (Bentall et al. 1994, Bentall 2003). But the pre-occupation with meaning, and the profoundly felt level of experience, which characterizes both pathological and benign psychosis, is not fully captured or explained by the concept of a defence mechanism. Moller and Husby (2000) report an in-depth, retrospective qualitative study of the initial prodromes of 19 people who later received a diagnosis of schizophrenia. Two themes emerged as the most consistent and central features of each prodrome were 'pervasive disturbances in the perception of "self"', and 'preoccupation with over valued ideas, supernatural, mystical or symbolic theories'. These 'seeing of meaning' experiences occurred before the onset of frank psychosis, strongly suggesting that such experiences are a primary feature of psychosis, rather than a secondary consequence.

Psychological models of psychosis

Recent cognitive models of psychosis aim to construct explanations for psychotic phenomena, using theoretical concepts drawn from non-psychotic disorders (Morrison *et al.* 1995; Bentall 2003; Garety and Freeman 1999; and see Kinderman's chapter in this volume) such as intrusive thoughts, externalizing and threatening appraisals, underlying negative schema about the self or the world, maladaptive metacognitions, and avoidance based 'safety behaviours'. These models have been supported by experimental research, and they have contributed useful insights for the process of cognitive therapy. In drawing on models of neurosis, they strongly support the notion of a psychosis continuum, and indeed there is an explicit goal of breaking down the distinction between psychosis and other disorders in much psychological theory, and in the normalizing approach of cognitive behavioural therapy (CBT). However, to varying extents, in their focus on explanations drawn from the clinical domain, these models are arguably restricted to a quasi-dimensional conception of the psychosis continuum, and limited by the pathologizing bias described in the introduction. They offer relatively little insight or comment into the benign aspects of psychotic disorder, or into benign psychosis occurring outside the context of disorder.

This is illustrated in the debate over the role of cognitive dysfunction in psychosis, which concerns the extent to which it is necessary to invoke uniquely psychotic processes that are qualitatively different to the processes involved in neurotic disorders. For example, Garety and Freeman (2001) propose that primary psychotic experiences, such as hallucinations and referential experiences, involve underlying 'cognitive disruption', which is triggered by the influence of acute stress on a vulnerable individual. Cognitive disruption involves processes such as 'a weakening of the influences of stored memories of regularities of previous input on current perception', leading to unstructured and ambiguous perceptual experiences (Hemsley 1993), or deficits in a self-monitoring mechanism, leading to the experience of intentional acts such as thoughts, as being alien (Frith 1992). The appraisal of these experiences by the individual as external (and usually threatening) is seen as a necessary step in generating a psychotic symptom, and some symptoms, such as paranoid delusions do not require anomalous experiences or cognitive disruption. Nevertheless, key psychotic experiences such as hearing voices and referential experiences depend on the presence of cognitive disruption.

By contrast, Morrison *et al.* (1995) propose a theory of auditory hallucinations on which their externality is explained entirely in terms of appraisal. On this model, 'normal' intrusive thoughts become auditory hallucinations when they create high levels of cognitive dissonance, either because they are strongly ego-dystonic, or because the sufferer has strong meta-cognitive beliefs about the need to control such thoughts. In these situations, intrusive thoughts are appraised as externally sourced, as a strategy to reduce cognitive dissonance. Such culturally unacceptable appraisals isolate the individual and define their experience as psychotic. There is no requirement on this account for any abnormal process of cognitive disruption, which would set psychosis apart from other disorders.

The benign psychosis examples fit these models in so far as they can also involve strong external appraisals for auditory hallucinations, which are, to different extents, culturally unacceptable. However, the experiences described do not have the characteristics of intrusive thoughts, and they are not apparently ego-dystonic. Although they involve anomalous experiences, the benign nature and the functional value of the hallucinations and insights described is not adequately explained by concept of 'cognitive disruption'.

An alternative theoretical approach is suggested in the spiritual experience literature, where a number of commentators have proposed that these phenomena illustrate a basic, adaptive psychological process, which is also observed in examples of artistic and scientific creativity (James 1902; Hadamard 1945; Kris 1952; Jung 1960; Prince 1979; Batson and Ventis 1982; Grof and Grof 1986; Storr 1996). Prince, for example, viewed religious experience as a 'homeostatic, self-healing mechanism', which the brain has evolved to resolve acute stress. Persinger (1983) suggested that the capacity for such experience has 'evolved as a species specific buffer against death anxiety'.

Batson and Ventis (1982) developed these ideas using a model of creative problem-solving proposed by Wallas (1926). This distinguishes four stages of a basic psychological process underlying 'inspirational' creative thinking. First, 'preparation' involves becoming aware of a problem, exploring and working on it, and arriving at an 'impasse' situation, in which it seems impossible to make any further progress. This generates cognitive or emotional tension, and is followed by a period of withdrawal from the problem, or 'incubation', during which conscious attention is diverted away. The unresolved tension triggers an 'illumination', the emergence of the 'happy idea' from the unconscious, which resolves the impasse, often by modifying the experient's explanatory framework, or creating a paradigm shift. This is characteristically in 'primary process' form, involving a sense of authority and meaning, symbolic hallucinations, and ecstatic feelings, and it tends to be experienced as coming from outside the subject. Finally, 'verification' involves systematizing the illumination in rational terms and testing its validity empirically. This is accompanied by the resolution or release of the cognitive tension that initiated the process.

Wallas's model, although clearly not applicable to all instances of creative thought, is based on the introspective reports of some acclaimed creative thinkers in the arts and the sciences (see also Harding 1964; Storr 1989). Some of the best-known scientific examples are Kekule's discovery of the structure of the benzene ring; Poincare's development of the Fuschian equations; and Archimedes discovery of the principle of specific gravity (the original 'Eurcka!' experience). Harding (1948) discussed a similar process in the creative work of distinguished composers, writers, poets and artists, such as Mozart, Tschaikovsky, and Blake. These are rich with variants on the theme that the critical idea appears to come from beyond the individual:

> I have written this poem from immediate dictation, twelve or sometimes twenty or thirty lines at a time, without premeditation, and even against my will
>
> (Blake on writing Milton, quoted in Harding 1964, p. 14.)

Batson and Ventis suggest that spiritual experience involves the same underlying problem solving process, triggered by existential rather than intellectual or aesthetic concerns. On this account spiritual experiences are viewed as a useful product of unconscious processing or 'incubation' of life problems, which appear fully formed and vividly in conscious experience, and are not experienced as being self-generated. This process is seen as an involuntary psychological response to high levels of stress, which is essentially adaptive rather than pathological. The suggested role of high levels of stress in triggering the process fits smoothly with the vulnerability stress model of psychotic disorders. The fully dimensional psychotic continuum could be conceptualized as one of individual differences in the level of stress required to trigger 'psychotic' problem solving processes.

An important element of this account is that the psychotic features of benign experiences can be see as necessary components of the process, in providing the sense of authority needed to induce a 'paradigm shift' in existing cognitive structures. Following a bereavement, for example, if I do not believe in life after death, I am unlikely to be convinced or reassured by considering intellectual arguments for survival. However, my scepticism and grief can be transformed by a deeply felt experience of my deceased relative's presence.

The general concept that psychotic experience involves 'solutions', in the more limited sense of containing symbolic information that is potentially useful to the subject, is central in psychodynamic theories of psychosis, such as 'regression in the service of the ego' (Kris 1952). Although he regarded it as regressive, Freud (1911), for example, in his classic study of Schreber's psychosis, suggested that 'the delusional formation, which we take to be the pathological product, is in reality an attempt at recovery, a process of reconstruction'. Depth psychology and transpersonal theorists have developed these ideas in more detailed (and speculative) accounts of this 'reconstructive process' in benign spiritual experience (Wilber 1980; Grof and Grof 1986) and in psychosis (Bateson et al. 1956; Perry 1974; Lukoff 1988), although these ideas have received little consideration in mainstream theories of psychosis.

Recovery from psychotic disorder

The possibility of viewing psychosis as a potentially benign or constructive process is perhaps absurd from the clinical perspective. Clearly, for many sufferers, psychotic disorders are largely negative experiences with devastating impact on their well-being and ability to function. But psychotic disorders are heterogeneous, and the growing literature on recovery illustrates the possibility of benign resolution (Boisen 1936; Custance 1952; Chadwick 1997; May 2000). One example from the interview study described above 'Penny', is briefly presented here.

Penny experienced her first of three psychotic episodes following the early death of her husband, and soon after the birth of her fourth child. She became preoccupied with death:

> I'd gone too deep in there and there was a danger that I couldn't get out again .... So I had a lot of images, a lot of symbolism going on in my mind... and at one point I felt very strongly that I was going to die, I had a whole lot of... as we'd say 'synchronist' kind of conditions which seemed to suggest to me that I was definitely going to die on a certain day.

She was 'sectioned' and treated for hypomanic disorder, but she relapsed again soon after being discharged. She began to develop messianic delusions:

> ... an absolutely overwhelming sense of being... as we say 'God', I mean I felt that I was a God-person'.

Behaviour associated with this belief led to a second involuntary admission, and within a year, a third, longer but voluntary admission. At the time of our interview, she had been stable for a period of 12 years, during which she had led an independent, constructive, and altruistic life. Penny strongly felt that a critical factor in her recovery was the discovery of a religious framework that made sense of, and valued, her psychotic experiences. She became a Bahai, from which perspective she viewed her experience of being a God-person as 'an awakening'.

> I think what I was doing was somehow to mistake a consciousness of God within me as God's consciousness, but I understand that there's a difference. I'm not the sun but I can be a mirror that reflects it, there's a difference.

> So I read words like 'turn unto thyself and find me'—(whatever me is)— 'standing within thee mighty and powerful and self-subsisting', those words sort of make sense of the fact that I have a self which is not myself, which is larger and which is more expanded and which is total.

> .. in religious terms.... the people that I have to do with understand these things, I mean the amazing thing is that those things which before seemed so bizarre and out of place, now have a place.

Her case (and others in the recovery literature) illustrates how what appear to be pathological psychotic meanings can be transformed and integrated into more benign and socially acceptable constructs. This process is facilitated by the availability of a sympathetic explanatory model, and a validating social context. Organized religions or spiritually oriented groups can offer a cultural bridge across which it is sometimes possible to communicate about psychotic experience, and to promote a process of integration (Jung 1960). This provides an opportunity for the fourth stage of Wallas's problem-solving process, in which the creative inspiration is tested and validated in consensual reality, resolving the stress which precipitated its emergence.

This level of resolution is perhaps unusual in psychotic disorders. Typically, where the psychotic individual has a subjective sense of revelation and insight, it is considered by others as madness, a symptom of illness, and this may lead to dramatic consequences such as social conflict, involuntary hospitalization and compulsory medication—as it did for Penny. Rather than resolving any triggering existential concerns, a situation of radical and threatening social dislocation is likely to exacerbate them, precipitating a positive feedback cycle of further 'insights' and increasing stress. In this way, an otherwise benign, self-limiting process could become an acute psychotic episode (Jackson 1991, 2001). Stabilization following an acute episode, will often involve withdrawal from social interaction or discussion of delusional beliefs, which protects the individual from repeating the cycle. People with psychotic disorders tend to be isolated by their delusional beliefs, and this 'semantic isolation' in turn, acts as a maintaining factor for their beliefs. (This can also be observed in benign psychosis, as illustrated by 'Sean', who strategically kept his beliefs and experiences to himself.)

On this speculative view of psychosis, therapy has a clear role in providing an opportunity for integration of psychotic experiences. The emphasis on personal meanings in psychosis suggests the importance of respect and openness towards delusional beliefs and psychotic experiences, and a willingness to explore the client's perspective on their meaning, as well as developing alternatives. This collaborative approach to therapy is a core feature of CBT for psychosis (Fowler *et al.* 1995).

A further issue raised by Penny was the potential therapeutic value of techniques for managing altered states, which have been developed within spiritual traditions:

> I'd learnt to meditate in the middle of all this—the meditation seemed, as I said, like a thread which held me together through the various circumstances there were, and eventually out of it so that I felt that whatever experience I was having, including the synchronicity, including the very high-peak feelings of elation and perhaps even of a very... extended joy, would come back to me without danger, without fear, and without me communicating in a totally bizarre and unacceptable way.

Despite recent developments in using mindfulness meditation therapeutically in chronic depression (Teasdale *et al.* 2000), its application in psychosis has as yet received little attention (May 2000; Mills 2001; Chadwick *et al.* 2005). Grof and Grof (1986) have developed the concept of using other spiritually based techniques in 'spiritual emergencies' (and see also Brett (2002) for a discussion of Hindu and Buddhist approaches).

Conclusions

The clinician's illusion focuses our attention on the pathological end of the psychosis spectrum, and on theoretical explanations that deal largely with dysfunction. This obscures the central question that arises from a fully dimensional view: What distinguishes those for whom psychosis is an occasional, brief, life-enhancing experience, from those for whom it is a curse? Why do some find 'seraphs' and others 'snakes'?. This suggests a radical agenda for research in which the study of pathological psychotic phenomena is routinely informed by comparisons with benign examples. This would enable a clearer distinction between factors that may be involved in the process of psychosis generally, and factors that are specifically associated with pathology in psychosis.

Three related hypotheses are suggested by the problem solving process model.

1. The psychosis continuum may map variations in the threshold of stress required to trigger psychotic processes, with more vulnerable (and creative) individuals requiring lower levels of stress. If the process is too easily triggered, it becomes less adaptive, and more likely to lead to psychotic disorder.

2. The process described by Wallas is self-limiting, in that it resolves the tension that acts as the trigger, and in this sense it is a homeostatic, negative-feedback process. If, however, it fails to resolve the 'impasse'— perhaps by increasing social pressure on the individual– it could become more of a positive-feedback process, resulting in a increasingly chaotic spiral of 'illuminations', which would constitute a psychotic disorder. Alternatively, as in systematized paranoid delusions, the individual may be forced to isolate themselves socially, in order to maintain their sense of resolution.

3. The contents of psychotic experiences are presumably determined by previous experience. The nature of a 'sense of presence'—whether it is experienced as benign or threatening—may derive from previous attachments or current relationships in the individual's life (Birchwood *et al.* 2002). This explanation is consistent with recent findings that voice hearers

with psychotic disorders are relatively likely to have experienced bullying and victimization (Morrison *et al.* 2003), or physical/sexual abuse (Meuser *et al.* 1998).

A number of clinical implications emerge from the consideration of benign psychosis, and recovery from psychotic disorders. The importance of profound personal meanings in psychosis strongly suggests the need to approach such experiences with respect, sensitivity, and an open mind. This may be a critical factor in CBT for psychosis and, particularly, for new clinical initiatives, which aim to detect pre-psychotic 'At Risk Mental States', in order to prevent first episodes of psychotic disorder (Morrison *et al.* 2004). The role of psychological techniques developed in religious traditions, particularly meditation, in gaining control over psychotic experiences, and promoting recovery, is as yet, relatively unexplored. The potential value of spiritual traditions in facilitating a recovery process in some people with psychotic disorders is also under-researched. Clearly, involvement with religious groups and spiritual practices has the potential to be harmful for some people with psychotic disorders. Exorcism, for example, may be an unhelpful response to auditory hallucinations; and cultish or fundamentalist religious groups may exacerbate paranoid beliefs. Whether they are helpful or harmful, such beliefs and practices also present a challenge to the values and assumptions of mental health professionals and systems. Improved understanding of these issues could be fostered by active collaboration between spiritual organizations and mental health services (C of E/Mentality/NIMHE 2004), in training, and in the provision of support.

References

Arieti, S. (1976). *Creativity: the magic synthesis*. New York: Basic Books.

Bateson, G., Jackson, D.D., Haley, J., and Weakland, J. (1956). Towards a theory of schizophrenia. *Behavioral Science,* **1**: 251–264.

Batson, C.P. and Ventis, L.W. (1982). *The religious experience*. Oxford University Press.

Beardsworth, T. (1977). *A sense of presence*. Oxford/Lampeter: Religious Experience Research Centre.

Bentall, R.P. (2003). *Madness explained*. London: Penguin.

Bentall, R.P., Claridge, G.S., and Slade, P. (1989). The multidimensional nature of schizotypal traits. *British Journal of Clinical Psychology,* **28**: 363–375.

Bentall, R.P., Kinderman, P., and Kaney, S. (1994). The self, attributional processes and abnormal beliefs: Towards a model of persecutory delusions. *Behaviour Research and Therapy*, **32**: 331–341.

Berkson, J. (1946). Limitations of the application of fourfold table analysis to hospital data. *Biometrics*, **2**: 47–53.

Birchwood, M., Meaden, A., Trower, P., and Gilbert, P. (2002). Shame, humiliation, and entrapment in psychosis: a social rank theory approach to cognitive intervention with voices and delusions. In: *A casebook of cognitive therapy for psychosis* (ed. A.P. Morrison), *pp.* 108–131, New York: Brunner-Routledge.

Boisen, A.T. (1936). *The exploration of the inner world.* Chicago: Willet Clark.

Boisen, A.T. (1947). Onset in acute psychoses. *Psychiatry*, **10**: 159–167.

Boisen, A.T. (1952) Mystical identification in mental disorder. *Psychiatry*, **15**: 287–297.

Brett, C. (2002). Spiritual experience and psychopathology: dichotomy or interaction? *Philosophy, Psychiatry and Psychology*, **9**:

Buckley, P. (1982). Mystical experience and schizophrenia. *Schizophrenia Bulletin*, **7**: 516–521.

Callahan, S. (1986). *Adrift.* New York: Bantam Press.

Campbell, J. (1972). *Myths to live by.* New York: Viking.

Chadwick P., Newman Taylor, K , and Abba, N, (2005). Mindfulness groups for people with Psychosis. Behavioural and Cognitive Psychotherapy, **33**, 351–359.

Chadwick, P.K. (1997). Recovery from psychosis: learning more from patients. *Journal of Mental Health*, **6**: 577–588.

Claridge, G.S. (1997). *Schizotypy: implications for illness and health.* Oxford: OUP.

Claridge, G.S. and Beech, A.R. (1994). Fully and quasi-dimensional constructions of schizotypy. In: *Schizotypal personality* (ed. A. Raine, T. Lencz, and S.A. Mednick). Cambridge: Cambridge University Press.

Claridge, G.S. and Broks, P. (1984). Schizophrenia and hemisphere function I. Theoretical considerations and the measurement of schizotypy. *Personality and Individual Differences*, **5**: 633–648.

Claridge, G.S., Pryor, R., and Watkins, G. (1990). *Sounds from the bell jar. Ten psychotic authors.* Basingstoke: Macmillan.

C of E/Mentality/NIMHE (2004). *Promoting mental health. A resource for spiritual and pastoral care.* http://www.nimhe.org.uk/downloads/Parish%20Resource.pdf

Cohen, P. and Cohen, J (1984). The clinician's illusion. *Archives of General Psychiatry*, **41**: 1178–1182.

Custance, J. (1952). *Wisdom, madness and folly.* New York: Pellegrini and Cudahy.

Delespaul, P. and van Os, J. (2003). In debate. *British Journal of Psychiatry*, **183**: 285–286.

Freedman, B. and Chapman, L.J. (1973). Early subjective experiences in schizophrenic episodes. *Journal of Abnormal Psychology*, **82**: 46–54.

Freud, S. (1911) (standard edition, 1958). *Notes on a case of paranoia*, vol. XII. (trans. J. Strachey). London: Hogarth Press.

Frith, C. (1992). *The cognitive neuropsychology of schizophrenia.* Hove: LEA.

Garety, P. and Freeman, D. (1999). Cognitive approaches to delusions: a critical review of theories and evidence. *British Journal of Clinical Psychology*, **38**: 113–154.

Greeley, A.M. and McCready, W.C. (1974). *The mystical, the twice born and the happy: an investigation of the sociology of religious experience.* Chicago: NOPR.

Grof, S. and Grof, C. (1986). Spiritual emergency: the understanding and treatment of transpersonal crises. *Re-Vision*, **8**: 7–20.

Hadamard, J. (1945). *The psychology of invention in the mathematical field.* New Jersey: Princeton University Press.

Harding, R.E.M. (1964). *An anatomy of inspiration.* Cambridge: W. Heffer and Sons.

Hardy, A.C. (1966). *The divine flame*. London: Collins.

Hay, D. (1987). *Exploring inner space* (2nd edn). Harmondsworth: Penguin.

Hay, D., and Morisy, A. (1978). Reports of ecstatic, paranormal or religious experience in Great Britain, and the United States—a comparison of trends. *Journal for the Scientific Study of Religion*, **17**: 255–268.

Hemsley, D. (1993). A simple (or simplistic) cognitive model for schizophrenia. *Behaviour, Research and Therapy*, **31**: 633–645.

Jackson, M.C. (1991). A study of the relationship between spiritual and psychotic experience. Unpublished D.Phil thesis, University of Oxford.

Jackson, M.C. (1997). Benign schizotypy? The case of spiritual experience. In: *Schizotypy. relations to illness and health* (ed. G.S. Claridge). Oxford: Oxford University Press.

Jackson, M.C. (2001). Psychotic and spiritual experience: a case study comparison. In: *Psychosis and spirituality: exploring the new frontier* (ed. I. Clarke). London: Whurr Publishers Ltd.

Jackson, M.C. and Fulford, K.W.M. (1997). Spiritual experience and psychopathology. *Philosophy, Psychiatry and Psychology*, **4**: 41–90.

James, W. (1902). *The varieties of religious experience*. New York: Longmans.

Jaspers, K. (1963). *General psychopathology* (trans. J. Hoenig and M.W. Hamilton). Manchester: Manchester University Press.

Johns, L.C. *et al.* (2004). Prevalence and correlates of self-reported psychotic symptoms in the British population. *British Journal of Psychiatry*, **185**: 298–305.

Joseph, S. and Peters, E. (1995). Factor structure of schizotypy with normal subjects. *Personality and Individual Differences*, **18**: 437–440.

Jung, C.G. (1960). On the psychogenesis of schizophrenia. In: *The collected works of C.G. Jung*, vol. 3 (ed. H. Read, M Fordham, and G. Adler) (trans. R.F.C. Hull). London: Routledge and Kegan Paul.

Kendler, K.S., Gallagher, T.J., Abelson, J.M. *et al.* (1996). Lifetime prevalence, demographic risk factors, and diagnostic validity of nonaffective psychosis as assessed in a U.S. community sample. The National Comorbidity Survey. *Archives of General Psychiatry*, **53**: 1022–1031.

Kris, E. (1952). *Psychoanalytic explorations in art*. New York, International Universities Press.

Lenz, H. (1983). Belief and delusion: their common origin but different course of development. *Zygon*, **18**: 117–137.

Liddle, P.F. (1987). The symptoms of chronic schizophrenia: a re-examination of the positive negative dichotomy. *British Journal of Psychiatry*, **151**: 145–151.

Lukoff, D. (1988). Transpersonal perspectives on manic psychosis: creative, visionary and mystical states. *Journal of Altered States of Consciousness*, **20**: 111–139.

Mason, O., Claridge, G.S., and Jackson, M. (1995). New scales for the assessment of schizotypy. *Personality and Individual Differences*, **18**: 7–13.

Maxwell, M. and Tschudin, V. (1990). *Seeing the invisible: modern religious and other transcendent experiences*. London: Penguin.

May, R. (2000). Routes to recovery from psychosis: the roots of a clinical psychologist. *Clinical Psychology Forum*, **146**: 6–10.

Meuser, K.T., Goodman, L.A., Trumbetta, S.D. *et al.* (1998). Trauma and posttraumatic stress disorder in severe mental illness. *Journal of Consulting and Clinical Psychology*, **66**: 493–499.

Mills, N. (2001). The experience of fragmentation in psychosis: can mindfulness help? In: *Psychosis and spirituality: exploring the new frontier* (ed. I. Clarke). London: Whurr Publishers Ltd.

Moller P. and Husby, R. (2000). The initial prodrome in schizophrenia: searching for naturalistic core dimensions in experience and behaviour. *Schizophrenia Bulletin*, **26**: 217–232.

Morrison, A.P., Haddock, G., and Tarrier, N. (1995). Intrusive thoughts and auditory hallucinations: a cognitive approach. *Behavioural and Cognitive Psychotherapy*, **23**: 265–280.

Morrison, A.P., Frame, L., and Larkin, W. (2003). Relationships between trauma and psychosis: A review and integration. *British Journal of Psychology*, **42**: 331–353.

Morrison, A.P., French, P., Walford, L. *et al.* (2004). Cognitive therapy for the prevention of psychosis in people at ultra-high risk: randomized controlled trial. *British Journal of Psychiatry*, **185**.

Perry, J.W. (1974). *The far side of madness*. Dallas: Spring Publications.

Persinger, M.A. (1983). Religious and mystical experiences as artefacts of temporal lobe function: a general hypothesis. *Perception and Motor Skills*, **57**: 1255–1262.

Peters, E., Joseph, S., and Garety, P. (1999). Measurement of delusional ideation in the normal population: Introducing the PDI. *Schizophrenia Bulletin*, **25**: 553–576.

Prince, R. (1979). Religious experience and psychosis. *Journal of Altered States of Consciousness*, **5**: 167–181.

Roberts, G. (1991). Delusional belief systems and meaning in life: a preferred reality? *British Journal of Psychiatry*, **159**(suppl. 14): 19–28.

Romme, M.A.J., and Escher, A.D.M.A.C. (1989). Hearing voices. *Schizophrenia Bulletin*, **15**: 209–216.

Sims, A. (1994). 'Psyche': spirit as well as mind? *British Journal of Psychiatry*, **165**: 441- 446.

Sims, A. (1997). Commentary on 'spiritual experience and psychopathology'. *Philosophy, Psychiatry and Psychology*, **4**: 79–81.

Simpson, J (2004). *Touching the void*. London: Vintage.

Slade, P.D. and Bentall, R.P. (1988). *Sensory deception: a scientific analysis of hallucination*. London: John Hopkins University Press.

Starbuck, E. (1901). *The psychology of religion*. London: Walter Scott.

Storr, A (1989). *Solitude*. London: Flamingo.

Storr, (1996). *Feet of clay. A study of gurus*. London: Harper Collins.

Teasdale, J., Williams, J.M.G., Soulsby, J.M. *et al.* (2000). Prevention of relapse/ recurrence in major depression by mindfulness based cognitive therapy. *Journal of Consulting and Clinical Psychology*, **68**.

Underhill, E. (1930). *Mysticism. A study in the nature and development of man's spiritual consciousness* (12th edn, revised). London: Methuen and Co.

Valla, J-P, and Prince, R. (1989). Religious experiences as self-healing mechanisms. In: *Altered states of consciousness and mental health* (ed. C.A. Ward). London: Sage.

van Os, J., Hanssen, M., and Bijl, R. (2000). Strauss (1969) revisited: a psychosis continuum in the general population? *Schizophrenia Research*, **45**: 11–20.

Verdoux, H. and van Os, J. (2002). Psychotic symptoms in non-clinical populations and the continuum of psychosis. *Schizophrenia Research*, **54**: 59–65.

Wallas, G. (1926). *The art of thought*. New York: Harcourt.

Wapnick, K. (1969). Mysticism and schizophrenia. *Journal of Transpersonal Psychology*, **1**: 49–68.

Watson, J.P. (1982). Aspects of personal meaning in schizophrenia. In: *Personal meanings* (ed. E. Sheperd and J.P. Watson). London: Wiley.

Wilber, K. (1980). The pre/trans fallacy. *Re-Vision*, **2**: 51–72.

Wing, J.K., Cooper, J.E. and Sartorius, N. (1974). *The measurement and classification of psychiatric symptoms*. London: Cambridge University Press.

Winters, K.C. and Neale, J.M. (1985). Mania and low self-esteem. *Journal of Abnormal Psychology*, **98**: 282–290.

Wootton, R.J. and Allen, D.F. (1983). Dramatic religious conversion and schizophrenic decompensation. *Journal of Religion and Health*, **22**: 212–320.

13 Defining persecutory paranoia

Jennifer Radden

Abstract

The classification and definitions of psychiatric disorders and their symptoms have been subject to recent conceptual critique. Long anomalous, the category of persecutory paranoia, as distinct from paranoid schizophrenia, is here assessed in light of such critique, of new awareness of the limiting legacy of faculty psychology in psychiatric classification, and of recent findings in neuroscience. An intensional definition is proposed emphasizing the attitude of mistrust in persecutory paranoid subjectivity.

Introduction

Anomalies and ambiguities in the concept of paranoia have long been acknowledged. These contribute to confusion over the relationship between paranoid schizophrenia and other paranoid states. Recent work on the overarching psychiatric category of delusion, and findings in neuroscience, together with new suspicion over the misleading legacy of faculty psychology, provide additionally urgent reasons for the research task embarked on here— some conceptual groundwork for a revised classification and definition of persecutory paranoia, as a first step in clarifying the relationship between paranoia and paranoid schizophrenia.

In contrast to the puzzles over the concept of paranoia, a stable and relatively easily identified clinical condition seems to exist, a condition revealing *mistrust of other persons or agencies in a mono-symptomatic, non-dementing state involving systematically organized ideas and attitudes.* Moreover these symptom descriptions are marked by a quite strong measure of validity, as well as reliability. Under the encompassing term 'melancholia' certain types of case have recurred since ancient times. One is an apparently mono-symptomatic or partial insanity whose sufferers complain of being the subject of others' ill-intended attention. Greek and Roman, and later Medieval, Renaissance, and eighteenth-century descriptions of the symptoms of melancholia repeatedly reveal this picture of the person convinced of others' malice toward him (repeatedly, but not always, for 'melancholia' was an umbrella term covering several disorders more sharply distinguished today; Jackson 1986).

Even if we restrict ourselves to some American and European classifications and their antecedents, the condition whose definition is our focus here (henceforth PP for 'persecutory paranoia'), appears to have several names. In Kraepelin's system it was an example of 'paranoia' although at the time he was writing it was also known as a type of 'non-hallucinating' or 'true' paranoia, not to be confused with the term 'classic paranoia' (indicating a notably elaborate and extensive delusional system).[1]

It has also been classified as one of several paranoid disorders (APA 1968); one of several paranoid states (APA 1980; WHO 1992); and one of several delusional disorders, vis., DDPT (Delusional Disorder Persecutory Type) (APA 1994).

Some might judge what is here identified as PP to be a manifestation not of delusion at all but of Jasperian delusion-like ideas, or over-valued ideas, precisely because of the absence of hallucination, so the adoption of none of the above variations is entirely theoretically unproblematic; nor, in fact, is their equation incontestable.[2]

However, the present discussion will proceed on the assumption— plausible, if not unassailable—that these different names all refer to one and the same condition.

While its clinical presence may be relatively unproblematic, PP raises a number of puzzles for the psychiatric classifier, which perhaps go some way to explaining this variation in nomenclature. Some of this category's recalcitrance is well known, even infamous; other anomalies will be identified here. I will emphasize the following problems:

(1) PP is not to be conflated with paranoid schizophrenia and, though often classified as a psychotic disorder, eludes the neurotic/psychotic rubric more generally;

(2) it similarly eludes the Kraepelinian division between schizophrenic and manic-depressive conditions;

(3) it is characterized, paradoxically, as strong in the area of functioning—the cognitive—wherein its deficiency is said to reside; and, because of that

(4) it wants for a satisfactory explanation of its disorder status.

1. Persecutory paranoia (PP) is not to be conflated with the psychotic condition of paranoid schizophrenia. Like paranoid schizophrenia, PP is judged a severe disorder, and in that respect different from the trait-based personality disorder known as paranoid personality, which is characterized by long-term attitudes of mistrust and aloof suspiciousness (Mcissner 1987). Moreover, to the extent that delusion is often treated as the hallmark of psychosis, and that paranoid beliefs rank as actual delusions, paranoia must by definition be a psychotic condition. Yet PP is mono-symptomatic, not

manifesting the (other) cognitive defects, nor the deficient reality testing associated with the hallucinations and bizarre, improbable delusions of the schizophrenias. More serious than neurosis, yet without these marks of psychosis, PP is recalcitrant to the division between psychotic and neurotic conditions despite its frequent classification as a functional psychosis.

2. Persecutory paranoia was separated from the broad Kraepelinian-derived division between schizophrenic disorders and manic-depressive disorders, as neither the one nor the other. Persecutory paranoia was a relatively stable condition, varying and deteriorating little or none in its course. And for Kraepelin's system as it emerged in later versions (for example, the eighth edition of the *Textbook*) this feature was critical: mono-symptomatic and unvarying 'pure'(persecutory) paranoia, where patients had relatively systematized delusions (most commonly on persecutory themes) without hallucinations in a condition whose course did not lead to eventual dementia, needed to be distinguished from *dementia paranoides* (paranoid dementia), a condition exhibiting delusions and hallucinations and the same dementing course and other characteristics as dementia praecox.(Kraepelin later added the intermediate group of paraphrenias to describe those conditions whose delusions and hallucinations did not lead to eventual dementia.)[3]

More recent attempts to mark the difference between paranoid disorder and paranoid schizophrenia have emphasized in addition the non-bizarre content and the mood congruence of the delusions of paranoid disorder (Winokur 1985; Butler and Braff 1991).

3. Similarly problematic is the status of PP as a disorder characterized merely by delusions understood as false, irrational, falsely held, and/or irrationally acquired beliefs. (This narrow characterization is relatively recent: pre-nineteenth century descriptions of paranoia sometimes included reference to the visual and auditory hallucinations now said to be absent; Hoff 1995.) Because the reasoning of PP is notably logical, the customary categorization of this condition as a disorder of cognition, in the framing faculty psychology of psychiatric classification, seems paradoxical today when its (alleged) source in inherited degeneracy, a nineteenth-century mainstay in accounts of paranoia, is no longer mentioned.

4. The status of PP as a disorder must be controversial for another reason. Kraepelin defined paranoia as the insidious development of a permanent and unshakable delusional system resulting from internal causes, accompanied by '*perfect preservation of clear and orderly thinking*, willing and action', the patient remaining 'permanently *sensible, clear and reasonable*' (Kraepelin 1920, pp. 212–213, 115, my emphasis). This emphasis on the intact cognitive processes of its sufferer requires us to question why PP is classified as a disorder at all. If, without hallucinations, these patients

reason logically to their beliefs, where is the incapacity, dysfunction, or disability in their condition?

One way out of this set of dilemmas and puzzles over defining and classifying PP is proposed here, with emphasis on mistrustful attitudes (though the following discussion provides only partial groundwork for a classificatory revision). Mistrust is at the heart of PP subjectivity. Mistrust is not a belief, however, but an attitude, in which both belief and affective elements are entwined.

Focusing on paranoid mistrust in defining this disorder appears to offer several nosological and definitional advantages, each of which will be explored in the following pages. (1) This emphasis supports the mood-congruence feature of paranoid disorders, a trait by which they are distinguished from paranoid schizophrenia; it thus serves to clarify the relationship between paranoid states and paranoid schizophrenia. Emphasis on mistrust avoids the traditional narrowly cognitive analysis of paranoia in terms of delusions, and in so doing side-steps (2) the several difficulties associated with defining delusion, as well as (3) the fact that there appears to be no cognitive incapacity with which PP can be consistently identified. To privilege this attitudinal feature of PP subjectivity is to adopt an analysis of PP in terms of its propositional content-type, rather than epistemic structure. Such an analysis is (4) interestingly consonant with recent findings in neuroscience. Finally, this focus seems to reveal a further advantage to the classifier: (5) it exposes an implicit norm, explaining our warrant in pathologizing persecutory paranoid behaviour and response.

One point of method must be stressed at the outset. The task at hand is a purely theoretical one: that of reconsidering PP in the sense of clarifying its meaning or intension. It is not, or is not primarily, to enhance our understanding of the extension of PP by redrawing the class of its sufferers, or developing a more accurate criterion to help the clinician diagnose such sufferers. These respective concerns over the term's extension and intension are separable. Clinicians may diagnose effectively in the absence of an intensionally adequate definition (and in fact little in this paper will be new to those familiar with paranoia from diagnostic and clinical experience). Sometimes—as seems to be so with PP here—the task of redefinition is to retain the extension and find a matching intensional description (Spitzer 1990).

Approaches to the classification of delusional disorders

PP is usually classified as a delusional disorder, and confusions and differences in its classification can be introduced by looking at approaches to the classification of all disorders marked by delusional symptoms.

Delusions may be understood generically, with a definition that captures the common epistemic structure (allegedly) shared by all delusions. Alternatively, delusions may be understood in terms of the sorts of thing their subjects are deluded about. An epistemic structural classification of delusion arranges according to defects of delusory cognition, while a content- type classification arranges delusions according to a characterization of their propositional content-type. Content-type is often used for sub-classifications, so strictly speaking, a 'content-type' classification is one in which the sole or the initial criterion for analysis appeals to content type. An example of the epistemic structural approach is found in a definition such as DSM-IV's classification of delusional disorder, which notes the characteristics of all delusions (APA 1994). Examples of the content-type approach is reflected in disorder categories such as the now unused lycanthropy (delusory belief that one is a wild animal), and Cotard's syndrome or *délire des negations* (delusory belief that one is dead), whose status as a delusion has been challenged (Berrios 1995), as well as others with more current acceptance: the delusion of parasitosis or acarophobia (the delusional conviction of infestation), anosognosia (the delusional denial of a real physical disability), and Capgras (the delusion that a familiar person is unknown to one).

Because the classificatory approaches contrasted here are sometimes combined, classifications may merely vary in the extent to which they privilege or emphasize the epistemic-structural over the content-type, using the latter to distinguish sub-categories. Thus, although his primary classificatory criterion is not based on content-type, Kraepelin introduces a secondary, content-type based organization: all paranoid delusions, he believed, either develop as ideas of exaltation or as ideas of injury (Kraepelin 1920, p. 220). A more common content-type classification distinguishes delusions of persecution from those with jealous, grandiose, and erotic content (see, for example: Freud 1922; Cameron 1963); to which is sometimes added somatic content (APA 1980). Such content-type analyses have been dismissed as antiquated and superficial (Garety and Hemsley 1994). Following Maher's influential rejection of content-based analyses on the grounds that they failed to yield useful prognoses, or aetiological associations, researchers in the last decades of the twentieth century exhibited a trend away from content-based analyses (Maher 1988; Garety and Hemsley 1994). Emphasis was placed instead on the epistemic-structural features allegedly shared by all delusions independent of content.

This dismissal of content-based analyses may have been premature, however. Despite the trend privileging the epistemic-structural over the semantic, recently identified difficulties inherent in epistemic-structural definitions of delusion, together with some findings in neuroscience, appear to favour a return to emphasis on propositional content-type.

Reasons to privilege content-type

At least as they have been construed thus far, analyses based on epistemic-structural features are conceptually flawed, and this constitutes the first reason to turn to classificatory principles and analyses emphasizing content-type. Definitions that presuppose the structural approach vary in emphasis and details, but they usually turn on three elements.

1. Delusions are beliefs or thoughts. When narrowly defined to cover present thoughts, beliefs and ideas, together with those cognitive states derived from seeming perceptual experience (yielding delusional perception or hallucination), and from past experience (yielding delusional memory), the cognitive does not extend to affective or volitional states.

2. Delusions are false, implausible or at least unshared factual beliefs. Their content is 'impossible,' is Jaspers's rather extreme way of asserting this, but other definitions range across the considerable latitude separating attributions of falsity, implausibility and merely of idiosyncracy (Jaspers 1963, p. 96).

3. Delusions are beliefs derived or maintained through faulty or inadequate methods of reasoning.

Included in 3 (above) are two of the features in Jaspers's analysis: delusions are held with extraordinary certainty, and are impervious to correction (Jaspers 1963, pp. 95–96, 104–10). The features outlined in 1–3 are true of standard analyses found in the literature (psychiatric and philosophical) on delusions; that said, the innovations introduced by Stephens and Graham in the present volume, which separate the believer's intentional states towards their beliefs from the beliefs themselves, may avoid some of the conceptual difficulties rehearsed below.

In contrast to the three criteria identified here French nosological traditions have distinguished separate 'delusional mechanisms': those which are (a) hallucinatory, (b) interpretive (logically coherent delusions based on the misinterpretation of correctly perceived facts), and (c) imaginative (fantastically imaginative delusional themes; Pichot 1990). But while the French system is also broadly epistemic and shares with the English-speaking classificatory traditions an assumption that delusions are beliefs or cognitive states, the French nosology emphasizes a different set of features. Moreover, the French term *délire* does not contain the same narrowly cognitive connotations, which its common translation as 'delusion' conveys (Berrios 1995). So the French classifications are not as vulnerable to the difficulties associated with classifying and defining delusions.

Long before recent challenges to the general category of delusion, persecutory delusions were identified as anomalous because they were logically impeccable. The patient suffered an apparent disorder without exhibiting the usual criterion of disability widely believed to distinguish mental disorder from normal psychological variation. More recently has come recognition that systematic and non-dementing delusions, such as those of persecution, were not alone in contradicting most generalizations made about delusions understood as a broad class. Both conceptual and empirical studies have revealed serious difficulties in traditional essentialist epistemic structural accounts of delusions defined in terms of false or irrationally acquired or maintained beliefs.

In summarizing these difficulties, we may distinguish three points. First, earlier definitions are insufficient because delusory beliefs are not always 'false factual' beliefs. Delusions are sometimes true, it has been illustrated (Jaspers 1902, p. 106; Moor and Tucker 1979; Fulford 1994; Gillet 1995). The so-called Othello syndrome is a well-known example of this, where delusions of possessive jealousy are not grounded in, but happen to conform to, fact (Schmiedeberg 1953). Sometimes, moreover, these beliefs are non-empirical and thus non-factual and non-falsifiable. This will be so when they concern religious and metaphysical content (Jaspers 1963; Radden 1985; Walkup 1990), and when they concern the kind of inner felt states usually supposed incorrigible, such as claims about one's inner sensations (Spitzer 1990).

Second, nor, it appears, can we use the method of acquiring or maintaining deluded beliefs to define them. Delusions are not more ill-formed, or reached through more flawed reasoning than the beliefs of ordinary reasoners, themselves rather flawed, Maher has established (Maher 1988, 1992). And despite the commonly held view that delusions are maintained with an unrelenting tenacity, recent work has shown this not to be so. Conviction fluctuates, even with so-called 'fixed' delusions (Garety and Hemsley 1994).[4]

(It is conceivable that some of this apparently fluctuating conviction can be explained away with a more sophisticated, hierarchical model such as Stephens and Graham sketch; only empirical research employing that model will tell, however.)

What then do delusional states, structurally understood, share in common? One useful discussion recognizes that 'nothing' may be the answer to this question (Oltmanns 1988; Fulford 1989). Delusion, Oltmanns suggests, may best be conveyed in terms of a number of features, no one of which is necessary to its characterization. Oltmanns's list includes seven items, e.g. 'The balance of evidence for and against the belief is such that other people consider it completely incredible'; 'The belief is not shared with others'. For some of the purposes to which definitions are put, Oltmanns's list will probably suffice. It has the limitation of being narrowly cognitive, however, with no place for delusions, which are, or rest on, value judgements, for example.

Third, nor are delusions all merely beliefs. Some delusions are value-judgements, for example (Fulford 1991, 1994). And while value-judgements—and other judgements—are constituted by beliefs in that they contain belief elements, they are not reducible to mere beliefs. They are more complex states comprising volitional and emotive as well as belief elements.[5]

While delusions may be clinically recognizable then, standard intensional definitions of them are insufficient. And these concerns over delusion in general are very serious. Delusion is a—Jaspers would say *the*—core psychiatric category. The presence of delusions, for instance, is at the centre of current notions about what distinguishes serious mental disorder. If we cannot satisfactorily define delusion, then not only is the category of delusion itself in trouble, so too is that of mental disorder.

Neuroscience

A second reason to eschew epistemic-structural classificatory principles in psychiatry and to seek content-type analyses seems to be suggested by findings in the closely related field of neuroscience, where correlations appear to link identifiable deficits with content-specific 'delusions'. It should be emphasized, however, that nothing in the argument that follows puts causal emphasis on this use of 'correlation': an exacting methodology would be required to transform correlations between cognitive or other functional deficits and brain defects as causally related, and such ambitions, fortunately, are beyond the scope of this discussion.

Correlations between organic conditions and particular delusions identified by way of content-type, such as the alleged link between alcoholism and delusional jealousy (now in some doubt), have long been claimed (Kolle 1932; Shepherd 1961). Other such correlations are today more widely accepted. Some content-type categories such as parasitosis have known correlations with cocaine caused brain toxicity (Siegel 1994), and, indeed, as far back as Kraepelin's time, cocaine was also implicated in delusions of jealousy. Delusions of jealousy have actually been associated with a number of brain diseases and disorders, including pre-senile dementia, cerebral arteriosclerosis, Huntington's chorea, Parkinson's disease, general paralysis of the insane, cerebral tumor, secondary carcinoma, Alzheimer's disease, pan-hypopituitarism, disseminated sclerosis, and temporal lobe epilepsy as a post-ictal phenomenon (Shepherd 1961).

Reviewing the evidence for these correlations in work through the early 1980s, Cummings made use of a content-based classification in noting the presence of four general types of 'false belief'(Cummings 1985): simple persecutory; complex persecutory; grandiose; and those associated with specific neurological defects (such as anosognosia). He used the word 'delusion' to characterize these states, and he emphasized that while they may coexist with other symptoms of CNS dysfunction, they may also be the sole manifestation of such dysfunction. Cummings's list includes not only delusional jealousy but: thought insertion, thought broadcasting, thought blocking, and external-influence delusions like those associated with schizophrenia; Capgras syndrome; Fregoli syndrome (where the patient identifies his persecutors in several, changing identities); intermetamorphosis syndrome (the belief that others have taken on the physical appearance of others); infestation; lycanthropy; and de Clerambault syndrome (the belief that one is secretly loved by another).

In the more than twenty years since Cummings wrote, additional evidence of such correlations has emerged. Some conditions, such as Capgras and anosognosia, are now known to result from brain disorder and disease, and others are more strongly suspected of such association (Joseph 1986; Joseph *et al.* 1986; Young *et al.* 1992; Damasio 1999). Destruction of the parietal regions has been shown to lead to forms of visuo-spatial neglect (failure to acknowledge and attend to the left or right side of space) and consequent delusional beliefs (McCarthy and Warrington 1990; Roland 1993; Anderson *et al.* 1997; Jeannerod 1997; Maguire 1997). Lesions of the corpus callosum have been found to result in 'alien limb' phenomena (Feinberg *et al.* 1992), where the patient complains of experiencing 'disownership' in relation to a limb, or experiences the presence of an additional phantom limb (Hari *et al.* 1998). Thus, for example, a patient with epileptic activity in a right-sided parietal lesion described a left-sided alien limb, which, she reported, 'felt it belonged to someone else and wanted to hurt me because it moved towards me'(Leiguarda *et al.* 1993). Those suffering schizophrenia similarly often believe themselves subject to alien control and various other forms of identity confusion and 'disownership' of their experiences (Radden 1996, 1998; Stephens and Graham 2000). They are hypothesized to suffer a deficit in 'internal monitoring' function (Frith and Done 1989), which PET scans have correlated with the right inferior parietal lobe and the cingulate gyrus (Spence *et al* 1997; Spence 1999).

Caution is in order as we evaluate these findings. It seems unlikely, for instance, that a single area or function of the brain can account for any one of these delusions (Roberts 1992). More likely, these disorders arise from a widely distributed system of interconnected brain regions (Spence, 1999, p. 25; Damasio 1999, pp. 209–215).

Moreover, linguistic variations require acknowledgement. Unlike Cummings, researchers in the last two decades speak more commonly of 'deficits' and 'experiences' or neglect syndromes than of 'delusions' in characterizing the bizarre, subjective states they describe, apparently presupposing disanalogies between these 'delusions' and the common delusions of functional psychiatry.

The actual extent of analogy here is arguably closer than these variations in nomenclature suggest, nonetheless, as a review of some points of comparison reveals. First, the 'delusions' of neuroscience are more than purely cognitive phenomena. The 'delusions' of neuroscience often affect not only belief but function and, with that, accompanying mood and attitude. More generally, they are not beliefs detachable from their subjective surround. If I believe myself infested, for example, I also loathe the idea (an attitude or emotion) and am eager to remedy the situation (a volitional state). This characteristic will not serve to distinguish such 'delusions' from common delusions for, as we have seen, common delusions also have extra cognitive features. Second, these 'delusions' may not be entertained in the same way, as are ordinary delusions. The problem here, also, is that recent studies have exploded the traditional structural characterization about how ordinary delusions are entertained. Moreover, some authorities ascribe typically 'delusion-like' aspects to these beliefs. Speaking of anosognosia, Damasio remarks on the tenacity of its sufferer's false belief, a tenacity that 'allows someone to hold a *persistent false belief* in spite of having received information to the contrary' (Damasio 1999, p. 212, my emphasis). Also, some research suggests that these 'delusions' are secondary products, derived from a prior experience of incapability or deficit. Thus the initial, non-cognitive experience of alienated control brought about, perhaps, by a deficit in internal monitoring function, is hypothesized to give rise to the schizophrenic belief that a sinister alien agency directs one's actions (Frith and Done 1989; Spence *et al.* 1997; Spence 1999). Although this feature is not customarily proposed in the case of ordinary delusions, we shall see (below) that some accounts of ordinary delusions have hypothesized a causal account importantly analogous to this.

A final point of comparison was noted earlier: these neurological 'delusions' sometimes occur as the sole manifestation of organic disorder and in this respect resemble the characteristically mono-symptomatic condition of PP.

Despite what may be differences between the delusions of psychiatry and the 'delusions' of neuroscience, the recent research on the concept of delusion reviewed earlier leaves us without a definition of delusion sharp enough to exclude these as instances of 'delusions'. Moreover correlations may emerge from further brain scientific research linking persecutory paranoid delusions (and other common delusions) with features of the brain's structure or function, as some researchers hypothesize (Butler and Braff 1991, p. 636). At the very least, then, these are some sorts of delusions, albeit delusions formed only after what seems likely to be some kind of non-cognitive experience of deficit or dysfunction.[6]

If these findings presage a special brain location or state as the source of content-type specific delusions, then in the interests of the eventual unification of psychiatry and brain science, we may perhaps be expected to decide to favour a content-type classification over an epistemic one.

This is not to claim that findings in brain science will in any way alter the phenomenological or functional facts about particular delusions, or vice versa. Whatever actual correlations emerge between brain disorder and psychological dysfunction cannot be affected by matters of description. But description and classification can affect the ease and speed with which these correlations are discovered. Deficit studies, where functional deficits are correlated with an identifiable brain disorder, provide the model for such mapping between brain states and psychological states. And when deficit studies are developed to confirm the aforementioned hypotheses linking psychological dysfunction and brain disorder, they may be expected to portray the appropriate deficit in these content-based terms, as, for example, delusory ideas of persecution, or jealousy. Unless a significant body of hypotheses and or findings is to be dismissed (and certainly this approach is not without its serious critics, such as William Utall), then this is the course future study, and the eventual unification of psychiatry and neuroscience seems likely to take (Utall 2000).

A content-based analysis of persecutory paranoia

Two considerations, outlined in the previous section, invite or at least permit a content-based approach to the analysis and classification of paranoia: the first, negative (analyses based on epistemic-structural features are conceptually flawed); the second, positive (some findings in brain science have seemed to support content based categories). A definition of PP will now be attempted through appeal to the mistrustful attitudes characterizing PP subjectivity.

The separation of cognition from affection and volition, a legacy from faculty psychology, has probably contributed to the neglect of paranoid subjectivity in segregating psychic functioning. Thus, previous analyses of PP focused on its manifestation in delusions, cognitively defined, at the exclusion of its other experiential and phenomenological features. Yet what makes, and marks, PP a disorder may not be a solely cognitive failing. (A more textured analysis of the subjectivity of delusion which confirms this last point, is provided by Sass (1997).) This may be because not all delusions are usefully seen as beliefs—or because, however broadly we understand delusions, PP is better characterized by something entirely other than the delusions to which it gives rise. Either way, we need to return to the (persecutory) paranoid frame of mind and see what else, in addition to unlikely and allegedly false or irrational beliefs, resides there. To do so is to work in a more piecemeal fashion than do theorists who concern themselves with delusions in general (Maher 1988, 1992; Fulford 1989; Maher and Spitzer 1992; Gillet 1995). It is also to violate the spirit of Jaspers's stricture that the 'content' (propositional content-type) of delusions is always 'a secondary product' (Jaspers 1963, p. 96) in the sense of a response triggered by, rather than initiating, the original delusional idea. (I shall return to Jaspers's thesis at the end of this paper.) But perhaps by thus breaking away from accepted assumptions and adopting this piecemeal approach we can discover a useful criterion for defining and characterizing the particular disorder of PP in which we are interested.

In contrast to the delusions of paranoid schizophrenia, we saw earlier, the delusions of paranoid disorders are typically mood congruent as well as non-bizarre, and this mood congruence is central to the approach adopted here. By emphasizing the attitude of mistrust, with its combination of extra-cognitive and cognitive elements, the present analysis captures the integration of mood and affective states with thought content which explains the mood congruence feature of PP.

Some passages from Kraepelin's description nicely illustrate the composite set of beliefs, feelings, suspicions, doubts, and concerns, apperception and response comprising paranoid mistrust (Kraepelin 1920, pp. 225–226):

> The patient, who already for a long time has perhaps felt himself neglected, unjustly treated, oppressed, not sufficiently valued, makes the observation, that on some or other occasion people ... avoid him, and in spite of many, as he says, hypocritical proofs of friendship, will have nothing more to do with him. In consequence of this his irritability and his distrust increase; he begins to ... find numerous indications that people are systematically planning to injure him in every way, to undermine his position, to make him impossible.... He is watched and spied on, detectives are sent after him, whose duty it is to keep their eye on him and collect material against him ... Harmless remarks are full of concealed malice; ... everywhere there is hounding and backbiting, jeering and chicanery.

Rather than a narrowly a cognitive belief set, the frame of mind here portrayed must be understood as a set of attitudes.

Interestingly, some of this complexity has been identified by French nosologists, who distinguish within delusional states those that are more 'intellectual' and 'emotional' (Pichot 1990), from those that are more hypersensitive and vindictive, for example. It seems undoubtedly true that the frames of mind of those suffering persecutory paranoid disorder vary in these ways distinguished in the French taxonomy. But to continue to emphasize these contrasts is to risk missing the composite quality of the states we entitle attitudes. These particular kinds of delusions (hypersensitive, vindictive, etc.) are manifestations of what must be seen as a larger whole, the attitude itself.

Attitudes are neither solely cognitive nor solely affective or volitional. They comprise elements from each faculty, and are identifiable by the particular mix of such elements they do comprise. Attitudes are not alone in this composite nature. Judgements, arguably, are more than merely cognitive, as we saw in the earlier example of value judgements. And indeed, many insist that since emotions themselves have cognitive and volitional elements as constituents, emotions belie faculty psychological legacies, which would sharply distinguish the cognitive from the affective parts of mental life (Sartre 1962; Solomon 1976; Turski 1996). As was noted earlier, the same composite nature is to be found in the concept captured by the French term *délire* (Berrios 1995), a point concealed by the mistaken practice of translating '*délire*' into the English 'delusion' with its more cognitive or 'intellectualist' semantics, Berrios argues.

The general attitude with which we are concerned, then, is improper or injudicious interpersonal mistrust—more accurately, mistrust of persons, other animate beings, and other inanimate sources of agency. And such mistrust bears further analysis. Recent research on trust, the contrary of mistrust, allows us to draw a number of conclusions (Govier 1992, 1993a, 1993b; Baier 1994; Brothers 1995; Jones 1996; Radden 1996, 1997) First, the evaluative norm we are concerned with here is judicious or proper trust, not trust simpliciter. It is neither prudent, nor virtuous, nor mentally healthy to trust too much, or injudiciously—any more than it is to trust too little as the paranoid does. But judicious trust entails judicious or proper mistrust. Knowing when to trust is knowing when to withhold trust. Thus, strictly speaking, the evaluative norm is judicious or proper trust/mistrust.

Second, the exercise of trusting rests on a number of social and relational responses such as a degree of empathic understanding. Trust requires the social and relational capabilities of empathy and identification, which serve an epistemic role: together they yield understanding of, as a basis for prediction about, others. While necessary for any trust, these epistemic responses will also be required for the judicious trust/mistrust we value. There is also a normative structure to the exercise of trust (as of judicious trust/ mistrust). Trusting is not merely a calculated prediction about the other's behaviour; it is also something closer to a kind of faith in the other.[7]

With this clarification of the attitude of proper trust, we can turn to the lack of this attitude in persecutory paranoia. Persecutory paranoia may now be defined, negatively but more fully, as a want not only of trust but also of a set of social or relational responses, a deficiency in the social practices of empathy, identification and understanding.

'Anomalous experience' analyses and Jaspers' criteria

Many theories, including that of Jaspers, have introduced the notion that delusions are a response to some kind of anomalous, inexplicable experience (Jaspers 1963; Maher 1988, 1992; Maher and Spitzer 1992; Roberts 1992). Maher's is typical: what delusional states share in common, he hypothesizes, is likely something fairly obscure, such as being triggered by anomalous experiences, themselves arguably resulting from anomalous brain disorder.

Jaspers's version of this hypothesis will be introduced here because in developing it, Jaspers comments on analyses derived from the attitude of mistrust, such as the one introduced earlier. Whether Jaspers would rank the delusions of PP as delusions proper, or merely as delusion-like ideas, or over-valued ideas is debatable. Nonetheless, Jaspers explicitly repudiates the idea that mistrust ('distrust') is important in the delusions proper he associates with paranoid schizophrenia. So his discussion requires comment here even if it was directed at the delusions of paranoid schizophrenia rather than to PP.

Any attempt to define delusion as Jaspers puts it, 'from preceding affects, *the affect of distrust*, for instance,'(my emphasis) is, on his view, mistaken.

His reasoning is that, 'There is no clear delineation here of the specific phenomenon, the actual delusional experience; we are only offered an understandable context for the emergence of certain stubborn misconceptions'. Since the paranoid experience does not originate in the 'affect' of distrust, Jaspers is concluding here, we cannot introduce that distrust as a key to what he names the 'essential nature' of delusion (Jaspers 1963, p. 97).

Jaspers emphasizes that an initiating feeling of unease is associated with delusion formation. But Jaspers' insistence that mistrust is a mere outcome or causal product of the delusion formation fails to acknowledge the process by which paranoid delusions occur, so effectively illustrated in the passage from Kraepelin quoted above. While perhaps initiated by feelings of unease, a feedback system appears to integrate mistrustful attitudes that in turn select and highlight the connections and perceptions organized to form a coherent belief system. Rather than a separable by-product, mistrustful attitudes would stand as central constituents of this organizational achievement.

There is a limitation in these 'anomalous experience' analyses of delusion. Neither Jaspers' nor other accounts, such as Maher's, explains why delusion should rank as a disorder of, rather than a variation on, normal experience. Although the customary structural definitions of delusion portrayed as false or irrationally acquired or maintained beliefs have other difficulties, such definitions make abundantly clear why to have a delusion was to suffer a disorder, for delusions were defined as a form of cognitive incapacity or dysfunction. At least until it is possible to 'cash out' the neurological story explaining the feeling of unease, or anomalous experience posited by these kinds of theories, Jaspers's and Maher's definitions reveal no such grounding for the ascription of disorder status.

This weakness allows us to recognize a final virtue of the analysis of PP in terms of the attitude of mistrust concerns the mental health norms inherent in (warranted) psychiatric diagnosis. Analysing PP as mistrust allows us to see why it is a mental disorder rather than a variation on normal behaviour—why we judge it an illness. We suppose the mistrustful attitudes and behaviour of the person suffering PP to be undesirable features of that person's psyche and features we find abhorrent, regrettable, or in need of treatment. This seems to reveal that judicious or proper trust/mistrust functions as a mental health norm here. Not only does it under gird the classification of PP by providing some component at least of an intensional definition. It may also serve as our warrant in 'pathologizing' persecutory behaviour and response—classifying it as ill health.

Conclusion

The need for a revised definition and classification of persecutory paranoia has been illustrated here through an analysis of persecutory paranoia as a want of proper trust and mistrust. This discussion focused on the intension and not the extension of persecutory paranoia: for although persecutory paranoia is a condition readily distinguished from the other forms of psychiatric disorder, confusion surrounds the classification and definition of the category. By rejecting an epistemic-structural analysis of persecutory paranoia and focusing instead on the attitude of mistrust at the heart of paranoid subjectivity, it was shown, we resolve or avoid certain anomalies and ambiguities in the concept, such as the overly cognitive interpretation of persecutory paranoid delusion. We appear to discover a psychiatric classification more consonant with some of the findings and categories of neuroscience. We emphasize features of paranoid disorder that render it distinct from paranoid schizophrenia. And finally, in the mistrustful attitude of the person suffering persecutory paranoia we seem to gain recognition of an implicit mental health norm, which in turn accounts for the judgement that disorder status is appropriate.

Endnotes

1. Delusion-like ideas (Jaspers) and over-valued ideas (Wernicke 1900) are set in contrast to delusions proper in two respects. They are related to longer term character patterns, rather than occurring abruptly or out of the blue. And they are mono-symptomatic. True, Jaspers recognizes his distinction between delusions proper and delusion-like ideas to be a soft one, with intermediate variations, permitting us to say that the delusions we are concerned with reside between the two categories, in being abrupt rather than characterological, while yet forming a mono-symptomatic disorder.
2. 'True paranoia' was used, for example, by Robertson, the editor of an English translation of Kraepelin's Textbook in its influential 1920 eighth edition.
3. The term 'paraphrenia' has not continued to reflect Kraepelin's usage, at least in the USA. Little studied, and inconsistently used, 'paraphrenia' is sometimes applied to late onset and mild schizophrenia (Roth 1955; Berger and Zareit 1978; Davison and Neale 1986).
4. Interestingly, Freud observed this as long ago as 1922: 'The new thing I learned from studying him [the paranoid patient]' he remarks, 'was that classical persecutory-ideas may be present *without finding belief or acceptance*. They flashed up occasionally during the analysis, but he regarded them as unimportant and invariably scoffed at them' (my emphasis). This may occur in many cases of paranoia, Freud goes on, 'and it may be that the delusions which we regard as new formations when the disease breaks out have already long been in existence'(Freud 1922, p. 238).
5. In a closely argued critique of Jaspers's definition of delusion, Spitzer has introduced an additional reason to question the classification of delusions as beliefs. Patients' delusions usually have the subjective certainty of knowledge, he insists, rather than belief. And viewed objectively, the notion that delusions are beliefs has no empirical meaning, at least when they concern subjective experience (Spitzer 1990). A weakness in Spitzer's reasoning lies with its dubious assumption that

'belief' is univocal, however, a claim belied by the difference between 'I believe he was the man I saw, but I'm not certain' and 'I believe God loves us...'.

6. It is interesting to note that the term delusional disorder that came to denote the functional disorders was reserved in DSM-III for such organic conditions.

7. A fuller account of the social and relational responses necessary for trust (as for the judicious trust/mistrust we value) can be drawn from self-psychology. For Kohut, emphasis is placed on empathy or 'vicarious introspection', which is both a strictly information gathering activity, and the source of an emotional bond between people (Kohut 1971, 1977, 1984.) Sharing these Kohutian views about empathy, the psychoanalyst Doris Brothers has more recently explored the role of empathy in the development of trusting. On Kohut's and Brothers's analyses, empathy plays two roles, only the first of which is epistemic. By 'vicariously introspecting' the other's subjectivity, a person acquires the knowledge-base for her trust judgements. In addition, the knowledge (acquired by her own empathic vicarious introspection) that she is known by the other (through her empathic vicarious introspection of her), also permits her to trust the other. It is the awareness of this reciprocal empathy that allows her not only to predict the other's behaviour and reliability, but also, when that is appropriate, to experience the additional normative component of trust, the other's constancy, competence, and good will. Summing up then: these theorists illustrate the way empathic and identificatory responses are required for trusting others and serve not only to provide information about others, but also, when empathy is reciprocal, to develop identificatory emotional bonds.

Acknowledgements

For help with earlier drafts of this paper I gratefully acknowledge members of the Philosophy Department at La Trobe University; members of the Nordic Network of Philosophy and Psychiatry; the audience and fellow panelists at the Boston University Colloquium for the Philosophy of Science; members of PHAEDRA Jane Roland Martin, Susan Franzosa, Ann Diller, Barbara Houston, Janet Farrell Smith and Beatrice Kipp Nelson, Marshal Folstein, John Sadler, and Louis Sass. In addition, George Graham provided a thoughtful critique and I benefited from reading Stephens and Graham's own contribution to this volume entitled 'The delusional stance'.

References

American Psychiatric Association (1968). *Diagnostic and statistical manual of psychiatric disorders* (2nd edn). Washington DC: American Psychiatric Press.

American Psychiatric Association (1980). *Diagnostic and statistical manual of psychiatric disorder* (3rd edn). Washington DC: American Psychiatric Press.

American Psychiatric Association (1994). *Diagnostic and statistical manual of psychiatric disorder* (4th edn).Washington DC: American Psychiatric Press.

Anderson, R.A. *et al.* (1997). Multimodal representation of space in the posterior parietal cortex and its use in planning movements. *Ann. Rev. Neurosci.* **20**: 303–330.

Baier, A. (1994). *Moral prejudices: essays on ethics*. Cambridge, Mass: Harvard University Press.

Berrios, G.E. and Luque, R. (1995). Cotard's delusion or syndrome? A conceptual history. *Comprehensive Psychiatry,* **36**(3): 218–223.

Bridge, T.B. and Wyatt, R.J. (1980). Paraphrenia: paranoid states of late life. *Journal of the American Geriatrics Society,* **28**: 210–215.

Brothers, D. (1995). *Falling backwards: an exploration of trust and self-experience*. New York: W.W. Norton & Co.

Butler, R.W. and Braff, D.L. (1991). Delusions: a review and integration. *Schizophrenia Bulletin,* **17**(4): 633–647.

Cummings, J. (1985). Organic delusions: phenomenology, anatomical correlations, and review. *British Journal of Psychiatry,* **146**:184–197.

Damasio, A. (1999). *The feeling of what happens: body and emotion in the making of emotion*. San Diego: Harcourt.

Davison, G.C. and Neale, J.M. (1986). *Abnormal psychology: an experimental approach,* (4th edn). New York: John Wiley & Sons.

Feinberg, T.E. *et al.* (1992). Two alien hand syndromes. *Neurology,* **42**: 1924.

Freud, S. (1911). Psycho-analytical notes upon an autobiographical account of a case of paranoia (Dementia Paranoides). In: *The collected papers of Sigmund Freud,* vol. III (trans. A. and J. Strachey), pp. 390–470. London: The Hogarth Press.

Freud, S. (1922). Certain neurotic mechanisms in jealousy, paranoia and homosexuality. In: *The collected papers of Sigmund Freud,* vol. III (trans. A. and J. Strachey), p. 232. London: The Hogarth Press.

Frith, C.D. and Done, D.J. (1989). Experiences of alien control in schizophrenia reflect a disorder in the central monitoring of action. *Psychological Medicine,* **13**: 779–86.

Fulford, K.W.M. (1989). *Moral theory and medical practice*. Cambridge: Cambridge University Press.

Fulford, K.W.M. (1995). Thought insertion, insight and Descartes' Cogito: Linguistic analysis and the descriptive psychopathology of schizophrenic thought disorder. In: *Speech and language disorders in psychiatry* (ed. A. Sims). London: Gaskell.

Garety, P.A. and Hemsley, D.R. (1994). *Delusions: investigations into the psychology of delusional reasoning*. Oxford: Oxford University Press.

Gillett, G. (1995). Insight, delusion and belief. *Philosophy, Psychiatry and Psychology,* **1**(4): 227–236.

Govier, T. (1992). Trust, distrust and feminist theory. *Hypatia,* **7**: 1.

Govier, T. (1993a). Self-trust, autonomy, and self-esteem. *Hypatia,* **8**: 99–120.

Govier, T. (1993b). An epistemology of trust. *International Journal of Moral and Social Studies,* **8**: 155–174.

Hari, G. *et al.* (1998). Three hands: fragmentation of bodily awareness. *Neurosci. Lett.,* **240**: 131–4.

Heinroth, J.C. (1957). *A textbook of disturbances of mental life: or disturbances of the soul and their treatments* (2 vols) (trans. J. Schmorak, introduction by G. Mora). Baltimore: Johns Hopkins Press.

Hoff, P. (1995). Kraepelin. In: *A history of clinical psychiatry: the origin and history of psychiatric disorders* (ed. German Berrios and Roy Porter), pp. 261–279. New York: New York University Press.

Jackson, S. (1986). *Melancholia and depression: from Hippocratic times to modern times*. New Haven: Yale University Press.

Jaspers, C. (1963). *General psychopathology* (translated from the German Seventh Edition of 1913 by J. Hoenig and M. Hamilton). Manchester, England: Manchester University Press.

Jeannerod, M. (1997). *The cognitive neuroscience of action*. Oxford: Blackwell.

Jones, K. (1996). Trust as an affective attitude. *Ethics*, October 1996.

Joseph, A.B. (1986). Cotard's syndrome in a patient with co-existent Capgras' syndrome, syndrome of subjective doubles, and palinopsia. *Journal of Clinical Psychiatry*, **47**: 605–606.

Joseph, A.B. and O'Leary, D.H. (1986). Brain atrophy and interhemispheric fissure in Cotard's syndrome. *Journal of Clinical Psychiatry*, **47**: 518–520.

Kahlbaum, K. (1973). *Catatonia* (trans. G. Mora). Baltimore: Johns Hopkins University Press.

Kohut, H. (1971). *The analysis of the self*. New York: International Universities Press.

Kohut, H. (1977). *The restoration of the self*. New York: International Universities Press.

Kohut, H. (1984). *How does analysis cure?* Chicago: University of Chicago Press.

Kolle, K. (1932). Uber eifersucht und eifsuchtswahn bei trinkern. *Monatsschr. f. Psychiatrie u. Neurol.* **83**: 128.

Kraepelin, E. (1920). *Textbook of psychiatry* (8th edn) (trans. R. Mary Barclay) (ed. G. Robertson. Birmingham: The Classics of Medicine Library, 1989.

Kraft-Ebbing (1891). Uber eifersuchtswahn beim manne. *Jahrb.f. Psychiatrie*, **10**: 221.

Leiguarda, R. *et al.* (1993). Paroxysmal alien hand syndrome. *J. Neurol. Neurosurg. Psychiatry*, **56**: 788–92.

Maguire, E.A. (1997). The cerebral representation of space: Insights from functional imaging data. *Trends Cog.Sci.*, **1**: 62–8.

Maher, B. (1988). Anomalous experience and delusional thinking: the logic of explanations. In: *Delusional beliefs* (ed. T.F. Oltmanns and B.A. Maher). New York: Wiley-Interscience.

Maher, B. (1992). Models and methods for the study of reasoning in delusions. *Revue Europeene de Psychologie Appliquee*, 2 trimestre 1992, **42**:97–102.

Maher, B.A.. and Spitzer, M. (1992). Delusions. In: *Comprehensive handbook of psychopathology* (2nd edn) (ed. H.E. Adams and P.B. Sutker). New York: Plenum.

McCarthy, R.E. and Warrington, E.K. (1990). *Cognitive neuropsychiatry*, San Diego, CA: Academic Press.

Meissner, W.W. (1986). *Psychopathology of the paranoid process and treatment*. New York: Jason Aronson.

Moor, J.H. and Tucker, G.J. (1979). Delusions: analysis and criteria. *Comprehensive Psychiatry*, **20**, L388–93.

Mullen, P. (1979). Phenomenology of disordered mental function. In: *Essentials of post-graduate psychiatry* (ed. P. Hill, R. Murray and G. Thorley), *pp.* 25–54. London: Academic Press.

Oltmanns, T.F. (1988). Approaches to the definition and the study of delusions. In: *Delusional beliefs* (ed. T.F. Oltmanns and B.A. Maher), pp. 3–11. New York: Wiley.

Pichot, P. (1990). The diagnosis and classification of mental disorders in the French-speaking countries: background, current values and comparison with other classifications. In: *Sources and traditions of classification in psychiatry* (ed. N. Sartorius, A. Jablensky, D. Regier, J.*et al.*), *pp.* 7–57. NY: Hogrefe & Huber Publishers.

Radden, J. (1985). *Madness and reason*. London: George Allen & Unwin.

Radden, J. (1996). *Divided minds and successive selves: ethical issues in disorders of identity and personality*. Cambridge, MA: MIT Press.

Radden, J. (1998). Pathologically divided minds, synchronic unity and models of the self. *Journal of Consciousness Studies,* **5**: 658–672.

Roberts, G. (1992). The origin of delusion. *British Journal of Psychiatry,* **161**: 298–308.

Roland, P.E. (1993). *Brain activation*. New York: Wiley-Liss.

Roth, M. (1955). The natural history of mental disorder in old age. *Journal of Mental Science,* **99**: 141–50.

Sartre, J-P. (1962). *The emotions: outline of a theory* (trans. H. Barnes). Chicago: Gateway.

Sass. L. (1995). *The paradoxes of delusion*. Ithaca: Cornell University Press.

Schmiedeberg, M. (1953). Some aspects of jealousy and feeling hurt. *Psychoanalytic Review,* **1**: 1.

Siegel, R. (1994). *Whispers: the voices of paranoia*. New York: Crown Publishers, Inc.

Solomon, R. (1976). *The passions*. Notre Dame, Ind: University of Notre Dame Press.

Spence, S. *et al.* (1997). A PET study of voluntary movement in schizophrenic patients experiencing passivity phenomena (delusions of alien control). *Brain,* **120**: 1997–2011.

Spence, S. and Frith, C.D. (1999). Towards a functional anatomy of volition. *Journal of Consciousness Studies,* **6**:11–29.

Spitzer, M. (1990). On defining delusions. *Comprehensive Psychiatry,* **31**: 377–397.

Spitzer, M (1995). Conceptual development in the neurosciences relevant to psychiatry. *Current Opinion in Psychiatry,* **8**(5): 317–329.

Stephens, L. and Graham, G. (2000). *When self-consciousness breaks*. Cambridge, MA: MIT Press.

Turski, W.G. (1994). *Toward a rationality of emotions: an essay in the philosophy of mind*. Athens, Ohio: Ohio University Press.

Utall, W. (2001). *The new phrenology: the limits of localizing cognitive processes in the brain*. Cambridge, MA: MIT Press.

Vauhkonen, K. (1968). On the pathogenesis of morbid jealousy. *Acta Psychiatrica Scandinavica Supplementum,* **202**: 1968. Munksgaard. Copenhagen.

Walkup, J. (1990). On the measurement of delusions. *British Journal of Medical Psychology,* **63**: 305–8.

Wernicke, C. (1900). *Grundriss des psychiatrie*. Verlag von Georg Thieme.

Winokur, G. (1985). Familial psychopathology in delusional disorder. *Comprehensive Psychiatry,* **26**: 241–248.

World Health Organization (1992). *International classification of diseases*. Geneva: WHO.

Young, A.W., Robertson, I.H., Hellawell, D.J. *et al.* (1992). Cotard's delusion after brain injury. *Psychological Medicine,* **22**: 799–804.

14 The functions of delusional beliefs

Peter Kinderman and Richard P. Bentall

Only the paranoid survive.

(Andrew Grove, CEO of the Intel Corporation; quoted in the *New York Times*, 18 December 1994.)

Why do we believe what we believe? It is tempting to regard the investigation of delusional beliefs as significant only to psychopathologists. We shall see, however, that a proper analysis of the nature of delusions means that we need to think more generally about the nature of 'belief'.

The German philosopher and psychiatrist Karl Jaspers (1913/1963) suggested that delusions differ from normal beliefs and attitudes because they are 'ununderstandable', by which he meant they are unamenable to empathy and cannot be understood by reference to the patient's background and experience (for a detailed discussion of Jasper's position see: Walker 1991). This account, which implies a fundamental difference between normal beliefs and those of psychotic patients, has important therapeutic implications. If delusions are ununderstandable and do not emerge from the kinds of psychological processes involved in normal beliefs and attitudes, it follows that the ordinary technologies of belief manipulation (discussion, debate, and psychotherapeutic intervention) are likely to be ineffective with deluded patients, and that engaging them in mature discussion about their beliefs will be a pointless exercise.

This attitude has been implicitly embraced by many influential modern psychiatrists—for example, by Kurt Schneider, who observed that:

> Diagnosis looks to the 'How?' (form) not the 'What?' (the theme or content). When I find thought withdrawal, then this is important as a diagnostic hint, but it is not of diagnostic significance whether it is the devil, the girlfriend or a political leader who withdraws the thoughts.

Quoted in Hoenig (1982) and explicitly adopted by others, for example, by German Berrios (1991), who asserted that delusions are, 'Empty speech acts, whose informational content refers to neither world or self. They are not the symbolic expression of anything'.

One problem with Jaspers' position, of course, is that the extent to which a belief seems understandable will depend on the efforts made to understand it.

In this chapter, in contrast to the conventional psychiatric approach, we will argue that delusions have meaningful psychological content. Indeed, we will claim that they appear to be very much like many ordinary beliefs and attitudes.[1]

Are delusions beliefs?

In one of the most influential attempts to define delusions, Jaspers (1913/ 1963) argued that, in addition to being ununderstandable, they are held with extraordinary conviction, are impervious to other experiences or counter-arguments, and have bizarre or impossible content. These ideas are reflected in modern definitions; for example, that given in the fourth edition of the American Psychiatric Association's Diagnostic and Statistical Manual (DSM-IV; American Psychiatric Association 1994), where a delusion is defined as (p. 765):

> A false personal belief based on incorrect inference about external reality that is firmly sustained in spite of what almost everyone else believes and in spite of what usually constitutes incontrovertible and obvious proof or evidence to the contrary. The belief is not one ordinarily accepted by other members of the person's culture or sub-culture (e.g. It is not an article of religious faith). When a false belief involves a value judgement, it is regarded as a delusion only when the judgement is so extreme as to defy credibility. Delusional conviction occurs on a continuum and can sometimes be inferred from an individual's behaviour. It is often difficult to distinguish between a delusion and an overvalued idea (in which case the individual has an unreasonable belief or idea, but does not hold it as firmly as is the case with a delusion).

A number of commentators have expressed both logical and empirical doubts about this kind of definition (Harper 1992; Heise 1988).

Falsity

False statements about the world can be expressed without the believer being castigated as delusional. Indeed, many people express, most waking hours of their lives, beliefs that are held to be 'incorrect inferences about external reality' by many other people and yet they are not regarded as mentally ill. Examples would include not only those who hold minority political and religious beliefs, but also those who make widely disputed assertions about the present world (for example, that aliens are regularly abducting human beings for purpose of experimentation) or about the past (for example, that the Holocaust did not take place).

Ironically, perhaps, the truth of a belief is not always sufficient to ensure that it is *not* delusional. In a bizarre consequence of the twin practical needs to help distressed people and to classify psychiatric problems, delusional (or morbid) jealousy is sometimes diagnosed even if the spouse is, indeed, unfaithful (Enoch 1991; Enoch and Trethowan 1979; Soyka *et al*. 1991), so long as the patient's belief that this is the case is deemed unreasonable. This judgement might seem appropriate, for example, if the patient's constant pre-occupation with the spouse's unfaithfulness has driven the spouse into the arms of another.

To an extent, these objections are anticipated in the DSM-IV definition's caveat that relates to sub-cultural beliefs. Beliefs are only defined as delusional if other members of the sub-culture do not share them. However, far from offering a solution to the difficulty of defining delusions, this approach creates many more problems. Cross-cultural researchers have argued about the degree to which delusions vary between cultures, some noting marked differences when specific belief contents are analysed (Westermeyer 1988) and others noting similarities across cultures when general themes are examined (paranoid beliefs, for example, appear to be the most common type of delusion reported by patients in most countries; see Ndetei and Vadher 1984). However, it is often forgotten that there is at least as much cross-cultural variation in the range of beliefs that are considered *not* to be delusional.[2] Hence, over-reliance on cultural incongruence as a defining feature of delusions will raise the interesting possibility that a person could be judged mentally ill in one culture and then cease to be delusional by the simple expedient of embarking on an aeroplane journey.

A further complication is that it is easy to under-estimate the degree to which beliefs vary in their acceptability within a culture. For example, it has been estimated that about one-quarter of USA citizens believe in ghosts (Gallup and Newport 1991) and that, amazingly, several million USA citizens believe they have had personal contact with aliens (Newman and Baumeister 1996). Indeed, when epidemiologists have given psychiatric interviews to random samples of the population of Western countries, much larger proportions of the samples have turned out to be delusional than might be expected from psychiatric admission data—in a study carried out in Holland, van Os *et al*. (2000) reported that 3.3% of the general population held 'true delusions', while 8.7% reported delusions that were not associated with distress and did not require treatment. Similarly, Poulton *et al*. (2000) found 20% of a general population sample in New Zealand expressed paranoid beliefs.

Incorrect inference

Because delusions appear illogical to the observer, many authors have suggested that they result from some kind of impairment of the individual's ability to think logically or deductively. This is reflected in the DSM-IV definition's reference to beliefs that are 'based on [an] incorrect *inference* about external reality'.

This idea has a long history. For example, Bleuler (1950) argued that the disruption of normal associative links is a fundamental feature of schizophrenia and that, in the absence of coherent, logical, associations, affective influences become dominant, thereby leading to the generation of delusional ideas. Von Domarus (1944) later studied syllogistic thinking in schizophrenia patients, and suggested that they mistake similar sounding premises for premises with logical equivalence. A further development of this model was proposed by Arieti (1974), who suggested that, for people with a diagnosis of schizophrenia, an association between concepts equals a causal relationship. Modern researchers have sometimes attributed these presumed deficits in thinking to more fundamental neurological problems; for example, arguing that delusions might be the consequence of some kind of frontal lobe abnormality, leading to an inability to weigh evidence appropriately (Benson and Stuss 1991) or to utilize real world knowledge (Cutting and Murphy 1988).

In fact, however intuitively appealing this kind of theory might sound, the evidence for it is at best inconclusive. Maher (1988) famously pointed out that the studies of logical reasoning in psychotic patients have failed to find consistent evidence of abnormality, but missed the more important point that ordinary people typically perform very badly on formal logical tasks anyway (Johnson-Laird 1983). It seems that, instead, we tend to make use of mental short-cuts or 'heuristics', which lead to efficient reasoning and problem-solving in most circumstances, but irrational conclusions under some conditions (Tversky and Kahneman 1974). When the reasoning strategies of deluded patients are compared with those of ordinary people, similarities are more evident than differences. For example, deluded patients appear to test their hypotheses in the same way as other people (Bentall and Young 1996) and, when assessed for their use of heuristic strategies, perform like anyone else, with the exception that they seem to attend excessively and give more weight to threatening information (Corcoran et al. 2006). Moreover, a direct role for neurological dysfunction in delusions seems unlikely because neuropsychological functions seem to be preserved in deluded patients, and there appears to be no correlation between positive symptoms and deficits in neurocognitive test performance (Green 1998).

Of course, these observations do not necessarily mean that there is nothing unusual about the reasoning abilities of patients who are judged to be deluded. Perhaps, while remaining as logical as anyone else, they show some kind of bias in the way that they attempt to make sense of their environment. For example, a number of studies have reported evidence that patients diagnosed as deluded tended to 'jump to conclusions' when placed in a position in which they can either form a belief on the basis of uncertain information or search for new information (e.g. Garety et al. 1991; John and Dodgson 1994).

The standard paradigm for investigating this phenomenon is Garety's 'beads in a jar' task, in which experimental participants are shown two jars of, say, red and yellow beads, with the yellow beads predominant in one jar and the red beads predominant in the other. Participants are then shown a sequence of beads and, at any point in the sequence, can either decide which jar the beads have been drawn from or choose to see more beads in the sequence. Most studies have reported that deluded patients decide earlier in the sequence than ordinary people (Garety and Freeman 1999). Ironically (from the present perspective) this seems to be because ordinary people are overly cautious when judged against a mathematical model of optimum judgement in this situation (Bayes' theorem), whereas psychotic patients are not.

Firmly sustained in spite of incontrovertible and obvious proof or evidence to the contrary

Delusions are typically regarded as impervious to counter-argument. However, many widely voiced beliefs would appear to have this characteristic, whereas recent evidence has suggested that the beliefs of psychotic patients may not be as fixed as has often been thought.

The most obvious types of everyday beliefs that typically defy even the most vigorous counter-arguments are political and religious convictions.[3]

In fact, several investigators have conducted formal comparisons between deluded psychiatric patients and people with strong religious beliefs. In a famous comparison of deluded psychiatric patients, recovered patients, Anglican ordinands, and ordinary people, Glen (Roberts 1991) found that the currently deluded patients and the ordinands reported a strong need for meaning in their lives, whereas the recovered patients and the ordinary people did not. (Interestingly, in this study, the majority of the deluded patients reported that they would rather not receive evidence that their beliefs were wrong, even though the beliefs were often a source of distress). In a more recent study, Peters *et al.* (1999) compared members of New Age religions, committed Christians, people without religious convictions, and psychotic patients on measures of delusional beliefs. The members of the New Age religions could not be differentiated from psychotic patients, except on measures of distress.

The best evidence that delusions need not be completely incorrigible has emerged from trials of cognitive therapy, a type of psychological treatment that involves the use of Socratic questioning and simple experiments to help patients question the validity of their beliefs. This type of treatment has shown some success with patients suffering from quite severe psychotic conditions (Chadwick and Lowe 1990; Garety *et al.* 1994; Kuipers *et al.* 1998; Sensky *et al.* 2000; Tarrier 1997; Tarrier *et al.* 1993). Indeed the first national clinical guidance issued by NICE—the UK National Institute for Clinical Excellence (2002)—on the treatment of psychotic patients stated that; 'cognitive behavioural therapy (CBT) should be available as a treatment option for people with schizophrenia' (p. 16). The success of such psychological treatments for delusional beliefs necessarily implies that psychiatric patients' conviction in their delusional beliefs is not always absolute.

A psychological approach

Given the apparent difficulty, perhaps impossibility, of constructing a definition that satisfactorily distinguishes between delusions and other kinds of beliefs, it seems sensible to try and construct an account that subsumes them within the family of propositional attitudes. One way of beginning this task is to think of the various properties along which beliefs in general seem to vary. In fact, phenomenological studies show that both delusional and ordinary beliefs can be classified along a number of continua; for example, their bizarreness to others, the conviction with which they are held, and the extent to which the individual is preoccupied or distressed by them (Garety and Hemsley 1987; Kendler *et al.* 1983). Of course, as we have already seen, we should not assume that delusions are the only beliefs that occupy extreme positions along these dimensions. Many religious and political convictions appear to be bizarre to others, are held with great conviction, pre-occupy the believer and may even be the source of considerable distress (think of those intensely religious people who believe that their chances of entering heaven are slim, and that they must spend large portions of the day in prayer or acts of atonement).

This dimensional approach has some pretty clear advantages over the conventional psychiatric approach that preceded it: it brings delusions back into the realm of psychological inquiry; it also allows us to accommodate the fact that large numbers of the population hold beliefs that are held to be 'crazy' by the majority, or even delusional by psychiatric experts; and it nonetheless enables us to ask whether these people have psychological characteristics that make them different from everyone else.

Two clues will help us to begin to address the last of these questions. First, it is fairly obvious that extreme and unusual beliefs of any kind, whether or not they are regarded as delusional, are associated with strong emotions. Efforts to challenge political or religious beliefs typically evoke discomfort, even anger, in the recipient of these efforts. There is evidence that the positive symptoms of psychosis, in general, are associated with high levels of affect (Norman and Malla 1991) and that delusional thinking specifically is associated with the experience of negative emotion (Myin-Germeys *et al.* 2001). Second, it is equally obvious that the most common delusional themes reported by psychiatric patients (persecution, grandiosity, or guilt) seem to reflect an intense pre-occupation with the individual's position in the social universe (Bentall 1994).

Putting together these observations, it seems reasonable to hypothesize that the holding of delusional beliefs is intimately related to the process of self-evaluation. Paranoid beliefs, which we will now consider in some detail, seem to exemplify this principle.

The paranoid worldview

As noted earlier, paranoid or persecutory beliefs appear to be the most common type of delusion reported by psychiatric patients in many different regions of the world (Garety *et al.* 1988; Jorgensen and Jensen 1994; Ndetei and Vadher 1984). Typically, patients who are diagnosed as suffering from this kind of delusion say that they are the target of some kind of organized conspiracy to cause them harm, although patients vary in the agencies to who they attribute this intention (which may be specific persons, religious or ethnic groups, or organizations such as the CIA. or MI5). It is also worth noting that psychiatric patients are by no means the only people to hold these kinds of beliefs, and that conspiracy theories are widely held within the general population (for example, about who really shot John Kennedy, whether or not the US government is covering up evidence of extraterrestrial life, or why Britain went to war with Iraq).

Trower and Chadwick (1995) have argued that paranoid delusions can be divided into two main types. According to their theory, 'poor-me' paranoia is said to be experienced when the individual feels unjustly persecuted by others, and 'bad-me' paranoia is experienced when the individual believes persecution is deserved. Trower and Chadwick argue that the former type of delusion is associated with normal or high self-esteem, whereas the latter type is associated with low self-esteem. However, the validity of this distinction has been drawn into question by a recent study which found that most paranoid patients experience 'poor-me' paranoia, and that some patients fluctuate in their conviction that they deserve to be persecuted, believing themselves to be unjustly persecuted on some occasions and deserving persecution on others (Melo *et al.*, 2006).

Social cognition and paranoid delusions

Psychologists' attempts to understand paranoia have mostly focused on the question of whether patients with severe paranoid delusions have any peculiar cognitive characteristics that might be plausibly linked to their beliefs. As described earlier, there is some evidence that deluded patients in general, in comparison with people with less colourful beliefs, have a tendency to jump to conclusions when formulating theories on the basis of sequentially presented information. However, the psychological process that has been most thoroughly investigated with respect to paranoid delusions is 'attribution'.

Social psychologists use the term 'attribution' to refer to a statement of causality (a statement that either contains or implies the word 'because'). People generate an extraordinary number of attributions in their daily lives—it has been estimated that an attribution can be found in every hundred or so words of ordinary speech (Zullow *et al.* 1988). Not surprisingly, clinical psychologists have wondered whether different styles of generating attributions might be linked to different kinds of mental health problems.

Abramson *et al.* (1978) famously suggested that depression arises from making pessimistic attributions for negative events. Using a three-dimensional typology of attributions, they suggested that a vulnerability to depression was associated with a tendency to make attributions for negative events that were internal (to do with the self, as opposed to external attributions, which are to do with other people or circumstances), stable (unchangeable, as opposed to unstable) and global (likely to affect all areas of life, as opposed to specific). For example, a student failing an exam would be likely to become depressed if he or she attributed this failure to low intelligence, as this is an internal cause, which is also stable (a person who lacks intelligence today is likely to lack intelligence in ten year's time) and global (low intelligence is likely to affect a wide range of life activities). A very large body of empirical research using a variety of methods, but most commonly by asking people to complete questionnaires such as (Peterson *et al.* 1982) Attributional Style Questionnaire (ASQ) have reported this style of generating attributions in people who are depressed (Sweeny *et al.* 1986). However, note that, according to the most common formulation of the attributional theory of depression, a pessimistic attributional style is viewed as a trait that is relatively fixed and that precedes the onset of depression. In fact, the evidence from prospective studies that a pessimistic style precedes (rather than accompanies) the onset of depression is rather mixed (Alloy *et al.* 1999; Robins and Hayes 1995).

The first study of attributional style in paranoid patients using the ASQ was reported by Kaney and Bentall (1989), and found that, like depressed patients, they had a tendency to attribute negative events to causes that are stable and global. However, in contrast with depressed patients, their explanations for negative events also tend to be highly external, a finding that has now been replicated many times (Candido and Romney 1990; Fear *et al.* 1996; Lee 2000).

Using a slightly different approach, Kaney and Bentall (1992) experimentally engineered experiences of success and failure to see what kinds of attributions depressed and paranoid patients would make afterwards. They required participants to make repeated forced-choices on two computer games, which were rigged, one so that the participants would think that they had done well and the other so that they would think they had done badly. Depressed patients believed that they had little control over either of the games—they were sadder but wiser. Non-patient controls claimed greater control following the 'win' game than the 'lose' game, and this bias was significantly greater for paranoid patients.

More recently Lee *et al.* (2006) asked paranoid patients to talk about good and bad things that had happened in their lives, and analysed their speech for attributions. In this study, paranoid patients made many more external attributions for negative events than the controls.

As ordinary people tend to make more internal attributions for positive events than for negative events (Campbell and Sedikides 1999), it seems reasonable to view the pattern of attributions observed in paranoid patients as an exaggeration of the normal 'self-serving bias'. However, paranoid patients differ from ordinary people not only in the degree to which they avoid attributing negative events to themselves, but also in the kinds of external attributions made for those events. Whereas ordinary people often resort to situational explanations in these circumstances ('I'm sorry I'm late but the traffic was dreadful'), patients usually attribute unpleasant experiences specifically to the intended actions of others (Kinderman and Bentall 1997) ('I'm sorry I'm late but the police deliberately set the traffic lights to red in order to stop me from getting here on time').

It is easy to see how this style of explaining events might be linked to the paranoid worldview. If a person experiences a series of negative, uncontrollable events in their life, and repeatedly attributes those events to the intentions of other persons, they are likely to develop ever more elaborate conspiracy theories to account for their misfortunes. However, it is less obvious how an individual might acquire this attributional style in the first place. In fact, several different processes may play a role.

Self-esteem and attributional style in paranoia

There is compelling evidence from a wide range of studies that the self-serving bias in ordinary people serves the function of maintaining self-esteem in the face of adversity (Campbell and Sedikides 1999). By assuming that the cause of an unpleasant event is external to the self ('I failed the exam because I was badly affected by other stressors in my life') we minimize the extent to which we feel bad about ourselves when something goes wrong. On this view, it seems reasonable to hypothesize that the exaggerated self-serving bias observed in paranoid patients results from over-vigorous attempts to preserve self-esteem. Although this idea has guided much of our own research (Bentall et al. 1994), it is not original to us: similar accounts of paranoia have been proposed on the basis of clinical experience by a number of previous writers, some of whom were clearly influenced by psychoanalysis (Colby 1977; Zigler and Glick 1988).

It is fair to say that some other researchers have viewed this idea as controversial. For example, Freeman et al. (1998) have objected that the theory predicts that self-esteem should be high in paranoid patients (because they are vigorously defending themselves from feelings of low self-esteem) when, according to them, it is more often low. In fact, the evidence on self-esteem in paranoia is contradictory. Candido and Romney (1990), for example, have reported that self-esteem is low in depressed patients (as everyone knows), high in paranoid patients who are not depressed, and intermediate in paranoid patients who are depressed. It might be argued that these findings are consistent with Trower and Chadwick's (1995) theory that there are two types of paranoia, one associated with high self-esteem and one associated with low self-esteem. However, even this may be an over-simplification because, as we have already seen, some patients fluctuate between 'poor-me' and 'bad-me' paranoid beliefs (Melo *et al.* 2006).

We have recently argued that all of these observations can be accommodated within a dynamic model that attempts to explain how paranoid thinking changes over time (Bentall *et al.* 2001). As we have seen, it is widely recognized that the kind of attributions that people make has an impact on how they feel about themselves; for example, that on blaming ourselves for something that goes wrong we feel bad. However, there is also compelling evidence that how we feel about ourselves influences the kinds of attributions we are likely to make (for example, when we are especially likely to attribute exam failure to ourselves if we lack confidence in our abilities). Attributions and beliefs about the self therefore seem to influence each other in a complex way. Furthermore, the kind of attribution we choose to make on any particular occasion will depend on a number of circumstantial factors; for example, the nature of the event that requires an explanation and whether or not anyone else is involved. In this kind of dynamic system, it might be expected that the paranoid patient's efforts to find an external cause for negative events will lead to fluctuations in self-esteem, rather than self-esteem that is either consistently high or consistently low (for a full exposition of this model and some of the experimental evidence that supports it, see: Bentall *et al.* 2001).

Overall, then, the available evidence available is consistent with the idea that paranoid beliefs arise partly as a consequence of excessive efforts to maintain a positive view of the self. However, this does not seem to be the whole story.

Cognitive deficits and attributional style in paranoia

Whereas the idea that paranoid patients are struggling to maintain a fragile self-esteem helps to explain their tendency to make external attributions, it does not explain why their external attributions specifically implicate other people.

This tendency may be related to a problem with mentalizing or 'theory of mind' (ToM; a not very helpful term employed by psychologists to describe the ability to infer the beliefs, attitudes, and intentions of other people). Frith (1994) has argued that problems with ToM may be implicated in a wide range of psychotic symptoms, especially persecutory delusions. According to this theory, patients misattribute malevolent intentions to others because they cannot read minds. In fact, there is considerable evidence that people with psychotic symptoms, when acutely ill, perform poorly on ToM tasks (Corcoran 2000; Corcoran *et al.* 1997), although whether this type of deficit is specifically related to paranoid symptoms remains doubtful (Drury *et al.* 1998; Sarfati *et al.* 1997).

One possibility is that ToM deficits affect the kinds of attributions that people make. When confronted by a person who treats us with unexpected rudeness, our first instinct is often to assume that they do so because they are preoccupied with their own problems or labouring under some kind of stress, and, of course, in order to make this assumption we have to temporarily mentally simulate the other person's point of view. For this reason, we might be more prone to attribute malevolent intentions to others when our ToM faculties are temporarily impaired. Consistent with this idea, in a study of healthy university students, we found a strong association between poor performance on a ToM task and a tendency to make paranoid attributions (Kinderman et al. 1998).

Clearly, impaired ToM is not sufficient to cause paranoid thinking. If this were the case, patients with autism and Asperger's syndrome (a relatively mild autistic spectrum disorder), who have marked ToM deficits, would be indistinguishable from paranoid patients. In fact, paranoid and Asperger's patients seem to perform similarly poorly on ToM tasks, but the Asperger's patients do not exhibit the attributional biases typically seen in paranoid patients (Blackshaw et al. 2001; Craig et al. 2004). This evidence therefore suggests that both attributional biases and ToM deficits contribute to paranoid thinking.

Attention to threat

A final psychological process that we will consider here is attention to threat. There is good evidence, collected using a wide range of methods, that paranoid patients selectively attend to information related to their beliefs. For example, if asked to name the print colours of words written in multiple colours (a method of testing known as the emotional Stroop technique), paranoid patients, compared to other groups, are slow at colour-naming words relating to threat (Bentall and Kaney 1989) or low self-esteem (Kinderman 1994) (this effect is caused by their difficulty in ignoring the meaning of the words). When given memory tests, paranoid patients also excessively recall threat-related information (Bentall et al. 1995; Kaney et al. 1992). Assessment of patients' eye movements suggests that they home in quickly on this kind of information, and then rapidly divert their gaze elsewhere, perhaps because they are on alert for further threats elsewhere (Phillips and David 1997a, 1997b). Interestingly, these kinds of biases result in paranoid patients being better at detecting some kinds of information than ordinary people. For example, paranoid patients seem to be very sensitive to negative facial expressions in other people (Davis and Gibson 2000; LaRusso 1978).

It makes sense for people who are surrounded by threats to become gradually more hyper-vigilant for threat-related information. After all, early detection of threat will enable them to take action to ensure their own safety. Unfortunately, this kind of bias in processing information will tend to lead to the maintenance of paranoid beliefs once established (Morrison 1998). By noticing only information that supports their beliefs, and by avoiding situations associated with threat (and hence the opportunity to discover that their beliefs are not realised) the paranoid patient has very little chance of developing an optimistic understanding of other people's intentions.

The social origins of the paranoia

The account we have given so far gives some indication of the breadth of psychological research that has been carried out into paranoid thinking over the last couple of decades. It has not been exhaustive; in order to keep the story as simple as possible we have focused only on those research findings which, to our minds, seem most important. The overall impression that emerges from this research is that paranoid delusions are far from ununderstandable. Although there are psychological differences between paranoid patients and ordinary people, these differences, in fact, make delusions all the more intelligible. The paranoid worldview becomes easier to understand once we realise that paranoid interpretations of events are fuelled by fragile self-esteem, that the paranoid patient has some difficulty understanding how other people think, and that he or she notices threats that other people would be oblivious to.

Of course, the identification of cognitive peculiarities in patients who harbour theories about malevolent conspiracies against them is only the starting point of the attempt to explain how these beliefs come about. In order to adequately account for these beliefs, it is necessary to trace their origins during the development of the individual. Very little research has addressed this issue, but there are some intriguing clues in the available literature.

Since the work of John Bowlby (1969), it has become widely recognized that early attachment relations can profoundly affect individuals' feelings about themselves and their capacity to form trusting relationships with others in adulthood. Developmental psychologists have recently demonstrated that early disruptions of attachment relations can impair the development of ToM skills in children (Meins *et al.* 1998; Meins *et al.* 2001), an observation that is of great interest to the psychopathologist because, as we have seen, ToM skills seem to be impaired in psychotic adults. In fact, studies of both clinical (Dozier *et al.* 1991) and general population samples (Cooper *et al.* 1998; Mickelson *et al.* 1997) show a relationship between paranoid symptoms and insecure, and especially dismissive-avoidant attachment styles. Perhaps this association should not be surprising; after all, the emotional theme underlying the dismissing-avoidant style is mistrust.

There is also some evidence to suggest that paranoid beliefs often arise in a context of actual victimization. When, in 1973, Henry Kissinger commented to Golda Meir (the Israeli Prime Minister) that the Israelis were paranoid about the Arabs, she famously retorted that, 'Even paranoids have enemies' (Schneider 1998). In a survey of the residents of Jaurez in Mexico and El-Passo in the USA, sociologists Mirowsky and Ross (1983) found that paranoid beliefs were associated with social circumstances that they characterized as leading to feelings of victimization and powerlessness. Fuchs (1999) found that elderly patients with paranoia were more likely than others to report discriminating, humiliating, and threatening experiences in earlier life. In a large-scale epidemiological study, Janssen et al. (2003) found that reports of discrimination predicted the future development of paranoid symptoms. More generally, these is some evidence that the onset of positive symptoms of psychosis often follows 'intrusive' life events in which some other person tries to exercise a high degree of control over the sufferer (Day et al. 1987; Harris 1987).

The cognitive biases exhibited by paranoid patients become quite easy to understand in the context of these findings. In particular, the assumption that negative experiences are caused by others and the paranoid patient's attention to threat-related information seem reasonable responses to a life in which other people cannot be trusted and threats are often experienced.

Delusions and the nature of belief

To briefly conclude this chapter, it will be useful to consider the evidence we have just outlined in the context of our earlier examination of attempts to define delusional beliefs. It will be recalled that we argued that no satisfactory distinction could be drawn between delusions and other kinds of strongly held beliefs and attitudes. We also suggested that the strong emotional investment that people have in delusions and other strongly held beliefs might reflect, in some way, the role that these beliefs play in their evaluation of themselves. This certainly seems to be true of political and religious beliefs, which are often incorporated into individuals' definitions of themselves (as in, 'I am a Marxist' or 'I am a Christian'). It also seems to be true of paranoid beliefs. Although other common kinds of delusional systems have not been thoroughly investigated we suspect that this principle will extend to them also. This is perhaps obvious in the case of grandiose beliefs, in which the individual claims impossible identity ('I am the son of God'), talents or riches. However, it may be equally true of less common delusions, for example the erotomanic patient's conviction that he or she is loved by someone important and famous (we may judge ourselves partly according to the mate we believe we are able to attract).

Of course, self-definition, although an important function of belief systems, is not the only function. Presumably, the human capacity for generating prepositional descriptions of the world evolved because it allows us to predict events in our environment, make preparations accordingly, and regulate our response to them. This is why human beings have developed efficient but non-logical strategies for inferring what is going on around them (the 'heuristics') and build their theories of the world on the basis of experience. Again, the paranoid patient does not appear to be noticeably different from anyone else in any of these respects. Whether this is so in the case of other delusional systems is less obvious. It is difficult to think of circumstances that would feed grandiose patients' beliefs about themselves, for example. Perhaps in these cases, the quest for an emotionally acceptable self-definition outweighs the other functions that belief systems are ordinarily required to perform.

Even if this last speculation turns out to be true, the overall impression that emerges from psychological research into psychosis is that deluded patients belong to the same species as everyone else. They are more like the rest of us than different and belong to the same social world. By denying that delusions are beliefs, the conventional psychiatric approach treats patients with disrespect, and often denies them a voice in determining their own treatment (Bentall 2003). The clinical implications of the account we have offered of delusions are beyond the scope is this chapter; suffice it to say that we believe it is possibly to work with patients in a way that respects their theories and treats these theories as perhaps unlikely but just possibly true. By working with patients in this way, it is possible to engage them in a quest to discover the advantages and disadvantages of their way of thinking, and to encourage them to consider alternative beliefs systems. This approach lies at the core of the new cognitive behavioural treatments of psychosis (Morrison *et al.* 2003).

Endnotes

1. During the course of this discussion the term 'delusion' should be read as shorthand for 'a belief that would be considered delusional by a conventionally-trained psychiatrist' and the term 'deluded patient' as shorthand for 'a person in receipt of psychiatric treatment whose beliefs are regarded as delusional by a conventionally trained psychiatrist'.
2. What is the Western-trained psychiatrist to make of the Fataleka of the Solomon Islands, who maintain that the Earth occupies the fifth of nine parallel strata, that reflections are in stratum three, flutes are in stratum four, crocodiles are in stratum seven, and stratum eight is empty? See Sperber 1982.)
3. Readers may find it useful to count instances in which they have engaged in heartfelt political debate with individuals with opposing political viewpoints, and recall whether on any of these occasions they managed to change the opponents' views.

References

Abramson, L.Y., Seligman, M.E.P., and Teasdale, J.D. (1978). Learned helplessness in humans: critique and reformulation. *Journal of Abnormal Psychology*, **78**: 40–74.

Alloy, L.B., Abramson, L.Y., Whitehouse, W.G., Hogan, M.E., Tashman, N.A., Steinberg, D.L. *et al.* (1999). Depressogenic cognitive styles: predictive validity, information processing and personality characteristics, and developmental origins. *Behaviour Research and Therapy*, **37**: 503–531.

American Psychiatric Association (1994). *Diagnostic and statistical manual for mental disorders* (4th edn). Washington DC: Author.

Arieti, S. (1974). *Interpretation of schizophrenia*. London: Crosby Lockwood Staples.

Benson, D.F. and Stuss, D.T. (1991). Frontal lobe influences on delusions: a clinical perspective. *Schizophrenia Bulletin,* **16**: 403–411.

Bentall, R.P. (1994). Cognitive biases and abnormal beliefs: towards a model of persecutory delusions. In: *The neuropsychology of schizophrenia* (ed. A.S. David and J.Cutting), pp. 337–360. London: Lawrence Erlbaum.

Bentall, R.P. (2003). *Madness explained: psychosis and human nature*. London: Penguin.

Bentall, R.P. and Kaney, S. (1989). Content-specific information processing and persecutory delusions: An investigation using the emotional Stroop test. *British Journal of Medical Psychology*, **62**: 355–364.

Bentall, R.P. and Young, H.F. (1996). Sensible-hypothesis-testing in deluded, depressed and normal subjects. *British Journal of Psychiatry*, **168**: 372–375.

Bentall, R.P., Kinderman, P., and Kaney, S. (1994). The self, attributional processes and abnormal beliefs: towards a model of persecutory delusions. *Behaviour Research and Therapy,* **32**: 331–341.

Bentall, R.P., Kaney, S., and Bowen-Jones, K. (1995). Persecutory delusions and recall of threat-related, depression-related and neutral words. *Cognitive Therapy and Research*, **19**: 331–343.

Bentall, R.P., Corcoran, R., Howard, R., Blackwood, R., and Kinderman, P. (2001). Persecutory delusions: a review and theoretical integration. *Clinical Psychology Review,* **21**: 1143–1192.

Berrios, G. (1991). Delusions as 'wrong beliefs': a conceptual history. *British Journal of Psychiatry,* **159**(Supplement 14): 6–13.

Blackshaw, A.J., Kinderman, P., Hare, D., and Hatton, C. (2001). Theory-of-mind, causal attributions and paranoia in Asperger's syndrome. *Autism*, **52**: 147–163.

Bleuler, E. (1950). *Dementia praecox or the group of schizophrenias* (originally published 1911, trans. Zinkin E.). New York: International Universities Press.

Bowlby, J. (1969). *Attachment and loss: vol 1—attachment*. London: Hogarth Press.

Campbell, W.K. and Sedikides, C. (1999). Self-threat magnifies the self-serving bias: a meta-analytic integration. *Review of General Psychology*, **3**: 23–43.

Candido, C.L. and Romney, D.M. (1990). Attributional style in paranoid vs depressed patients. *British Journal of Medical Psychology*, **63**:355–363.

Chadwick, P. and Lowe, C.F. (1990). The measurement and modification of delusional beliefs. *Journal of Consulting and Clinical Psychology*, **58**: 225–232.

Colby, K.M. (1977). Appraisal of four psychological theories of paranoid phenomena. *Journal of Abnormal Psychology*, **86**: 54–59.

Cooper, M.L., Shaver, P.R., and Collins, N.L. (1998). Attachment style, emotion regulation, and adjustment in adolescence. *Journal of Personality and Social Psychology*, **74**: 1380–1397.

Corcoran, R. (2000). Theory of mind in other clinical samples: Is a selective 'theory of mind' deficit exclusive to schizophrenia. In *Understanding other minds:*

perspectives from developmental neuroscience (2nd edn) (ed. S. Baron-Cohen, H. Tager-Flusberg, and D. Cohen). Oxford: Oxford University Press.

Corcoran, R., Cahill, C., and Frith, C.D. (1997). The appreciation of visual jokes in people with schizophrenia: a study of 'mentalizing' ability. *Schizophrenia Research*, **24**: 319–327.

Corcoran, R., Cummins, S., Moore, R., Rowse, G., Bedford, N., Blackwood, N. *et al.* (2006). Reasoning under uncertainty: heuristic judgements in patients with persecutory delusions and patients with depression. *Psychological Medicine*, **36**, 1109–1118.

Craig, J., Craig, F., Hatton, C., and Bentall, R.P. (2004). Theory of mind and attributions in persecutory delusions and Asperger's syndrome. *Schizophrenia Research*, **69**: 29–33.

Cutting, J., and Murphy, D. (1988). Schizophrenic thought disorder: psychological and organic perspective. *British Journal of Psychiatry*, **152**: 310–319.

Davis, P.J. and Gibson, M.G. (2000). Recognition of posed and genuine facial expressions of emotion in paranoid and nonparanoid schizophrenia. *Journal of Abormal Psychology*, **109**: 445–450.

Day, R., Neilsen, J.A., Korten, A., Ernberg, G., Dube, K.C., Gebhart, *J. et al.* (1987). Stressful life events preceding the onset of acute schizophrenia: a cross-national study from the World Health Organization. *Culture, Medicine and Psychiatry*, **11**: 123–206.

Dozier, M., Stevenson, A.L., Lee, S.W., and Velligan, D.I. (1991). Attachment organization and familiar overinvolvement for adults with serious psychopathological disorders. *Development and Psychopathology*, **3**: 475–489.

Drury, V.M., Robinson, E.J., and Birchwood, M. (1998). 'Theory of mind' skills during an acute episode of psychosis and following recovery. *Psychological Medicine*, **28**: 1101–1112.

Enoch, D. (1991). Delusional jealousy and awareness of reality. *British Journal of Psychiatry*, **159** (Supplement 14): 52–56.

Enoch, M.D. and Trethowan, W.H. (1979). *Uncommon psychiatric syndromes* (2nd edn). Bristol: Wright.

Fear, C.F., Sharp, H., and Healy, D. (1996). Cognitive processes in delusional disorder. *British Journal of Psychiatry*, **168**: 61–67.

Freeman, D., Garety, P., Fowler, D., Kuipers, E., Dunn, G., Bebbington, P. *et al.* (1998). The London-East Anglia randomized controlled trial of cognitive-behaviour therapy for psychosis IV: self-esteem and persecutory delusions. *British Journal of Clinical Psychology*, **37**: 415–430.

Frith, C. (1994). Theory of mind in schizophrenia. In: *The neuropsychology of schizophrenia* (ed. A.S. David and J.C. Cutting), (pp. 147–161). Hove: Erlbaum.

Fuchs, T. (1999). Life events in late paraphrenia and depression. *Psychopathology*, **32**: 60–69.

Gallup, G.H. and Newport, F. (1991). Belief in paranormal phenomena among adult Americans. *Skeptical Inquirer*, **15**: 137–146.

Garety, P. and Freeman, D. (1999). Cognitive approaches to delusions: a critical review of theories and evidence. *British Journal of Clinical Psychology*.

Garety, P.A. and Hemsley, D.R. (1987). The characteristics of delusional experience. *European Archives of Psychiatry and Neurological Sciences*, **236**: 294–298.

Garety, P.A., Everitt, B.S., and Hemsley, D.R. (1988). The characteristics of delusions: a cluster analysis of deluded subjects. *European Archives of Psychiatry and Neurological Sciences,* **237**: 112–114.

Garety, P.A., Hemsley, D.R., and Wessely, S. (1991). Reasoning in deluded schizophrenic and paranoid patients. *Journal of Nervous and Mental Disease,* **179**(4): 194–201.

Garety, P.A., Kuipers, L., Fowler, D., Chamberlain, F., and Dunn, G. (1994). Cognitive behavioural therapy for drug-resistant psychosis. *British Journal of Medical Psychology,* **67**: 259–271.

Green, M.F. (1998). *Schizophrenia from a neurocognitive perspective: probing the impenetrable darkness.* Boston: Allyn and Bacon.

Harper, D.J. (1992). Defining delusions and the serving of professional interests: the case of 'paranoia'. *British Journal of Medical Psychology,* **65**: 357–369.

Harris, T. (1987). Recent developments in the study of life events in relation to psychiatric and physical disorders. In: *Psychiatric epidemiology: progress and prospects* (ed. B. Cooper), pp.81–102. London: Croom Helm.

Heise, D.R. (1988). Delusions and the construction of reality. In: *Delusional beliefs* (ed. T.F. Oltmanns and B.A. Maher), pp.259–272. New York: Wiley.

Hoenig, J. (1982). Kurt Schneider and anglophone psychiatry. *Comprehensive Psychiatry,* **23**: 391–400.

Janssen, I., Hanssen, M., Bak, M., Bijl, R.V., De Graaf, R., Vollenberg, W. *et al.* (2003). Discrimination and delusional ideation. *British Journal of Psychiatry,* **182**: 71–76.

Jaspers, K. (1913/1963). *General psychopathology* (trans. J. Hoenig and M.W. Hamilton). Manchester: Manchester University Press.

John, C.H., and Dodgson, G. (1994). Inductive reasoning in delusional thought. *Journal of Mental Health,* **3**: 31–49.

Johnson Laird, P.N. (1983) *Mental models,* Cambridge: Cambridge University Press.

Jorgensen, P., and Jensen, J. (1994). Delusional beliefs in first admitters. *Psychopathology,* **27**: 100–112.

Kaney, S. and Bentall, R.P. (1989). Persecutory delusions and attributional style. *British Journal of Medical Psychology,* **62:** 191–198.

Kaney, S. and Bentall, R.P. (1992). Persecutory delusions and the self-serving bias. *Journal of Nervous and Mental Disease,* **180**: 773–780.

Kaney, S., Wolfenden, M., Dewey, M.E., and Bentall, R.P. (1992). Persecutory delusions and the recall of threatening and non-threatening propositions. *British Journal of Clinical Psychology,* **31**: 85–87.

Kendler, K.S., Glazer, W., and Morgenstern, H. (1983). Dimensions of delusional experience. *American Journal of Psychiatry,* **140**: 466–469.

Kinderman, P. (1994). Attentional bias, persecutory delusions and the self concept. *British Journal of Medical Psychology,* **67**: 53–66.

Kinderman, P. and Bentall, R.P. (1997). Causal attributions in paranoia: Internal, personal and situational attributions for negative events. *Journal of Abnormal Psychology,* **106**: 341–345.

Kinderman, P., Dunbar, R.I.M., and Bentall, R.P. (1998). Theory of mind deficits and causal attributions. *British Journal of Psychology,* **71**: 339–349.

Kuipers, E., Fowler, D., Garety, P., Chizholm, D., Freeman, D., Dunn, G. *et al.* (1998). London-East Anglia randomised controlled trial of cognitive-behavioural therapy for psychosis III: follow-up and economic considerations. *British Journal of Psychiatry*, **173**: 61–68.

LaRusso, L. (1978). Sensitivity of paranoid patients to nonverbal cues. *Journal of Abnormal Psychology*, **87**: 463–471.

Lee, D., Randall, F., Beattie, G., and Bentall, R.P. (2006). Delusional discourse: an investigation comparing the spontaneous causal attributions of paranoid and non-paranoid individuals. *Psychology and Psychotherapy—Theory, Research, Practice*.

Lee, H.J. (2000). Attentional bias, memory bias and the self-concept in paranoia. *Psychological Science*, **9**: 77–99.

Maher, B.A. (1988). Anomalous experience and delusional thinking: the logic of explanations. In: *Delusional beliefs* (ed. T.F. Oltmanns and B.A. Maher), pp.15–33. New York: Wiley.

Meins, E., Fernyhough, C., Russell, J.A., and Clark-Carter, D. (1998). Security of attachment as a predictor of symbolic and mentalising abilities: a longitudinal study. *Social Development*, **7**: 1–24.

Meins, E., Fernyhough, C., Fradley, E., and Tuckey, M. (2001). Rethinking maternal sensitivity: Mothers' comments on infants mental processes predict security of attachment at 12 months. *Journal of Child Psychology and Psychiatry*, **42**: 637–648.

Melo, S., Taylor, J., and Bentall, R.P. (2006). 'Poor me' versus 'bad me, paranoia and the instability of persecutory ideation. *Psychology and Psychotherapy—Theory, Research, Practice*. **79**, 271–287.

Mickelson, K.D., Kessler, R.C., and Shaver, P.R. (1997). Adult attachment in a nationally representative sample. *Journal of Personality and Social Psychology*, **73**: 1092–1106.

Mirowsky, J. and Ross, C.E. (1983). Paranoia and the structure of powerlessness. *American Sociological Review*, **48**: 228–239.

Morrison, A.P. (1998). Cognitive behaviour therapy for psychotic symptoms of schizophrenia. In: *Treating complex cases: the cognitive behavioural therapy approach* (ed. N. Tarrier, A. Wells and G. Haddock), pp. 195–216. London: Wiley.

Morrison, A.P., Renton, J.C., Dunn, H., Williams, S., and Bentall, R.P. (2003). *Cognitive therapy for psychosis: a formulation-based approach*. London: Brunner-Routledge.

Myin-Germeys, I., Nicolson, N.A., and Delespaul, P.A.E.G. (2001). The context of delusional experiences in the daily life of patients with schizophrenia. *Psychological Medicine*, **31**: 489–498.

Ndetei, D.M. and Vadher, A. (1984). Frequency and clinical significance of delusions across cultures. *Acta Psychiatrica Scandinavica*, **70**: 73–76.

Newman, L.S. and Baumeister, R.F. (1996). Towards an explanation of the UFO abduction phenomenon: hypnotic elabouration, extraterrestrial sadomasochism, and spurious memories. *Psychological Inquiry*, **7**: 99–126.

Norman, R.M.G. and Malla, A.K. (1991). Dysphoric mood and symptomatology in schizophrenia. *Psychological Medicine*, **21**: 897–203.

Peters, E., Day, S., McKenna, J., and Orbach, G. (1999). Delusional ideation in religious and psychotic populations. *British Journal of Clinical Psychology*, **38**: 83–96.

Peterson, C., Semmel, A., Von Baeyer, C., Abramson, L., Metalsky, G. I., and Seligman, M.E.P. (1982). The Attributional Style Questionnaire. *Cognitive Therapy and Research*, **3**: 287–300.

Phillips, M. and David, A.S. (1997a). Abnormal visual scan paths: a psychophysiological marker of delusions in schizophrenia. *Schizophrenia Research*, **29**: 235–254.

Phillips, M. and David, A.S. (1997b). Visual scan paths are abnormal in deluded schizophrenics. *Neuropsychologia*, **35**: 99–105.

Poulton, R., Caspi, A., Moffitt, T.E., Cannon, M., Murray, R., and Harrington, H. (2000). Children's self-reported psychotic symptoms and adult schizophreniform disorder: a 15-year longitudinal study. *Archives of General Psychiatry*, **57**: 1053–1058.

Roberts, G. (1991). Delusional belief systems and meaning in life: a preferred reality? *British Journal of Psychiatry*, **159** (Supplement 14): 19–28.

Robins, C.J. and Hayes, A.H. (1995). The role of causal attributions in the prediction of depression. In: *Explanatory style* (ed. G.M. Buchanan and M.E.P. Seligman), pp. 71–98. Hillsdale, New Jersey: Lawrence Erlbaum.

Sarfati, Y.H.B., Nadel, J., Chavalier, J.F., and Widlocher, D. (1997). Attribution of mental states to others by schizophrenic patients. *Cognitive Neuropsychiatry*, **2**: 1–17.

Schneider, S. (1998). Peace and paranoia. In: *Even paranoids have enemies: new perspectives on paranoia and persecution* (ed. J.H. Berke, S. Pierides, A. Sabbadini and S. Schneider), pp. 203–218. London: Routledge.

Sensky, T., Turkington, D., Kingdon, D., Scott, J.L., Scott, J., Siddle, R. *et al.* (2000). A randomized controlled trial of cognitive-behaviour therapy for persistent symptoms in schizophrenia resistant to medication. *Archives of General Psychiatry*, **57**: 165–172.

Soyka, M., Naber, G., and Volcker, A. (1991). Prevalence of delusional jealousy in different psychiatric disorders. *British Journal of Psychiatry*, **158:** 549–553.

Sperber, D. (1982). *On anthropological knowledge: three essays*. Cambridge: Cambridge University Press.

Sweeny, P., Anderson, K., and Bailey, S. (1986). Attributional style and depression: a meta-analytic review. *Journal of Personality and Social Psychology*, **50**: 774–791.

Tarrier, N. (1997). *The Manchester Cognitive-Behaviour Therapy Trial for Chronic Schizophrenia*. Paper presented at the British Association for Behavioural and Cognitive Psychotherapy Annual Conference, Cantebury.

Tarrier, N., Beckett, R., Harwood, S., Baker, A., Yusupoff, L., and Ugarteburu, I. (1993). A trial of two cognitive-behavioural methods of treating drug-resistant residual psychotic symptoms in schizophrenic patients I: Outcome. *British Journal of Psychiatry*, **162**: 524–532.

Trower, P. and Chadwick, P. (1995). Pathways to defense of the self: a theory of two types of paranoia. *Clinical Psychology: Science and Practice*, **2**: 263–278.

Tversky, A. and Kahneman, D. (1974). Judgement under uncertainty: heuristics and biases. *Science*, **185**: 1124–1131.

van Os, J., Hanssen, M., Bijl, R.V., and Ravelli, A. (2000). Strauss (1969) revisited: a psychosis continuum in the normal population? *Schizophrenia Research*, **45**: 11–20.

von Domarus, E. (1944). The specific laws of logic in schizophrenia. In: *Language and thought in schizophrenia* (ed. J.S. Kasanin). New York: Norton.

Walker, C. (1991). Delusions: what did Jaspers really say? *British Journal of Psychiatry*, **159**(Supplement 14): 94–103.

Westermeyer, J. (1988). Some cross-cultural aspects of delusions. In: *Delusional beliefs* (ed. T.F. Oltmanns and B.A. Maher). Chicester: Wiley.

Zigler, E. and Glick, M. (1988). Is paranoid schizophrenia really camoflaged depression? *American Psychologist*, **43**: 284–290.

Zullow, H.M., Oettingen, G., Peterson, C., and Seligman, M.E.P. (1988). Pessimistic explanatory style in the historical record: CAVEing LBJ, Presidential candidates, and East versus West Berlin. *American Psychologist*, **43**: 673–682.

15 The logical basis of psychiatric meta-narratives

Rom Harré

Introduction

On being a nuisance

There are many 'discourses of psychiatry', relevant to the processes and practices of diagnosis, cure, and management of some of the ways in which people can be odd. There are many ways of being 'odd', only some of which attract the attention of psychiatrists. Is schizophrenia, as currently understood, just one genre of oddness? Do the layers of talk and writing within which this concept is embedded differ in any essential way from those in which concepts for other kinds of oddness are embedded? I believe that oddness concepts fall into two discursive patterns. There are those like 'ADHD', which are wholly socially constructed, existing only in certain discursive practices. Half a century ago some psychiatrists thought that 'schizophrenia' was such a concept. Then there are those like 'Alzheimer's Condition', which are embedded in a complex discourse genre with reference both to meanings and rules and to material mechanisms. I believe 'schizophrenia' is such a concept. Other 'oddness' concepts, such as Chronic Fatigue Syndrome are contested.

Psychiatric discourse and its congeners, such as counselling talk, display many layers of reflexive self-reference. Roughly we can start with the vernacular, nowadays heavily infected with material that draws on technical jargons. However, we will surely finish up far from common speech in various genres of high level meta-discourses of which this paper is an example. The higher level discourses seem to take the lower level discourses as topics. However, the interpenetration of these layers suggests that, at least to some extent, the discourse of psychiatrists, and indeed of those who practise the philosophy of psychiatry, use the vernacular as a resource.

It is an uncontroversial commonplace that the discursive procedures that result in diagnoses are driven from the vernacular via the application of criteria of deviant meanings and rules to lay discourse. However, some classificatory work will have already been done long before problematic examples of lay discourse are offered to the psychiatrist, either by a targeted individual or by some of those who know him or her. The primary diagnosis of oddness may be overlooked in our attempt to get at the root of the discourse of psychiatry. It may have already taken place in the home or the work place or the neighbourhood leisure facilities or the local police station and magistrates court long before the person comes into view on the periphery of the domain of the psychiatric services. Already, long before a history is taken, the boundaries that delineate proper and improper ways of being have been re-instituted and confirmed by being invoked, even if only implicitly.

However I think we need another lay category to get this preliminary to psychiatry right, that of 'being a nuisance'. Thus labelled a child can finish up muzzy with Ritalin to 'cure' his or her ADHD; a formerly tolerated rubber fetishist can be enjoying a course of cognitive behaviour therapy (Marks and Gelder 1967) and so on.

Are there studies of the lay procedures and practices of pre-psychiatry? I have not seen any. What ways of being a nuisance are there? What adjustments are implicit in the stability of social entities like families, which do not bring their nuisances to anyone's attention? Some of this can be found in the work of Pearce and Cronen (1980).

The abstraction of 'file-selves' from 'concrete-selves'

A human being progresses through the medical services accompanied by a flock of files. Sometimes the real self is substituted by a file self; for example' in a case conference in a psychiatric hospital or clinic. The fatefulness of the content of files prompts some deep questions. How are personal files created? What characteristics do they display? Let us call the person as presented in a file, a file-self. File-selves are in contrast to real-selves. Both are multiple in several dimensions. However, the dimensions of multiplicity of file-selves are not the same as those of real-selves.

The comments to follow come from a study I conducted in Oxford, using the files generated by the Warneford Hospital, which houses the university department of psychiatry (Harré 1983, pp. 69–74). A psychiatric file typically included the GP's case notes taken during interviews with the person who was destined to become a patient. They also included letters to and from the GP to a Consultant Psychiatrist. The study focused on the transformation of the description of the patient's troubles in the course of the exchange of letters within the hierarchy of the medical services.

Should the patient pass on from the GP's care to the psychiatric services the file-self generated by the letter writing process was a crucial element in the perception of the patient by the people who manned these services.

The phenomenon of a file-self standing in for the real-self is ubiquitous in contemporary advanced countries. For example, one's credit rating is determined by reference to a file-self or selves, never by reference to a flesh-and-blood person. The bulk of applicants for a post are considered not in interviews with real people but in the form of the file-selves created by the assembly of a file of documents according to some local rules and conventions. A person's first contact with a psychiatrist will be as a file-self, generated by the referral letter from GP to consultant.

How does the interaction between file-self and consultant or a member of a selection committee go on? Typically the bulk of the actual file is deceptive, since the reader usually looks for certain documents thought to be salient and skims or ignores the rest. A real person is a store of huge quantities of diverse reflexive information. A file-self's information content is confined to what the documents in the file contain, and further restricted by the choice of salient items by the psychiatrist.

Unlike a real-self, a person can be present as a file-self at many different locations and in many different situations simultaneously, most of which will be unknown to the real-self. In these circumstances the real-self or person can exert very little influence on how his or her file-self is interpreted by the relevant functionaries. Unlike a real-self, a file-self cannot refuse to answer. A file-self is never mute. A file-self cannot produce a tactical lie or a clever evasion or a significant elaboration. File-selves are neither conscious nor have they autonomous agency.

Clearly self-knowledge and self-mastery are limited by the file-selves with which a person is accompanied through the life course.

The study of Oxford psychiatric files showed how in the course of file construction a radical simplification and typification of the real-self took place. Let us first look at the vocabulary in use in the construction of a psychiatric file-self.

The most striking characteristic of the lexicon was the almost complete absence of words for long-term traits. The 'history' began with a moment of 'complaint', usually fairly recent. The vocabulary included the following categories of words: feelings ('disgust', 'heaviness at night'), moods ('low', 'no interest in anything'), cognitive states ('perplexed', 'feels she partly blames him'), current behaviour ('sits and stares', 'wakeful'), self-interventions ('shakes himself', 'builds a fantasy world').

The few trait terms that do appear are short-term such as 'gets bullied', 'wants to be a woman', and the like.

The file-self springs into being when the complaining starts and disappears when the complaining ceases. Whose complaints open and close the life course of a file-self? Rarely the person whose file-self we are examining. The complaints usually emanate from someone else, who appears as a shadowing but influential file-self in the consultancy process.

The process by which a general practitioner transforms the discourse of the consultant with the patient as real-self into a file-self can be followed in the conventions for the writing of the referral letter to the consultant. Vernacular terminology is replaced by terminology from a 'pop' psychological lexicon. For example 'represses his feelings' is rendered as 'unexpressed affect'. One who has lost his capacity to manage his life is described as suffering 'loss of self-esteem'. It is evident at a glance that the file-self terminology does not render the nuances of the real-self terminology. These, it should be noted, are real examples from real files.

To my surprise I found that letters from psychiatrists to general practitioners reverted to the vernacular, back translating the 'pop' psychology lexicon. Not surprisingly, more often than not, the back translation did not correspond with the original vernacular description, that had used the patient's own vernacular terminology for the most part. The cycle of translations not only resulted in massive loss of data, but also created an eventual file-self that deviated in important ways from the real-self from which it was ultimately derived.

Three Wittgensteinian grammars

The notion of a grammar on which I will be drawing comes from Wittgenstein (1953, pp. 371, 373). Meanings, he thought, were best made clear by describing how a word or other significant material thing is used. However, there are standards of correctness for the uses of meaningful devices, be they traffic lights, cocktail dresses, or words. Standards of correctness can be explicitly set out as sets of rules, expressing norms of meaning and use. A locally recognized set of such rules is a Wittgensteinian 'grammar'.

To my eye, there are three main grammars or sets of norms, conventions, and customs, to which contemporary common discourse conforms. I believe it is useful to distinguish one grammar from another by reference to the most basic or fundamental kind of entity, which their use presupposes. Thus, in talking about anti-oxidants, the greenhouse effect, and so on, lay persons freely make use of a grammar that presupposes that there are minute material particles chemists and physicists call 'molecules'. I will call this set of rules, the M-grammar. Here is an example of a statement that requires an M-grammar convention to make sense. A dispute between an oil company and the local community as reported by Ray (2002, p. 28), tells of a sign erected by the locals, which read as follows, 'If you can read this sign you are being exposed to toxic chemicals'. Nothing untoward could be seen or heard. The referents must be molecules. Causal explanations are appropriate for discourses within the constraints of the M-grammar. Molecular mechanisms are readily conjured up to account for well-established causal relations between events. Only if such a mechanism can be found or modelled can we describe a correlation between types of events as a generative relation between cause and effect.

However, another grammar is almost as ubiquitous. Discourses shaped by the O-grammar make use of lay versions of concepts such as 'organ donation', 'gene therapy', 'irritable bowel syndrome', and so on. The basic entity presupposed in the uses of the O-grammar is an organism. To think, to talk, and to write O-speak, the human organism is taken as the point of reference. Organic phenomena are usually explained by functional hypotheses, again requiring the support of control mechanisms, which, if unknown to observation, must be imagined with the help of iconic models.

The P-grammar presupposes that there are persons, active agents trying to carry through projects and whose performances are subject to moral and other forms of assessment. The P-grammar is in use in courts of law, in family life, in business, and everywhere that people undertake tasks and, for the most part, try to meet standards of correctness and propriety. In this way of talking and writing people are presumed to be aware of what they are doing, to be willing to take responsibility or their actions or, if not, explicitly repudiating them. People have their reasons. When an explanation is called for, reasons are often proffered in satisfaction of the demand. To explain what one has done causally is exactly to repudiate responsibility and cast oneself as a mere machine.

To attempt to deal with conduct, a P-grammar concept, by pharmacological intervention presupposes that there must be something involved in the production of that conduct that would or could be influenced through a chemical reaction. Should the pharmacology be targeted on some class of neurotransmitters, the O-grammar must be drawn on so that M-grammar descriptions of chemical reactions be locatable somewhere in the human body, the conduct of which is in question. Evidently we are employing a hybrid discourse genre. Cognitive psychology is just such a genre.

Hybrid psychological discourses can be created in various ways (Harré 2002). For our purposes the most important is the Task/Tool principle, allowing the M- and O-grammars to be absorbed into the P-grammar, as the rules for talking about the brain as a cognitive tool. According to this principle P-grammar defined tasks, that is tasks involving the management of meanings in accordance with local standards of correctness and propriety, are performed by the use of tools, the most important and useful of which is the actor's brain. How it functions is expressed in the M- and O-grammars. Tennis makes a nice parallel. People play the game, intent on playing good strokes, and winning games, sets, and matches. It is played with certain tools, in particular racquets and balls. To understand how they function requires the physics of elastic strings and the mechanics of ballistic missiles. The complete discourse of tennis is a hybrid.

In this essay I aim to identify the multi-layered discourse of 'schizophrenia' as a hybrid discourse constructed along the same lines as cognitive psychology and tennis talk. The description of the phenomena requires the P-grammar, which is linked via the Task/Tool metaphor to an M- and O-grammar description (usually via an iconic model) of the workings of the brain. That these are non-standard is a top down diagnosis from the application of oddness and nuisance concepts to someone's conduct.

The social construction of disorders

The implication of such socially defined concepts as 'oddness' and 'nuisance' in the criteria with which mental disorders are picked out in the P-grammar, reflects the fact that there is an irreducible element of social construction in the psychiatric phenomenon themselves. To create a 'disorder' the boundaries of acceptable conduct must be implicitly set in the practices of a community. If there are such boundaries they can, in principle, be reset.

The question of the ontological category of a disorder requires attention to how well the hybrid format for a psychology can be realized. Is there a state of the brain and/or other parts of the human body revealed by the use of the Task/ Tool metaphor to suggest an O- or M-grammar specification of a biological boundary of normal functioning? Alzheimer's Condition satisfies the 'hybrid' requirement since conduct that lies outside the boundary defining 'good linguistic performance' is matched by observable brain states that are thereby taken to be outside the boundary of 'healthy brain'. But for ADHD the hybrid requirement is not met. Furthermore, our suspicions are aroused by the historical fact that the boundaries of acceptable childhood conduct had to be redefined to make a certain range of conduct a nuisance in the sense of an abnormality to create ADHD. Let us look more closely at the social process of boundary revision.

Boundary revisions

ADHD: from failure of self-discipline to psychiatric disorder

It is not infrequent in the United States to have a student come up to one with the startling news that he, or more rarely she, has been diagnosed as suffering from a 'learning disorder'. This brings certain privileges with it. The most important from the point of view of the great grades race is that examinations are to be taken in the 'Learning Center' without which no US university would be complete.

Let us pause to examine an actual case. Let us call him 'Jake'. He was the brightest student in the class. He had a kind of eagerness about him. If the class were asked to provide an illustration or example of some abstract concept that was being introduced, Jake would come up with the most apposite. His mid-term exam script was a top A.

Where were the 'symptoms'? As we have noted, the concept of 'symptom' is relative to the setting of a base range defining 'normality'. Deviations from the local standard are 'symptoms'. It is not hard to work out how Jake attracted this 'diagnosis'. His secondary education had been in a third-rate high school, where the base range of normal classroom behaviour would have been resentful and sullen indifference. The eagerness of such a lad as Jake is a 'symptom'. Now, we follow Jake through the school counselling system to the psychiatrist and the prescription of Ritalin. As 'treatment' progresses Jake too displays sullen indifference, and fulfils the school's standards of a 'normal' male adolescence.

Jake is currently at a second-string US university, and doing very well. He has boldly chosen to write his examinations with his fellow students. He scores straight As. His eager attention is a great encouragement to those who teach him.

Tourette's: extending the domain of 'rights to a diagnosis'

In a recent study of the social context of Tourette's Syndrome (Hamilton 1999), an interesting extension of the right to claim to be a sufferer of the condition emerged. In 1885 Giles de la Tourette described a pattern of involuntary behaviour, which included inappropriate shouting and other 'tics'. The syndrome was soon expanded to include the involuntary shouting of obscenities.

In recent years two further dimensions have been added to the description of TS. There seems to be some evidence that certain neural pathways are implicated in the tendency to display the standard repertoire of 'tics' including the verbal aspect. Another link for which there is some evidence is to heredity. The tendency to develop TS may run in some families. Hamilton found that there were people attending the national congress for TS who declared themselves to be sufferers though they had never displayed any of the symptoms. Their grounds for the claim were membership of a family in which one or more members had suffered from TS. As yet inactivated genetic tendencies were offered as the material basis for membership of TS.

Let us look now at the social constructionist aspect of the second of these developments. Over the last few years active TS support groups have sprung up. They provide a social context in which sufferers from TS can shed the feeling of marginality that their tics invoke. These groups are also active in extending the scope of medical insurance to cover this disorder. Those claiming the attention of TS support groups now include symptomless members of families in which there have been one or more TS sufferers.

In this research Hamilton has shown how the scope of a syndrome can open out, driven by social forces, such as the need to belong.

Alzheimer's: tangled speech to tangled neural nets

In the case of Alzheimer's Condition the Task/Tool distinction is correctly applied, since the ontological hypothesis, that there will be a distinctive brain condition that can be smoothly located outside the reciprocally set boundaries of healthy brain states.

However, we need to bear in mind the Kitwood/Sabat reminder of widespread existence of 'malignant psychology'. This is the possibility that social constructions of 'mental incompetence', though rooted in the actual level of disorderly speech, may far exceed any 'objective' assessment of what the person so diagnosed can and cannot do. Even if the hybrid psychology principle is met, and the condition is not wholly the result of shifting social boundaries of what is odd and what is a nuisance, there may still be a tendency to shift boundaries to the detriment of the quality of life of the sufferer.

The working principles

Summing up this discussion we now have two major principles to guide us in trying to understand how a 'mental disorder' can be given a determinate status.

Principle 1

The current syndrome of a condition is a social construction based on social categorizations of someone's speech and actions.

Principle 2

The criterion by which a condition is classified as a disease is derived from the Hybrid Psychology thesis, by which an abnormality of conduct is related to an abnormality of brain function.

Two uses of models

These principles are not yet enough to guide the analyst in locating 'schizophrenia' or any other diagnostic term. A scientific approach to any domain involves building a working taxonomy and constructing models both of the phenomena (analytical models) and of their presumed generating processes (explanatory models). The latter are usually unobservable when a research programme begins. For example, Darwin's brilliant exposition of the phenomena of natural selection was based on the use of the techniques of stockbreeding as an analytical model to present the process of speciation. One-hundred years later, Watson and Crick constructed a successful explanatory model of the intracellular processes that underlay the processes of speciation.

It is a cardinal error in science to mistake an analytical model for an explanatory model. It is no less so in psychiatry, as we shall see. In general, in psychology and psychiatry, analytical models make use of the P-grammar, while M- and O-grammars are used to present explanatory models.

The schizophrenia enigma

Boundary revisions: history of first level meta-discourse

Emil Kraepelin's symptomology drew on an existing 'technical' vocabulary, in particular by the recovery of Morel's term 'dementia praecox'. This provided Kraepelin with a nice contrast to 'manic-depression'. In his memoirs (Kraepelin 1987) he offers the reader the working distinction, commenting on how he has been driven to take account of intermediate cases. In short, Kraepelin has created a boundary between two ways of being sufficiently odd to be a nuisance, a boundary he himself blurs in his endeavour to remain true to the phenomena. So far as I can discern there is no hint in what I have read of Kraepelin, of the application of the hybrid psychology principle to fabricate a suitable concept of a neural defect. It would have needed to be sufficiently well-defined to sustain a programme of post-mortem examinations of the brains of his patients. However, the next step along the line initiated by Kraepelin must surely be an application of the hybrid psychology principle.

R.D. Laing and the rejection of the Hybrid Psychology Principle

Laing's writings relevant to this discussion date from the 1960s during his co-operation with other 'existential psychiatrists'. A key passage from *The divided self* (Laing 1960) allows the reader to see very clearly where in the genesis of a psychological account of a psychiatric condition Laing stands. In commenting on one of Kraepelin's vivid descriptions of the odd and nuisance-making conduct of a patient, Laing queries Kraepelin's comment that though the patient has understood all the questions 'he has not given us a single piece of useful information . . . ' (quoted by Laing from Kraepelin 1905, pp. 79–80). Instead he suggests that the patient ' . . . is carrying on a dialogue between his own parodied version of Kraepelin, and his own defiant rebelling self' (Laing 1960, p. 30). The patient, says Laing, is objecting to being measured and tested. He wishes to be heard. But about what topic? How the world seems to him.

As Laing's analysis unfolds we remain entirely within a discursive world. He says of one of his former patients that she provides us with 'a clear statement of the phenomenology of her psychosis [Laing's 'false self' and 'true self' dichotomy] in straightforward simple language. When however one is dealing with a patient who is actively psychotic, one has to take the risk of translating the patient's language into one's own, if one is not to give an account that is itself in schizophrenese' (Laing 1960, p. 177).

Though this was written half a century ago it illustrates very well the embodiment of the phenomena exclusively in a discursive domain. In the absence of the hybrid psychology principle linking discursive oddness to malfunctioning of the organic tools for living, there is only a place for the oddness of life narrative, the living out of which has an external nuisance value. It must reside wholly in the discursive domain. Repairing one's discourse to conform to the style and manner of the circumambient society is 'cure'. Kraepelin's patient might one day learn to reply to the doctor's queries politely and submissively.

Laing's account of schizophrenia is based on a model. He imagines a pair of selves, the relations between which underlie both what someone does that merits the diagnosis of 'schizophrenia' and what brings it about that the person acts thus, and so. This was an analytical model, a way of presenting the phenomena both overt and phenomenological to an interested reader or listener. Applying the Hybrid Psychology Principle requires the insertion of an explanatory model into the discourse. Eventually Laing did this, but, as we know, turned back to the social world for it. It too was presented in the P-grammar.

Applying the Task/Tool metaphor institutes the discourse of medicalized 'cure'

To rephrase a famous aphorism: 'If it is broke, then fix it!' According to the Hybrid Psychology Principle the brain is best regarded as a tool with which a person carries out a variety of tasks and projects. In preparing the garden for spring sowing the gardener uses a spade to turn over the soil. Why should the brain be any different in principle from a spade? Furthermore blunt chisels and slack tennis racquets spoil the work of wood carving and inhibit the bullet serve. Should not the brain be looked at in the same light?

There is nothing very surprising about these anodyne remarks. However, the consequences of keeping the brain-as-tool concept in mind are profound. The Task/Tool metaphor does not sanction reductionism. Some of the disgraceful cases of consigning people to oblivion, highlighted by Kitwood and Sabat as 'malignant psychology', seem to me to depend on taking the evident applicability of the Task/Tool metaphor as indicative of a right to delete the Task side of the pair. The Tool is defective and so the Task performance is never given another thought, written off as unsalvageable. In Sabat (2001) there are a plethora of case studies to the contrary.

Reflexive application of the Hybrid Psychology Principle to re-revise boundaries at the vernacular level

The successful application of the Hybrid Psychology Principle in the last couple of decades is evidenced by the relative success of a pharmacological repertoire for the management of schizophrenia. From the point of the student of the meta-discourses of psychiatry it is evident that this has resulted in the drawing of a boundary within a boundary. While the wholesale use of Ritalin to discipline unruly children has expanded, though not without being contested, the boundary of the explanatory model 'brain as defective tool' to colonize the territory formerly occupied by a wholly social set of criteria for what is unacceptable, the widespread use of drugs to manage the oddness of those who are said to be 'schizophrenic' has actually shrunk the domain of usability of the generic explanatory model: 'brain as defective tool'.

Conclusions

The analysis of the meta-discourses of those who find themselves involved with people whose conduct breaches the local conventions of acceptability reveals a complex interplay between the social construction of a 'condition' and the creation of an explanatory model depending on the Hybrid Psychology Principle. Pharmacological or even surgical intervention to remedy oddness of conduct is made conceptually coherent to the extent that such a model can meet the criteria of empirical adequacy and ontological plausibility that the use of such models demands. Where the criteria are not met we have situations like the expansion of the populations 'with' ADHD and Tourette's Syndrome. The closest attention must be paid to the 'grammars' according to which the discourses directed to odd and unacceptable conduct.

At the same time, the conceptual error that led Laing to treat his analytical model as explanatory, needs to be remembered. Caution in slipping from a socially constructed condition to a medical syndrome should not inhibit the disciplined use of the Hybrid Psychology Principle to look for a defect in the cognitive tool-kit.

Since file-selves are fateful in the bureaucratized medical services of the modern state, it behoves the student of the practices of psychiatry to pay close attention to how file-selves are constructed. How important is the seeping away of information as the file-selves proliferate? At what point do the M- and O-grammars begin to dominate the order imposing principles that the content of file-selves intelligible and to whom?

References

Hamilton, G.S. (1999). Tourette's Syndrome, support groups and the transformation of a syndrome. Unpublished doctoral dissertation. Georgetown University.

Harré, R. (1983). *Personal being*. Oxford: Blackwell.

Harré, R. (2002). *Cognitive science: a philosophical introduction*. London: Sage.

Kraepelin, E. (1987). *Memoirs* (trans. C. Wooding-Deane). New York: Springer-Verlag.

Marks, I.M. and Gelder, M.G. (1967). Transvestism and fetishism. *British Journal of Psychiatry* **113:** 711–729.

Pierce, W.B. and Cronen, V. (1980). *Action, communication and meaning*. New York: Praeger.

Ray, J. (2002). Guardian of grand bois. *Sierra,* May/June: 26–30.

Sabat, S.E. (2001). *The experience of Alzheimer's*. Oxford: Blackwell.

Wittgenstein, L. (1953). *Philosophical investigations*. Oxford: Blackwell.

16 Suspicions of schizophrenia

Eric Matthews

Introduction

There would be widespread agreement that schizophrenia has played a key role in the development of the modern medicalized conception of 'mental illness' out of older, more popular, ideas of 'madness'. As is well known, Kraepelin's original conception of 'dementia praecox', the ancestor of the term 'schizophrenia' first introduced by Bleuler, was central to an attempt to make psychiatry into a branch of scientific medicine. The essence of this 'Kraepelinian revolution', according to Edward Shorter's *History of psychiatry*, consisted in 'Looking at outcomes in psychiatric illness, and differentiating distinct diseases on the basis of these outcomes' (Shorter 1997, p. 103). The diseases thus differentiated were believed to be natural disease entities, to be classified in the same way as ordinary organic diseases, and dementia praecox/schizophrenia was certainly so regarded.

It is in this regard that schizophrenia can be seen, to use a philosophical term, as a 'paradigm case' of a mental illness in the modern, medicalized, sense: that is, as an example that embodies the central defining features of the concept in question. Schizophrenia is, if anything is, a clear case of what we mean by a mental illness, and other alleged candidates for that title qualify to the extent that they are similar to schizophrenia. Calling certain kinds of disorders 'mental illnesses' is meant to emphasize the similarities between these conditions and the more familiar bodily illnesses, such as diabetes, hepatitis, or pharyngitis. The latter are generally taken to be objectively identifiable and distinguishable from each other, by a combination of their overt symptoms and the particular bodily organ that is affected. The word 'objectively' is used here to emphasize that their identification has nothing to do with the inner feelings of the patient who suffers from them: the patient may, indeed, be suffering from the illness without experiencing any relevant feelings at all.

As the etymology of the word 'patient' itself makes clear, an illness of this sort is something which one suffers, a kind of invader from outside oneself, which imposes itself upon one. The immediate cause of the symptoms that manifest the illness is taken to be the failure to function or inefficiency of functioning of the organ in question, which is itself caused by injury, infection, the consequences of abuse (overeating, excessive consumption of alcohol, etc.), and similar factors. These are external causes, in the sense that they operate independently of the choice or consciousness of the person affected. Because of this, it is pointless to try to treat such an illness by appealing to the patient's consciousness or will-power—by, for instance, talking to her. The only effective way to relieve the patient's suffering is to act directly on its causes, that is, to set right, by drugs, surgery, or similar means, the malfunction of the relevant organ: that is why specifically medical expertise is required for successful treatment.

Kraepelin's conceptualization of 'dementia praecox', and Bleuler's later reformulation of that concept as 'schizophrenia', are clearly intended to fit certain kinds of human problems of behaviour, emotion, and thought processes into the same pattern, thus reinforcing by a striking example the notion that there are 'mental' illnesses that are comparable in essential respects with the kinds of bodily disorders mentioned above. And schizophrenia is a good example to choose from this point of view: it undoubtedly does cause considerable human suffering, of a kind that the sufferer plainly does not choose for herself and that is therefore not amenable to being changed by simple persuasion or good advice. It is not surprising, therefore, that the conception of schizophrenia as a paradigm of 'mental illness' is widely accepted, not only by psychiatrists (who might be thought to have a vested interest in propagating this notion), but by society in general.

Nevertheless, there is also a tradition of scepticism about the concept of schizophrenia. And since schizophrenia, as just argued, can be regarded as a paradigm of the medicalized concept of mental illness, the most interesting of these suspicions also tend to be directed towards what they describe as the 'medical model' in general: they are an expression of the movement often called 'anti-psychiatry'. The anti-psychiatric movement is usually associated with a rather romantic rebellion against the modern world of science and technology. Some of its claims might well be regarded by working psychiatrists, busily engaged in attempting to provide therapy for the intense misery of mental disorder, as a mere trivialization of serious human problems. It is tempting therefore to dismiss it as a facile rebellion of the counter-culture against scientific medicine. This chapter, however, is written in the conviction that such a dismissal is too easy. I shall argue that we should not accept all the anti-psychiatrists' conclusions, and certainly should not abandon the practice of psychiatry as a science-based branch of medicine. But I shall try to show how, by their use of ideas and arguments drawn from philosophy, anti-psychiatrists draw our attention to some features of schizophrenia that are neglected in purely neuropsychiatric models. Their deficiencies lie, in my view, in the inadequacy of their grasp of this philosophical framework and the way it can be applied to the questions with which they are concerned. My aim in this chapter is to see how their work looks when it is based on a more adequate philosophical analysis, derived from the work of the French phe-nomenologist, Maurice Merleau-Ponty; in particular his concept of human beings as embodied subjects. This, I shall argue, will make it possible to extract the genuine insight from the rather confused romanticism that often surrounds it, and to show how it implies, not the rejection of any kind of medical model of schizophrenia, but a reinterpretation of what such a model involves.

For various reasons, I shall concentrate on two such critics, Thomas Szasz and R.D. Laing. One reason is that they are two of the best known represen-tatives of the anti-psychiatric movement. In a sense, they define what is meant by that term. Furthermore, they are or were practising psychiatrists themselves. But the most important reason is that their critique of schizophre-nia is also a critique of the more general concept of mental illness, and hence necessarily requires the philosophical framework spoken of above. Other critics of schizophrenia (and of the concept of mental illness in general), such as Michel Foucault (Foucault 1965) or Mary Boyle (Boyle 2002), direct their attack at external factors, such as the power structures of the society in which psychiatry functions or the desire of psychiatrists to gain the status of medical scientists. Szasz and Laing, by contrast, go to what seems to me the heart of the matter; namely, to the way in which we should respond to the people we call 'schizophrenics', and recognize that reflection on that issue is essentially philosophical in character. For this reason, what they have to say has a very concrete bearing on the actual practice of psychiatry and on the nature of its contribution to human welfare. My approach will be, first, to critically examine each of these thinkers in turn in their own terms, and then to present Merleau-Ponty's philosophical framework and to re-examine their work in the light of it.

Thomas Szasz

One of the best-known critics of the medical model of mental disorder is Thomas Szasz, who, in the title of his most notorious book, even dismissed the notion of mental illness as a 'myth' (Szasz 1972).[1]

His reasons for calling mental illness a myth are, however, far less clear than he seems to think. At times, he seems to be arguing, in a Popperian vein, that psychiatry is a 'pseudo-science', like alchemy or astrology (Szasz 1972, p. 17): in that case, presumably, mental illness would be a 'myth' in the sense that it did not belong as part of a genuinely scientific way of understanding human behaviour, so that the pretensions of psychiatry to be 'scientific' were ill-founded.

Another, and more characteristic, argument here is that mental illness is a 'myth' in that it is an *illegitimate use of an extended concept*. It is, of course, a normal, and unexceptionable, part of any living language that the meanings of terms get extended beyond their original use: metaphors are one obvious example of this practice. A word is originally used in one context, as, for instance, the term 'leg' originally applies to the limb of an animal: but then it is metaphorically extended to other cases that can be seen as similar in certain respects, so that we start speaking of the 'legs' of a table or a chair. (Whether or not this is historically correct, I cannot say, but it may still help to illustrate the point.) But suppose someone thought that it was indecent for human beings to display their uncovered legs to strangers, and concluded that the same must be true of any kind of legs, including table legs. (The Victorians are sometimes said, wrongly I understand, to have thought in this way.) Then that person would be making an illegitimate use of an extended concept in the sense I am trying to explain: she would, we might say, be taking a metaphor too literally.

We could apply this to interpret some of the criticisms that Szasz makes of the concept of mental illness. The primary use of the term 'illness', Szasz often seems to be saying, is to refer to a bodily condition. He claims that when we say we are ill, we normally mean that we believe ourselves to be suffering from an 'abnormality or malfunctioning of [our] body' (Szasz 1972, p. 11), of a kind for which we may voluntarily seek medical help. Modern medical science, he argues, is based on the premise that it seeks to correct such bodily abnormalities; and that also underpins the centrality to modern medical ethics of the principle of respect for patient autonomy, that is, that medical intervention is justifiable only with the patient's free consent. But terms like 'ill' or 'sick' are also, as he points out on the same page, widely used in metaphorical senses, as when we speak of 'sick jokes' or 'sick economies'. Here the meaning of the term is extended to cover other kinds of abnormalities than bodily malfunctions—abnormalities in the sense of deviations from socially acceptable norms ('sick jokes') or from socially desirable states of affairs ('sick economies'). Szasz's point seems to be that talk of someone's being 'mentally ill' is similarly metaphorical or extended: someone is called 'mentally ill', in his view, not because of any bodily abnormality or malfunctioning, but for another reason, more like the reason for calling a joke or an economy sick.

Why should this be thought a problem? No one would describe the notion of a sick joke as a myth: it is a useful metaphor. If Szasz chooses to characterize the concept of mental illness in this way, it must be because it involves taking the metaphor too literally. We do not seek medical help for sick economies, and no one would be tempted by this use of the word 'sick' to think that we should: but in the modern world we do consider mental illness to be a medical problem, and Szasz implies that this is a confused failure to understand the term's metaphorical character. This interpretation is borne out by his remark (ibid.) that the relationship between bodily illness and mental illness is the same as that between a defective television receiver and an objectionable television programme.

Szasz's argument here could be seen as an application of the later Wittgenstein's philosophy. Wittgenstein came to believe that it was a mistake to focus on the 'meaning' of expressions, which suggests that each expression gets its sense by referring to one and only one element of reality. Instead, we should concern ourselves with how expressions are used, and recognize that the same expression may be used in different ways in different contexts (in different 'language-games', as Wittgenstein puts it). Thus, 'sick' has a different use when talking about an economy, about a joke, or about a patient: and, Szasz is claiming, 'illness' likewise has a different sense when applied to hysteria from the one it has when applied to, say, bronchitis. Recognizing the difference between language-games, in Wittgenstein's view, enables us to avoid the kinds of philosophical confusions we get into when we assimilate one use of a term to another.

Having said this, let us go back to the comparison between a television receiver and a television programme. To say that a television receiver is 'defective' is to say that there is something objectively and identifiably wrong with its internal mechanisms, which is preventing it from fulfilling its function of enabling television transmissions to be seen by viewers. To say that a television programme is 'objectionable', on the other hand, is to say that it offends against moral, aesthetic, or other social norms. So the point of the comparison, as Szasz goes on to say, is to claim that 'psychiatric interventions are directed at moral, not medical, problems'. We might interpret this as follows: a person with a moral problem (for instance, someone who is inclined to be cowardly in her relations to those in authority) does not, if she understands what a moral problem is, regard herself as in need of medical help, but as someone who needs to make an effort of will to improve her behaviour and attitudes. If someone proposed to 'cure' her of cowardice by giving her drugs, say, she would not voluntarily consent to such 'therapy'. In this way, Szasz regards the concept of 'mental illness', as presently used, as ethically, as well as scientifically, misguided. It undermines the sense of personal autonomy. The diagnosis of someone as mentally ill is not, he says, the identification of a 'genuine disease' from which that person is suffering, but a 'stigmatizing label' (Szasz 1972, p. 12).

The use of a stigmatizing label is, of course, to identify someone as a person who has committed an offence, something for which they are to blame and for which they deserve punishment. Someone deserves punishment for something only if they have freely chosen to do it: so to identify someone as an offender is at least to recognize their autonomy, as someone capable of making choices for themselves. To call someone's condition a 'disease' or 'illness', however, is to recognize that it is something that happened to them, something for which they deserve compassion and help rather than punishment, something that is bad for them themselves and not (or at least not primarily) for others. An illness is something we ought to 'treat', in the hope of 'curing' it. Thus, to talk of 'mental illness', Szasz seems to be arguing, is to conflate the use of 'sick' as a stigmatizing label with its use as referring to an illness—to suggest that we should try to cure people of their offensive behaviour. But to talk in that way is to deny the human dignity of the 'mentally ill' by denying them their autonomy, their power to choose how they will behave. At the same time, it licenses psychiatrists to act as agents of social control, confining and manipulating those who deviate from social norms. Because of their pretensions to be doctors, however, psychiatrists perform this function in particularly dangerous ways, which, unlike ordinary imprisonment, even deny deviants the dignity of responsibility for their own actions. (In this respect, there is a certain similarity to the critique offered by Foucault.)

Szasz's argument is tangled. Even the account of it given above has required some reading between the lines in order to clarify what is going on, and more disentanglement will be needed if its force is to be properly assessed. The key assertion seems to be the claim that only bodily dysfunction, purely as such, can legitimately be described as 'illness'. All that I have been able to find in Szasz's own writings by way of supporting argument is the contention, referred to above, that what we normally mean when we say we are ill is that we believe ourselves to be suffering from some bodily abnormality or malfunction. But this is, to say the least, highly questionable. What we mean when we say we are ill surely has nothing to do with any beliefs we may have about the causes of illness: to say that one is ill is to say something about one's present state, rather than about the causes of that state. Most of us in the modern Western world may believe that most of our bodily ills are the result of bodily abnormality or malfunction, but people with different views do not necessarily mean something different by the word 'illness'. (This is a different question from that of the significance of illness in a particular culture, which may well be bound up with views about its causation). Szasz might, of course, want to say that in our culture, at least in recent times, we have generally identified 'illness' with 'bodily malfunction': but even if that is so, it does not necessarily follow that an extension of the concept to cover disorders of thought, emotion, mood or behaviour is illegitimate. To decide whether it is, we need to ask whether there is sufficient in common *of a relevant kind* between the two sorts of cases to justify the extension.

In view of the focus of this paper, we need to ask this particularly in the case of schizophrenia: whatever may be true of other conditions nowadays classified as 'mental illness', what matters to us is whether Szasz's critique applies to schizophrenia. Szasz says, as we have seen, that 'psychiatric interventions are directed at moral, not medical, problems'. The core of his argument that mental illness is a myth, is that mental disorders are deviations from social norms (of behaviour, thought, etc.) rather than the outcome of bodily malfunction. But why is this thought to be significant, apart from the dogmatic and mistaken claim that 'illness' is by definition synonymous with 'outcome of bodily malfunction'? The only other reason for thinking this is that part of the concept of illness is that an illness is an undesirable condition for which one is not to blame: one is clearly not to blame for the outcomes of bodily malfunction, but deviations from social norms are generally considered to be within one's control. Szasz significantly chooses to use the word 'moral'—significantly, because in our culture, and especially in the post-Kantian era, it is taken to be the mark of a moral issue that it is one in which one has a choice what to do ('ought implies can').

Now schizophrenics may sometimes behave in ways which, in others, would be regarded as immoral or even criminal: for instance, committing violent assaults against other people. But most of the characteristic symptoms of schizophrenia do not fall within our normal conception of what is morally blameworthy. They include such things as delusions, hallucinations, disorganized speech, grossly disorganized or catatonic behaviour, which are associated with marked social or occupational dysfunction (quoted from DSM-IV1994, pp. 273–274). In this sense, they are plainly undesirable, and undesirable because they are deviations from social norms: but they are not morally blameworthy, and it is at least not clear that they are the product of the person's choice, rather than of factors beyond her control.

In order to see how Szasz might deal with that point, we need to look further into his discussion. Taking conversion hysteria as his paradigm of a 'mental illness', he argues (Szasz 1972, p. 25) that it provides a good example 'of how so-called mental illness can best be conceptualized in terms of sign-using, rule-following, and game-playing...'. At the bottom of the same page, he extends the scope of his claims to other examples: 'Everything', he says there, 'that will be said about hysteria pertains equally, in principle, to all other so-called mental illnesses and to personal conduct generally'. And on the next page, he specifically includes schizophrenia in his claims by comparing the differences between hysteria, obsessions, paranoia and schizophrenia to the 'manifest diversity characterizing different languages'.

Thus schizophrenia, like hysteria, is treated as a 'language-game', a special form of communicative behaviour. It follows, Szasz claims, that it is 'meaningless to inquire into its "causes"' (Szasz 1972, p. 28). The only questions we can meaningfully ask about a language, he argues, are: how was it learned? And, what does it mean? If schizophrenia is a language, we cannot meaningfully say, on Szasz's view, that it is caused by brain disease, deficit, or injury (or indeed that it has any other kind of cause). We can only inquire how schizophrenics learned to use that particular form of language, and what it means (i.e. seemingly, what purpose it serves in their lives). The purpose of the schizophrenic use of language (as of other forms of mental disorder) is, according to Szasz, 'object-seeking and relationship-maintaining', rather than the communication of information (cf. Szasz 1972, pp.,137ff.).

Schizophrenic behaviour thus serves certain purposes that the schizophrenic person has. It is a 'strategy' for dealing with situations in which 'people feel unable to prevail by means of ordinary speech over the significant persons in their environment' (Szasz 1972, pp. 124ff.). In short, they are having problems in their dealings with specific individuals who are important to them (parents, lovers, etc.), and they seek to overcome them by pretending. 'To be able to speak the truth', Szasz declares, 'is a luxury which few people can afford' (Szasz 1972, p. 228). Only those who feel personally secure can afford it: those who feel oppressed or helpless, on the other hand, have to resort to a form of 'lying' or 'cheating', involving impersonating certain social roles, notably the sick role. When schizophrenics claim to be dying or dead, for example, this is 'best regarded as an impersonation of the dead role' (Szasz 1972, ibid.). 'Indeed', he concludes (same page), 'the label of psychosis is often used to identify individuals who stubbornly cling to, and loudly proclaim, publicly unsupported role-definitions'. Psychotic behaviour is thus a form of communication in which the person seeks both to preserve contact with others, and at the same time to maintain a 'psychological distance' from them.

How is this relevant to the claim that it is a 'myth' to think of schizophrenia as a 'mental illness'? Szasz's analysis seems to be that schizophrenic symptoms are a form of learned and purposive behaviour, for which (he says) it is meaningless to seek a 'cause', which are therefore not caused by anything outside the individual's own control, and so which cannot and ought not to be treated medically like a genuine illness. Behaviour of this kind may lead to difficulties in functioning as a member of society, for which the person may quite reasonably seek help: but the help cannot be medical in character, since the person is not a patient, a passive sufferer from factors beyond her control, but someone with 'problems in living', which she herself has created by her own purposive behaviour. She assumes a role to which she is not entitled, as a way of escaping from the sense of oppression felt at being unable to play the social game properly. The 'therapy' required, therefore, is not anything analogous to medical treatment, but rather to a process of 're-learning' to play the standard game. Szasz focuses particularly on psychoanalytic psychotherapy, which he describes as 'learning situations in which an attempt is made to acquaint the player ('patient') more fully with the penalties of his own strategies ('neurosis')' (Szasz 1972, p.,265). The aim of this is that such knowledge should motivate the 'patient' to wish to modify her own behaviour.

What are we to make of this position? The first thing that strikes one on reading Szasz is the number of assumptions that he makes and the number of logical leaps from one claim to another. He assumes, first, that hysterical hypochondriasis can be taken as a paradigm for all the conditions we nowadays call 'mental illness'—even psychoses like schizophrenia. But while it is more or less true by definition that hypochondriasis consists in simulating bodily illnesses, and in that sense 'playing games', it is not self-evident that schizophrenia does. It might be plausible to see the hypochondriac as playing a game in which she seeks, by adopting the 'sick role', to escape the demands of normal human relationships: it is far from plausible, and is indeed rather inhuman, to see the schizophrenic's delusions in the same way.

Again, even if one does treat hypochondriacs, at least, as playing language-games, it does not follow, as Szasz seems to think, that the playing of that game does not have a cause that is beyond the hypochondriac's own direct control. The concept of 'cause' is considerably more complex than Szasz allows. The explanation of why someone speaks French rather than English as a mother-tongue does not, of course, lie in the structure of their brains, but nevertheless it is clear that we can give an explanation (a cause) of this fact: it lies in the circumstances and location of their initial language-learning— something which they did not choose. Similarly, the explanation of why someone plays a deviant language-game must lie in circumstances beyond their own conscious control. For playing an unusual language-game, unlike having a particular mother-tongue, needs to be explained by factors affecting one individual but not others. Sometimes, such deviant behaviour is a result of conscious choice, as someone may decide to cheat at cards: but in that case, the behaviour can be understood as the pursuit of some rational goal, such as a desire to make money. ('Rational', in the sense of 'intelligible to most human beings'.) This rational intelligibility is precisely what is lacking in the schizo-phrenic's behaviour, which is why it seems right to attribute it to causes beyond the person's own control. Merely describing schizophrenics as playing games, in short, would not preclude saying that they are suffering from an illness, on even the narrowest interpretation of what that means.

R. D. Laing

Nevertheless, I want to argue that the conception of schizophrenic behaviour as purposive is worth pursuing further. This is a point of connection between Szasz and the other figure I want to concentrate on, R.D. Laing. Laing came to public notice a little later than Szasz, as part of the radical cultural questioning of the 1960s. Whereas Szasz is motivated by a libertarian ideology, a kind of conservative anarchism that asserts the rights of the individual against society, Laing is inspired rather by a much more leftist view, which criticizes the present structure of social institutions—in Laing's case, mainly the institution of the family—because of their malign influence on the individual. There are also important differences between the two in their philosophical approach. Whereas Szasz's method is essentially that of analytic philosophy in a broad sense of that term, in particular the work of Wittgenstein and Popper, Laing explicitly relates his own position to existential phenomenology, in particular to Sartre. Finally (particularly important for our present theme), whereas Szasz considers schizophrenia as only one example among many of 'so-called mental illnesses', schizophrenia is Laing's central pre-occupation.

In order to grasp what Laing is saying about schizophrenia, it is essential to understand how he conceives of his phenomenological starting-point. To be a phenomenologist about schizophrenia, as Laing sees it, is to regard it primarily as a particular way in which human beings experience the world, rather than as an externally observable condition, or a set of observable behavioural symptoms with their postulated internal causes. There are such observable symptoms, but they themselves need to be understood in terms of their meaning for the schizophrenic person, a meaning which is 'existential' in the sense of being related to the person's mode of being in the world. Thus, Laing says that the problems that constitute schizophrenia, and the schizophrenic's responses to them, cannot be understood by the methods of clinical psychiatry, but only by using an existential-phenomenological method to demonstrate 'their true human relevance and significance' (Laing 1960, p. 16). Laing explicitly rejects the Kraepelinian tradition, which sees the schizophrenic person as a 'case' in the normal medical sense, someone to be treated decently, but nevertheless to be considered as a 'patient', suffering from a 'disease'.

Seen from Laing's point of view, many of the characteristic behaviours of schizophrenics are not, as in classical psychiatry, 'signs' of a 'disease', but intelligible responses to being treated like a 'patient', an object to be dissected by the psychiatrist, rather than as a human being in distress who is asking for help. Laing cites a case from Kraepelin's own practice, in which the 'patient' is reported to make a number of utterances, which Kraepelin interprets as 'a series of disconnected sentences having no relation whatever to the general situation' (Laing 1960, p. 30). Laing, however, reads these utterances differently, as a form of rebellion by the 'patient' against Kraepelin's questioning him in this way: 'He probably does not see what it has to do with the things that must be deeply distressing him' (Laing 1960, p. 31).

It is worth considering for a moment both the similarities and the significant differences between Laing's approach and other writers' suggestions that schizophrenic symptoms are attempts to make sense of their experience. The Harvard psychologist Brendan Maher, for instance, argues for an analysis of the cognitive peculiarities of patients with schizophrenia (delusions in particular), which sees them as arrived at by processes that are not essentially different from those used by the general population. 'Delusional beliefs', he says, 'like normal beliefs, arise from an attempt to explain experience' (Maher 1999, p. 550). Where delusional beliefs differ from normal beliefs is mainly in 'the nature and intensity of the phenomenological experience that is being explained' (Maher 1999, p. 551). The experiences that give rise to delusional beliefs are 'anomalous': examples would be the sense that something about a situation is different from normal, or the (false) feeling of recognizing someone or something, or feelings of surprise, as when a sentence uttered by someone else ends differently from the way one would expect. Such anomalous experiences arise in everyday life as a result of real factors in the environment: delusion occurs, Maher hypothesizes, when the experience is endogenous, i.e. independent of external input. The feeling occurs because of the person's own thoughts and their associated images, which in turn originate from 'neuropsychological anomalies' (Maher 1999, p. 551). The delusional belief is then the attempt to make sense of this endogenous anomalous experience by finding 'meaning' in unrelated features of the external environment: Maher refers to a paper by Arthur, in which he cites as a classic example of a delusion 'the case of a patient who looked at the marble tables in a café and suddenly became convinced that they meant that the end of the world was coming' (Arthur 1964, p. 106).

This analysis is like Laing's in one respect: that it sees one kind of schizophrenic symptom as purposive, as an expression of a person's desire to make sense of experience. But then the two accounts diverge in significant respects. For Maher, the schizophrenic's delusions are purposive, in that they seek, as we all do, to make sense of an anomalous experience, but they are unintelligible to normal people because the experience in question would not be seen as anomalous by those normal people. The tables in the café would not be seen as puzzling by most of us, or requiring interpretation: above all, we would not interpret them as signs of the imminent end of the world. For Laing, by contrast, the schizophrenic's behaviour is not strictly delusive at all. For seeing the café tables (for instance) as signs of the approaching end of the world is not making sense of an anomalous experience, as we all do, but is an expression of another purpose, which is intrinsically intelligible to normal people. Schizophrenics are trying, as we all do, to cope (not merely intellectually, but existentially) with difficult and emotionally charged relationships with other people. The difference from the rest of us is that the experiences with which schizophrenics have to cope are so much more difficult and emotionally charged that they cannot really cope with them, and in the effort to do so lose their self-integrity. Because it has elements in common with general human experience, it is in principle possible for others to understand schizophrenic behaviour. But because it differs in degree of intensity from the experience of normal people, it requires great powers of imagination to understand it. In some ways, Laing seems to conceive of understanding schizophrenics as like understanding a very different human culture: one which shares our basic humanity with us, and so is in principle intelligible, but which expresses that humanity in such alien ways that it becomes very difficult to understand.

This implies that schizophrenia, or any other form of psychosis, is not, for Laing, a 'disease' that one either has or does not have: it is a way one is. It comes within the purview of the psychiatrist both because it is a 'deeply distressing' way to be and because it involves a 'strange and even alien view of the world' (Laing 1960, p. 35). But then Laing starts to talk in a different tone, describing the schizophrenic's view of the world as 'insane', and saying that the 'kernel of the schizophrenic's experience of himself must remain incomprehensible to us' (Laing 1960, p. 39). Nevertheless, he still wants to say that the psychiatrist is required, difficult though the task is, to endeavour to 'know' the schizophrenic 'without destroying him': but in doing so, 'We have to recognize all the time his distinctiveness and differentness, his separateness and loneliness and despair' (ibid.). That is to say, psychiatrists need, as far as possible, to try to enter into the psychotic's strange world and share it with him: by so doing, they are supposed in some way to help the patient to overcome his problems.

What is the nature of these problems? According to Laing, a schizophrenic person suffers from 'ontological insecurity': that is, he cannot, unlike normal people, 'encounter all the hazards of life from a centrally firm sense of his own and other people's reality and identity', and so has 'to become absorbed in contriving ways of trying to be real, of keeping himself or others alive, of preserving his identity, in efforts to prevent himself losing his self' (Laing1960, p. 44). In a later book, Laing further expands this characterization: the schizophrenic, he there says, 'lacks the usual sense of personal unity, a sense of himself as the agent of his own actions rather than as a robot, a machine, a *thing* [Laing's italics], and of being the author of his own perceptions, but rather feels that someone else is using his eyes, his ears, etc.' (Laing 1971, p. 51). His problems thus consist in the anxieties to which this loss of a sense of personal unity gives rise—the fear of the threats posed by any close relationship with another person, or indeed by being in the world at all.

If the psychiatrist is to help him, therefore, it must be by establishing a non-threatening relationship with him, in which the therapist, while remaining other, enters into the schizophrenic's world, so enabling the schizophrenic to reintegrate himself with his world, and his world with that of normal people. Laing cites approvingly Jung's statement 'that the schizophrenic ceases to be schizophrenic when he meets someone by whom he feels understood' (Laing 1960, pp. 179ff.). He (Laing) even speaks of 'the physician's *love* [my italics], a love that recognizes the patient's total being, and accepts it, with no strings attached' (Laing 1960, p. 180). Finally, in Laing 1971 he argues that those most likely to be diagnosed as schizophrenic are those who are extremely sensitive about being recognized as human beings, who need 'both to give and receive more love than most people' (Laing 1971, pp. 106ff.).

Having said this, it is clear from what Laing says that he offers no great hopes of being able to help the schizophrenic to recover in this way. He speaks of significant barriers to getting to know schizophrenics. The schizophrenic's language is said to be necessarily obscure both in content and in form, since it reflects the fact that his experience is split where ours coheres, and runs together elements that we keep apart. It is at this point that the romanticism already spoken of tends to enter Laing's account. For the alien character of schizophrenic experience now becomes, not so much a reason for compassion and psychiatric help, but something more like the superior insight of the prophet or seer, which may be a source of suffering, but which must be accepted as the price of pushing forward the boundaries of human thought. He says, for instance, that 'the cracked mind of the schizophrenic may *let in* light which does not enter the intact minds of many sane people whose minds are closed' (Laing 1965, p. 27). The psychiatrist becomes, not the healer who makes the sick person well, but more the channel by which this light is brought into sane people's intact minds. 'Psychiatry could be,' he says, 'and some psychiatrists are, on the side of transcendence, of genuine freedom, and of true human growth' rather than being 'a technique of brainwashing, of inducing behaviour that is adjusted, by (preferably) non-injurious torture' (Laing 1965, p. 12).

Schizophrenia as an existential problem

There is a clear inconsistency at the heart of Laing's whole approach to schizophrenia. The phenomenological approach implies that schizophrenia is an existential problem, rather than a result of a neurological disorder. Laing and his colleague, Aaron Esterson, say, 'We do not accept 'schizophrenia' as being a biochemical, neurophysiological, psychological fact...' (Laing and Esterson 1970, p. 12). For them, it is a problem in coping with stressful human experience. According to Laing's hypothesis, based on Bateson's concept of the 'double bind', people become schizophrenic if they are unfortunate enough to be embroiled in a confused conflict involving people to whom they are emotionally attached and on whom they are dependent. But we can understand this as a possible explanation of someone else's behaviour only if we can imagine how we ourselves might respond in a similar way to the same sort of stress. In terms of the linguistic metaphor, we can find the other person's behaviour meaningful and intelligible only if we can at least translate her language into our own. This is how we manage to make sense of the prima facie 'unintelligible' behaviour of people belonging to a different human culture. We find something in common between their thinking and ours that enables us to bridge the gap, and we can do this because we share a common humanity with them. But at the same time Laing also wants to say that schizophrenics are 'crazy' or 'insane', which implies that they are so alien from the rest of us that, even with the aid of unusual powers of imagination, it may be virtually impossible to make sense of their behaviour and utterances. Most of us humbler mortals may find this with the thoughts of the tortured geniuses to whom, as said above, Laing sometimes compares schizophrenics. But often he seems to mean that schizophrenics are 'crazy' in a much more straightforward sense. For instance, he says in chapter 1 of *The divided self*, 'In the following pages, we shall be concerned specifically with people who experience themselves as automata, as robots, as bits of machinery, or even as animals. Such persons are rightly regarded as crazy' (Laing 1965, p. 23). On this view, schizophrenics are alien, not in the sense that members of another human culture are, but more in the sense that Martians might be. The problem with the Martians is that they *ex hypothesi* do not share a common humanity with us, so that there is nothing to support our imagination in its attempt to make sense of what they say and do (indeed, we should have no way of knowing whether the sounds that they uttered were part of a meaningful language at all).

This also has moral relevance. Part of the attraction of Laing's position for many people (including himself) is its humanism: its insistence on treating schizophrenics as people like ourselves rather than as 'cases' or 'patients', as 'subjects' rather than 'objects'. But he ends by seeing them as aliens, in a very strong sense of that word, in other words by dehumanizing them. This conclusion is the theoretical reflection of the practical experience of therapeutic impotence, of the inability in fact to penetrate the minds of schizophrenics, as Laing's own theory suggested one could, in order to help them overcome their problems. I shall argue shortly that this indicates something of profound philosophical significance: but first I want to turn aside from Laing to reconsider Szasz.

Szasz too sees the behaviour of schizophrenics (and others who would nowadays be described as 'mentally ill') as a kind of language that we can make sense of, rather than as the symptoms of a disease that requires a causal explanation. But unlike Laing he does not appear to see any particular difficulty in making sense of this language: not only is it not completely impossible, like understanding the speech of Martians, it is not even as difficult as the attempts of a linguistically untalented Englishman to understand a French newspaper. The strategies adopted by those who are called mentally ill are just forms of cheating, in situations when most of us feel no need to cheat: but there is no difficulty for someone with even moderate powers of imagination in making sense of such minor deviations. Hence there is no difficulty either in finding ways to help those with such 'problems in living'. Szasz thus does not, like Laing, end up with the feeling of therapeutic impotence. But he does come to an equally unsatisfactory conclusion, in that he effectively denies the strangeness of psychosis and the sheer depths of human misery to which it leads: Laing, at least, avoids that kind of reduction of schizophrenic experience to the banal.

Merleau-Ponty and the mind

Szasz and Laing thus differ from each other in important respects: but what they have in common is at least as important. They agree in seeing schizophrenia as primarily a problem of meaning rather than of neurological dysfunction. For them, it is a matter of deviating from certain social norms, rather than from norms of a more biological kind. There is something right about this: for one thing, it coincides with the descriptions given in the official diagnostic manuals. To quote from ICD-10 (1992, p. 86):

> The schizophrenic disorders are characterized in general by fundamental and characteristic distortions of thinking and perception, and by inappropriate or blunted affect.... The disturbance involves the most basic functions that give the normal person a feeling of individuality, uniqueness, and self-

direction. The most intimate thoughts, feelings, and acts are often felt to be known to or shared by others, and explanatory delusions may develop, to the effect that natural or supernatural forces are at work to influence the afflicted individual's thoughts and actions in ways that are often bizarre.

Key words in this quotation seem to me to be 'distortions', 'inappropriate', 'blunted', 'bizarre'. These terms refer, not to biological norms, but to human or social standards. The schizophrenic's behaviour, affects, speech, beliefs, etc., are called 'disordered' in that they deviate from the way in which we think they ought to be, in a normal, rational, person in our society, not because they deviate from the normal biological functioning of the brain and nervous system.

This is a claim about the kind of problem this is, though it has implications about the way in which the problem is to be explained and treated. The contention is that the schizophrenic is a human being who has problems fitting into normal human society because of the way she thinks, feels, and so on. They are problems arising from how someone is as a person, rather than mechanical difficulties or deficiencies in bodily functioning. And clearly, what counts as an appropriate way of helping them with their problems will differ accordingly. So far, so good. But the extravagances of the anti-psychiatric position arise from the conclusions that both writers draw (wrongly, as I shall argue) from this insight. They wish to oppose the orthodox medical model, which regards mental disorders like schizophrenia, as stated above, as another form of bodily illness, specifically a brain disease, and adopts correspondingly physical modes of therapy for them. And so they deny all involvement of neurophysiology in the explanation, and all use of physical methods in the treatment, of schizophrenia. Schizophrenia must be explained, according to them, as a rationally intelligible response to existential problems. Its treatment must accordingly consist, for Szasz, in helping the schizophrenic to re-learn more appropriate responses. For the more romantic Laing, it is not clear whether schizophrenia itself needs treatment at all: the schizophrenic is someone who, through the sheer intensity of his or her emotional experiences, has achieved a greater insight into certain truths of life, and those who most need treatment are the 'normal' people who fail to recognize this insight, and so reject people with schizophrenia.

In saying that this conclusion is wrongly drawn, I do not wish to reinstate the traditional version of the medical model. Rather, I want to argue that the anti-psychiatrists and their opponents both go astray in basing their thinking on sharp dichotomies, on 'either/or' oppositions. Either we must see psychiatric conditions as illnesses (specifically, as bodily illnesses) or we must regard them as existential problems. Either we must treat mentally disordered human beings as mere objects, the passive victims of physical agencies intervening from outside themselves to whom we can apply our medical skills to make them 'better' in some objective sense, or we must regard them as purposive subjects who choose to live differently from the way most 'normal' people do, and who encounter problems as a result. The acceptance of these sharp dichotomies, I want to argue, results from philosophical presuppositions, and a satisfactory conclusion about the explanation and treatment of schizophrenia can be reached only if we question these presuppositions. This questioning will itself involve some philosophical work, and I propose to use as my tools in this work some of the central concepts in the thought of the French philosopher Maurice Merleau-Ponty (1908–1961), and especially in his conception of human beings as what has been called 'body-subjects' (see especially Merleau-Ponty 2002) The account of Merleau-Ponty's philosophy to be given here will necessarily be abbreviated and simplified, for reasons of space: more detailed discussion can be found in my book on Merleau-Ponty (Matthews 2002).

The dichotomies spoken of above are part of the lingering effect of Cartesian dualism, the conception of 'mind' and 'body' as distinct components of human beings, with utterly incompatible properties. The subjective, inner, purposive side of our humanity, our notions of value and meaning, belong to the 'mind', whereas the objective, visible, mechanistic side belongs to the 'body'. The subjective can be 'understood' in terms of the person's reasons for thinking, acting, feeling, or choosing as she does; but the objective or bodily cannot be understood in this sense, only causally explained in terms of regular sequences recorded in scientific laws, ultimately, the laws of physics. The subjective, on this view, is the realm of imagination and empathy, the objective the domain of science: so that, if one accepts the Cartesian dichotomy, one must regard a mental disorder in one of two, mutually exclusive, ways. *Either* it is a matter for scientific investigation and treatment, and so a bodily condition to be causally explained, without reference to any meanings it may have for the person suffering it. This is the approach of advocates of the traditional medical model, in a laudable desire to be scientific. *Or* it is something which has to be understood in terms of its meaning for the sufferer, and so is not a matter for causal explanation in terms of bodily processes, or indeed for science. This is the approach adopted by such writers as Szasz and Laing.

One way of interpreting Merleau-Ponty's version of phenomenology is as an attempt to return from the a priori presuppositions of traditional metaphysics to a more basic level of ordinary human experience. He says, 'one of the great achievements of modern art and philosophy . . . has been to allow us to rediscover the world in which we live, yet which we are always prone to forget' (Merleau-Ponty 2004, p. 39). Any science worthy of the name must, after all, start from our ordinary experience of the world, including ourselves and other human beings, and offer an explanation of that experience, rather than attempting to fit the phenomena into preconceived categories derived from metaphysics. Much of modern thought, however, in Merleau-Ponty's view, involves the latter rather than the former. It is, to use his term, 'objectivist' in that it sees the facts through the spectacles of the Cartesian sharp separation between 'subjective' experience and the 'objective' world which is experienced. Cartesian dualism implies that we, as subjects, are not part of the world, but contemplate it, as it were, from the outside (in somewhat the same way as the audience in a cinema contemplates the 'world' of the film they are viewing without being part of that world). Our own bodies, and the bodies of other people, become objects for us, parts of matter which, like all matter, functions in a purely mechanical way: one bodily process follows on from another in time, in a regular, but ultimately meaningless way. We can explain the movements of material things, like the body, by answering the question, 'How?' (How do they come about?), but it makes no sense to ask, 'Why?' (Why, for what reason, do they happen as they do?). The pumping of the heart causes the blood to circulate: but the heart has no reason for pumping, it just does (fortunately for us).

Treating mental disorder scientifically, on this view, means treating it objectively, thus in effect equating it with a bodily malfunction or disease, most likely a brain disease. That means regarding the person with a mental disorder as an object: the disorder is not really a problem *in* their personal lives (though it may like, say, liver disease cause problems *for* their personal lives), but a mechanical failure of a part of their body, needing to be causally explained and treated by putting right the cause. And then it seems as if we can introduce meaning into our conception of mental disorder only by abandoning science and physiology altogether and seeing mental disorder as necessarily something that is rationally intelligible in essentially the same way as normal, undisordered, behaviour.

Merleau-Ponty, as said above, aimed to get away from all such assumptions and to return to our pre-theoretical experience of the world and of human beings. How do we see ourselves and other human beings when we are not seeking to give a theoretical explanation of human existence? We do not see ourselves as in the position of the cinema audience in relation to what is happening on the screen: we are part of the world, and experience the other parts, not from the outside, but from our position within the world. The world is the place we inhabit, not an object to be contemplated. In particular, our own bodies are not experienced as objects, but as ourselves, as what gives us our position and point of view within the world. Other people, likewise, are experienced not merely as objects or bits of machinery, but as other subjects, beings with whom we can communicate and whose actions we can understand as expressions of the same kinds of reasons which we express in our own actions. Being part of the world in this way involves being both a subject (an experiencer) and an object (a body), in such a way that the subjectivity and the embodiment are inseparable: we subjectively experience the world through our bodily engagement with it, and our bodies are of such a kind that they make subjective experience possible. Merleau-Ponty is often said by commentators to hold the view that human beings are 'body-subjects', and though he himself does not ever seem to have used precisely that term, it is a useful short way of describing his conception.

One way of understanding the idea of human beings as body-subjects is to say that it is the view that human beings are essentially biological creatures, while at the same time reinterpreting what is meant by a 'biological creature'. The Cartesian view sees living matter, like all matter, as a mechanistic system: so biology is simply a branch of physics, and biological organisms differ from other physical systems only in being more complex. Instead, the body-subject idea sees living bodies (human and non-human) as we actually, pre-theoretically, experience them, as active and so purposive beings. Purposiveness, on this view, does not necessarily require consciousness, but only biological organization. Biological organisms function as wholes, not simply as collections of parts: for instance, it is meaningful to ascribe to them certain needs, which are needs of the whole organism, such as the need for food. If they have such needs, then we can explain their behaviour in terms of their pursuit of such needs; for example, we can explain the behaviour of a bird pecking away at a tree by saying it is looking for insects or other sources of food (and without implying that the bird is consciously pursuing this purpose). In the case of living beings, our attempts to explain their behaviour can thus be answers to the question 'Why?' as well as to the question 'How?', or, to put it differently, it can take the form of understanding their reasons for acting as they do, as well as the causes which bring it about that they act as they do. 'Cause' and 'reason' explanations are not rivals, but complementary: the causal explanation tells us what processes need to precede the behaviour we want to explain if it is to be possible at all, the reason explanation tells us why the animal behaves as it does, what purpose is achieved by so behaving.

But there is more to be said than this about the relation between cause and reason explanations. The causal explanation tells us how it can come about that behaviour in pursuit of a particular purpose is possible. We have the purposes we have at all only because our bodies, and particularly our brains, are structured in the way they are. This is true both at the level of the species and at the level of the individual. As members of the human species, we have certain needs and so purposes, which are characteristic of that species, e.g. we need to eat and drink, to engage in sexual activity, and so on. We have those needs as a species because human bodies are structured in the way they are (just as human beings, unlike some other animals, have colour vision because of the typical structure of the human eye). At the individual level, there are variations in the structures of the brain and other relevant parts of the body, some inherited, some the result of injury or disease, which constrain the purposes, and the ways of expressing those purposes, which are available to that individual.

But there is still another dimension to the relation between causes and reasons. If a human being acts 'rationally', that is, in pursuit of purposes that she shares with most normal members of her society, then citing those purposes is in most contexts all that is necessary for a satisfactory explanation of her behaviour. For example, if we were told that someone has given up smoking and we ask 'Why?', then the answer that she was afraid of dying of lung cancer if she did not, tells us all we need to know. All normal people will readily understand the desire to avoid a premature and painful death, and the connection of that desire with giving up smoking. We do not need in addition to be told about the way in which her brain behaved when she was formulating that desire or connecting it with her cigarette addiction (unless, of course, we are scientists with a specialist interest in normal brain functioning). On the other hand, if someone acts 'irrationally', that is, for reasons that most normal people cannot easily share, then citing her reasons, while necessary, will not be sufficient for a satisfactory understanding of her behaviour. For instance, suppose someone knows about the link between smoking and lung cancer, and is very much afraid of dying in that way, but nevertheless refuses to give up smoking. When we ask her why, she replies 'Because I find it so comforting to smoke'. That answer will only partly satisfy our need for explanation: we still have to ask why she, unlike most of us, gives a greater weight to the need for this kind of comfort than to the fear of premature and painful death. This second question will be answered by a causal explanation of how this unusual weighting of needs has come about (it may be in terms of something neurological, or of something in her past environmental conditioning, but some causal answer of that kind seems necessary if our desire for explanation is to be satisfied).

If we accept this account of human beings and their behaviour, then perhaps we can escape from the dichotomous thinking about the explanation and treatment of schizophrenia discussed earlier. The explanation of schizophrenic symptoms cannot be the kind of rational understanding that we offer for normal, chosen, human actions, like taking precautions against burglary when there has been a spate of such crimes in the district: we understand such actions because we can conceive of acting similarly ourselves in the same circumstances. Even Szasz accepts that schizophrenic behaviour is a result of an attempt to escape the demands of normal human relationships, i.e. of something normal people cannot straightforwardly understand. And Laing sees schizophrenics as having lost the normal sense of self, in terms of which we understand the behaviour of most human beings. What we want in the schizophrenic case is thus, as in any other case of irrational behaviour, a causal explanation of why the person has deviated from that intelligible pattern of behaviour or feeling. But a purely causal explanation will not suffice: schizophrenic symptoms, such as hearing voices, are not like reflex movements such as the knee-jerk response, in that they have an essentially intentional dimension to them. Distorted thinking is still thinking, involving the use of concepts just as undistorted thinking does. What has to be explained therefore is why the schizophrenic's use of concepts deviates from the normal in ways that cannot be rationally understood. This explanation cannot refer, as

Maher suggests, only to 'neurological anomalies'. It may well be that some human beings are predisposed by the way their brains function to develop unusual ways of thinking: but even if that is the case, it is not a complete explanation of why a subset of such people become schizophrenic (as opposed to, say, original thinkers). For that, some other kind of cause seems necessary, and a plausible candidate (to say no more) would be something to do with their problems in dealing with an emotionally complex human and social environment. If that is right, then there is an obligation on the psychiatrist who seeks to help schizophrenics to understand and deal with these environmental causes of the patient's condition, as well as with any neurological background.

Saying that schizophrenia has causes, whether neurological or social, which are beyond the person's control implies that Szasz is simply wrong to dismiss the idea of 'mental illness' as a mere myth. It runs counter also to Laing's sometimes romanticized conception of schizophrenics as tortured geniuses, whose very suffering is the birth-pangs of a superior insight: they are indeed 'patients', as much as sufferers from cancer are, the victims of conditions that they cannot control, and from which relief will be obtained by methods which require more than 'love'. But although Laing and Szasz were mistaken to be against a medicalized psychiatry as such, there is something ultimately right, and applicable as much to general medicine as to psychiatry, in their insistence on treating patients as human subjects with problems rather than simply machines to be repaired. What is needed is not the abandonment of any kind of 'medical model', but a reinterpretation of that model to take account of the humanity and subjectivity of patients.

Endnote

1. Szasz's primary example of a 'mental illness', it is true, is hysteria, but he has many references to schizophrenia in his works, and clearly regards it as an instance of the same broad kind as hysteria: I shall consider his critique only in so far as it is relevant to schizophrenia.

References

Arthur, A.Z. (1964). Theories and explanations of delusions: a review. *American Journal of Psychiatry*, **121**: 105–115.

Boyle, M. (2002). *Schizophrenia: a scientific delusion?* (2nd edn). London: Routledge.

DSM-IV 1994: *Diagnostic and statistical manual of mental disorders* (4th edn). Washington, DC: American Psychiatric Association.

Foucault, M. (1965). *Madness and civilisation: a history of insanity in the age of reason*. New York: Mentor Books.

ICD-10 (1992). *The ICD-10 classification of mental and behavioural disorders: clinical descriptions and diagnostic guidelines*. Geneva: World Health Organization.

Laing, R.D. (1960). *The divided self: a study of sanity and madness*, Chicago: Quadrangle Books.

Laing, R.D. (1971). *Self and others*, Harmondsworth: Penguin Books.

Laing, R.D. and Esterson, A. (1970). *Sanity, madness and the family*. Harmondsworth: Penguin Books.

Maher, B.A. (1999). Anomalous experience in everyday life: its significance for psychopathology. *The Monist*, **82**(4): 547–570.

Matthews, E. (2002). *The philosophy of Merleau-Ponty*. Chesham, Bucks: Acumen Publishing.

Merleau-Ponty, M. (2002). *Phenomenology of perception* (trans. C. Smith). London: Routledge (Classics edition).

Merleau-Ponty, M. (2004). *The world of perception* (trans. O. Davis). London: Routledge.

Shorter, E.(1997). *A history of psychiatry: from the era of the asylum to the age of prozac*. New York: John Wiley and Sons Inc.

Szasz, T. (1972). *The myth of mental illness: foundations of a theory of personal conduct*. St. Albans: Granada Publishing (Paladin edition).

Index

Note: 'n.' after a page reference indicates the number of a note on that page.